SPEECH OF THE HEARING IMPAIRED

Speech of the Hearing Impaired: Research, Training and Personnel Preparation is a volume in the **PERSPECTIVES IN AUDIOLOGY SERIES**—Lyle L. Lloyd, Ph.D., series editor. Other volumes in the series include:

Published:
Principles of Speech Audiometry edited by Dan F. Konkle, Ph.D., and William F. Rintelmann, Ph.D.
Forensic Audiology edited by Mark B. Kramer, Ph.D., and Joan Armbruster, M.S.
Aging and the Perception of Speech by Moe Bergman, Ed.D.
Communicating with Deaf People: A Resource Manual for Teachers and Students of American Sign Language by Harry W. Hoemann, Ph.D.
Language Development and Intervention with the Hearing Impaired by Richard R. Kretschmer, Jr., Ed.D., and Laura W. Kretschmer, Ed.D.
Noise and Audiology edited by David M. Lipscomb, Ph.D.
The Sounds of Speech Communication: A Primer of Acoustic Phonetics and Speech Perception by J. M. Pickett, Ph.D.
Hearing Assessment edited by William F. Rintelmann, Ph.D.
Auditory Management of Hearing-Impaired Children: Principles and Prerequisites for Intervention edited by Mark Ross, Ph.D., and Thomas G. Giolas, Ph.D.
Introduction to Aural Rehabilitation edited by Ronald L. Schow, Ph.D., and Michael A. Nerbonne, Ph.D.
Acoustical Factors Affecting Hearing Aid Performance edited by Gerald A. Studebaker, Ph.D., and Irving Hochberg, Ph.D.
American Sign Language and Sign Systems by Ronnie Bring Wilbur, Ph.D.

In Preparation:
Acoustic Amplification: A Unified Treatment by Harry Levitt, Ph.D.

Publisher's Note
Perspectives in Audiology is a carefully planned series of clinically oriented and basic science textbooks. The series is enriched by contributions from leading specialists in audiology and allied disciplines. Because technical language and terminology in these disciplines are constantly being refined and sometimes vary, this series has been edited as far as possible for consistency of style in conformity with current majority usage as set forth by the American Speech-Language-Hearing Association, the *Publication Manual of the American Psychological Association,* and the University of Chicago's *A Manual of Style*. University Park Press and the series editors and authors welcome readers' comments about individual volumes in the series or the series concept as a whole in the interest of making **Perspectives in Audiology** as useful as possible to students, teachers, clinicians, and scientists.

A Volume in the Perspectives in Audiology Series

SPEECH OF THE HEARING IMPAIRED
Research, Training, and Personnel Preparation

edited by
Irving Hochberg, Ph.D.
Professor and Executive Officer
Doctoral Program in Speech and Hearing Sciences
  Graduate School
City University of New York
Harry Levitt, Ph.D.
Professor
Doctoral Program in Speech and Hearing Sciences
  Graduate School
City University of New York
and
Mary Joe Osberger, Ph.D.
Research Associate
Boys Town Institute for Communication
  Disorders in Children

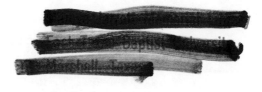

University Park Press
Baltimore

UNIVERSITY PARK PRESS
International Publishers in Medicine and Human Services
300 North Charles Street
Baltimore, Maryland 21201

Typeset by Maryland Composition Company, Inc.

Manufactured in the United States of America by
The Maple Press Company

Library of Congress Cataloging in Publication Data
Main entry under title:

Speech of the hearing impaired.

(Perspectives in audiology series)
Includes indexes.
1. Hearing disorders—Complications and sequelae.   2. Speech
perception.   3. Speech disorders.   4. Deaf—
Rehabilitation.   I. Hochberg, Irving.   II. Levitt, Harry.   III. Osberger,
Mary Joe.   IV. Series.   [DNLM: 1. Speech disorders.   2. Hearing
disorders.   3. Speech—Therapy.   WV 270 S742]
RF291.S66   1983   616.85′52   82-25818
ISBN 0-8391-1782-5

CONTENTS

103812

CONTRIBUTORS

Peter M. Blackwell, M.A.
Principal
Rhode Island School for the Deaf
Corliss Park
Providence, Rhode Island 02908

Arthur Boothroyd, Ph.D.
Associate Professor
Ph.D. Program in Speech and
Hearing Sciences
Graduate School and University
Center
City University of New York
New York, New York 10036

Diane Brackett, Ph.D.
Clinical Supervisor
New York League for the Hard of
Hearing
71 West 23rd Street
New York, New York 10010

Judith L. Braeges, M.S.Ed.
Center for Communications
Research
Rochester School for the Deaf
1531 St. Paul Street
Rochester, New York 14621

Laura Bulle, M.A.
Teacher
White Oak School
8014 Leefield Road
Baltimore, Md. 21234

Julia M. Davis, Ph.D.
Professor and Chair
Department of Speech Pathology
and Audiology
University of Iowa
Iowa City, Iowa 52242

Norman P. Erber, Ph.D.
Victoria College
Institute of Special Education
221 Burwood Highway
Burwood, Victoria 3125
Australia

John Fisher
Moray House, College of
Education
University of Edinburgh
Edinburgh, Scotland

Moise H. Goldstein, Jr., Sc.D.
Professor
Electrical Engineering and
Computer Science Department
Johns Hopkins University
Baltimore, Maryland 21205

Katherine S. Harris, Ph.D.
Professor
Ph.D. Program in Speech and
Hearing Sciences
City University of New York
Graduate School
33 West 42 Street
New York, New York 10036
Haskin Laboratories
270 Crown Street
New Haven, Connecticut 06510

Janet Head, M.A.
Speech Supervisor
Lexington School for the Deaf
30th Avenue & 75th Street
Jackson Heights, New York 11370

Ira Hirsh, Ph.D.
Central Institute for the Deaf
818 South Euclid
St. Louis, Missouri 63110

Irving Hochberg, Ph.D.
Executive Officer
Ph.D. Program in Speech and
Hearing Sciences
City University of New York
Graduate School
33 West 42 Street
New York, New York 10036

Lisa D. Holden, M.S.
Research Assistant
Sensory Communication Research
Laboratory
Gallaudet College
Washington, D.C. 20002

Robert A. Houde, Ph.D.
Center for Communications
Research
Rochester School for the Deaf
1531 St. Paul Street
Rochester, New York 14621

Angela King
Scientific and Technical
Department
Royal National Institute for the
Deaf
105 Gower Street
London, England

Harry Levitt, Ph.D.
Professor
Ph.D. Program in Speech and
Hearing Sciences
City University of New York
Graduate School
33 West 42 Street
New York, New York 10036

Nancy S. McGarr, Ph.D.
Research Assistant
Haskins Laboratories
270 Crown Street
New Haven, Connecticut 06510
Center for Research in Speech
and Hearing Sciences
City University of New York
Graduate School
33 West 42 Street
New York, New York 10036

Jean Maki, Ph.D.
Associate Professor
Speech and Hearing Clinic
Andrews University
Berrien Springs, Michigan 49104

János Mártony, Sc.D.
Department of Speech
Communication
Royal Institute of Technology
(KTH) S-100 44
Stockholm 70, Sweden

Antonia B. Maxon, Ph.D.
Assistant Professor
Communication Sciences
Department
University of Connecticut
Storrs, Connecticut 06268

Randall B. Monsen, Ph.D.
Research Associate
Central Institute for the Deaf
818 South Euclid
St. Louis, Missouri 63110

Raymond S. Nickerson, Ph.D.
Senior Vice President; Director
Information Sciences Division
Bolt Beranek and Newman Inc.
10 Moulton Street
Cambridge, Massachusetts 02238

Mary Joe Osberger, Ph.D.
Research Associate
Human Communication
Laboratories
The Boys Town Institute for
Communication Disorders in
Children
Omaha, Nebraska 68131

Ann Parker, M.C.S.T.
Scientific and Technical
Department
Royal National Institute for the
Deaf
105 Gower Street
London WC1E6AH, England

J. M. Pickett, Ph.D.
Director
Sensory Communication Research
Laboratory & Rehabilitation
Engineering Center
Gallaudet College
Washington, D.C. 20002

Adele Proctor, Sc.D.
Assistant Professor
Department of Speech Pathology
and Audiology
Northeastern University
Boston, Massachusetts 02115

Sally Revoile, Ph.D.
Associate Professor of Auditory
Research
Sensory Communication Research
Laboratory
Gallaudet College
Washington, D.C. 20002

Ann M. Rollins, M.A.
Scientist
Information Sciences Division
Bolt Beranek and Newman Inc.
10 Moulton Street
Cambridge, Massachusetts 02238

Claude Ruffin-Simon, Ph.D.
University College London
Wolfson House
4 Stephenson Way
London, NW1 2HE England

Joanna L. Schmidt, M.A.
Research Associate
Ph.D. Program in Speech and
Hearing Sciences
City University of New York
Graduate School
33 West 42 Street
New York, New York 10036

Neil T. Shepard, Ph.D.
Chief, Clinical Electrophysiology
Laboratory
Department of Otolaryngology
Henry Ford Hospital
Detroit, Michigan 48202

Hiroshi Shimizu, M.D., M.Sc.D.
Associate Professor
Department of Laryngology and
Otology
Director of Hearing and Speech
Center
Johns Hopkins Hospital
Baltimore, Maryland 21205

S. Richard Silverman, Ph.D.
Director Emeritus
Central Institute for the Deaf
818 South Euclid
Professor Emeritus of Audiology
Washington University
St. Louis, Missouri 63110

Rachel E. Stark, Ph.D.
Associate Professor
Department of Neurology
Johns Hopkins University School
of Medicine
Director
Hearing and Speech Division
John F. Kennedy Institute
Baltimore, Maryland 21205

Kenneth N. Stevens, Ph.D.
Professor of Electrical
Engineering and Computer
Science
Massachusetts Institute of
Technology
Cambridge, Massachusetts 02139

Carol Stoel-Gammon, Ph.D.
Research Assistant Professor
Department of Speech and
Hearing Sciences
University of Washington
Seattle, Washington 98195

Harvey Stromberg
Manager of Software
Development
Grumman Data Systems, Inc.
45 Grossway Park Dr.
Woodbury, NY 11797

Joanne Subtelny, Ph.D.
Professor
Special Assistant Research and
Curriculum
Communication Program
National Technical Institute for
the Deaf
Rochester Institute of Technology
Rochester, New York 14623
Adjunct Professor
Graduate School of Education and
Human Development
University of Rochester
Rochester, New York 14627

Terry L. Thies, Ph.D.
Program Coordinator, Audiology
Division of Special Education
Office of the L.A. County
  Superintendent of Schools
Downey, California 90242

Jane Trammell, M.A.
Program Specialist
Auditory Skills Project
Division of Special Education
Office of the L.A. County
  Superintendent of Schools
Downey, California 90242

Tekla Tunblad
Teacher
Manilla School for the Deaf
Stockholm, Sweden

Robert L. Whitehead, Ph.D.
Chairperson
Department of Communication
  Research
National Technical Institute for
  the Deaf
Rochester, New York 14623

Richard Wright, M.A.
Scientific and Technical
  Department
Royal National Institute for the
  Deaf
London, England

Victor Zue, Sc.D.
Assistant Professor
Department of Electrical
  Engineering and Computer
  Science
Massachusetts Institute of
  Technology
Cambridge, Massachusetts 02139

PREFACE TO PERSPECTIVES IN AUDIOLOGY

Audiology is a young, vibrant, dynamic field. Its lineage can be traced to the fields of education, medicine, physics, and psychology in the nineteenth century and the emergence of speech pathology in the first half of this century. The term "audiology," meaning the science of hearing, was coined by Raymond Carhart in 1947. Since then, its definition has expanded to include its professional nature. Audiology is the profession that provides knowledge and service in the areas of human hearing and, more broadly, human communication and its disorders. Audiology is also a major area of study in the professional preparation of speech pathologists, speech and hearing scientists, and otologists.

Perspectives in Audiology is the first series of books designed to cover the major areas of study in audiology. The interdisciplinary nature of the field is reflected by the scope of the volumes in this series. The volumes (see p. ii) include both clinically oriented and basic science texts. The series consists of topic-specific textbooks designed to meet the needs of today's advanced level student and of focal references for practicing audiologists and specialists in many related fields.

The **Perspectives in Audiology** series offers several advantages not usually found in most texts, but purposely featured in this series to increase the practical value of the books for practitioners and researchers, as well as for students and teachers.

1. Every volume includes thorough discussion of relevant clinical and/or research papers on each topic.
2. Most volumes are organized in an educational format to serve as the main text or as one of the main texts for graduate and advanced undergraduate students in courses on audiology and/or other studies concerned with human communication and its disorders.
3. Unlike ordinary texts, **Perspectives in Audiology** volumes will retain their professional reference value as focal reference sources for practitioners and researchers in career work long after completion of their studies.
4. Each volume serves as a rich source of authoritative, up-to-date information and valuable reviews for specialists in many fields, such as administration, audiology, early childhood studies, linguistics, otology, psychology, pediatrics, public health, special education, speech pathology, and/or speech and hearing science.

Speech development and intervention is one of the most critical aspects of aural rehabilitation and education of the hearing impaired. Meaningful speech is the only uniquely human aspect of communication. Therefore, *Speech of the Hearing Impaired: Research, Training, and Pesonnel Preparation,* edited by Irving Hochberg, Harry Levitt, and Mary Joe Osberger, is a major addition to the Perspectives in Audiology series. This book provides not only a major updating of this important area, but also a greater combined depth and breadth of research and application coverage than has been achieved in any previous volume on speech of the hearing impaired.

This book exemplifies many of the major features of the Perspectives in Audiology series. It is transdisciplinary, combining basic research with practical applications. It provides an authoritative and well-documented text on a critical area of concern in audiology—it will have an enduring reference value. Furthermore, it is unique in that as a basic text on research and application issues, it also addresses the critical area of personnel preparation.

Speech of the Hearing Impaired is based on papers originally presented at a national working conference organized by Hochberg, Levitt, and Osberger; but unlike many conference proceedings this volume has been extensively edited to make it a more functional text and reference.

Lyle L. Lloyd, Ph.D.

Chairman and Professor of Special Education
Professor of Audiology and Speech Sciences
Purdue University

PREFACE

Recent advances in several disciplines have had a substantial impact on our understanding of the acquisition of speech and language in the hearing impaired. Investigators from traditional and quite diverse backgrounds, including acoustic phoneticians, sensory psychologists, speech physiologists, engineers, and others in the speech, language, and hearing sciences have made significant contributions to our field. These advances have served to refine our thinking about the ways in which hearing-impaired children and adults perceive and produce oral language, and have important practical implications for educational and intervention programs.

A concurrent development with respect to the education of the deaf has been the merging of manual and oral philosophies of education into what is now referred to as *total communication*. Although the importance of speech is clearly recognized, the teaching of speech if often de-emphasized at many schools aspiring to the total-communication philosophy. This appears to be a result of neglect and/or logistic factors rather than ideology. There is a clear and present need to help educators provide more effective speech teaching. At the same time, with notable exceptions, personnel preparation programs in the education of the hearing impaired and speech-language pathology and audiology have not addressed the issues of teaching and remediating the speech problems associated with the deaf child, and have been graduating teachers of the hearing impaired and speech-language pathologists who are inadequately prepared to meet the oral communicative needs of these children. The result is that many hearing-impaired children do not receive effective speech training as part of their educational and habilitative program, and thereby are not able to reach their maximum potential for oral communication.

Given these circumstances, the time was propitious for a conference that would bring together individuals who have a commitment for the improvement of communication skills of the hearing impaired: researchers, who are contributing to our further understanding of the speech of the hearing impaired; practitioners, who are developing more effective methods of speech training; and educators, who would apply this knowledge towards improving the speech of the hearing impaired.

This book contains the papers and discussions of the participants at the "Conference on the Speech of the Hearing Impaired: Research, Training, and Personnel Preparation," which was held over a 3-day period in the Fall of 1979 at the City University of New York Graduate School. The papers presented at the conference were divided into seven areas: 1) speech production; 2) speech perception; 3) assessment procedures; 4) development of speech; 5) sensory aids and speech training; 6) auditory training; and 7) personnel preparation. Each session was followed by a discussion period involving both the participants and members of the audience.

An historical critique of the nature of speech training is set forth by S. Richard Silverman at the outset of the book. His remarks bring into focus the essential purpose of what is to follow, namely, the current status and future directions of speech training for the hearing impaired.

The first section is devoted to a series of research papers concerned with the physiological processes underlying speech production, and their consequent effects upon the phonation, articulation, and intelligibility of the speech training for the hearing impaired.

The abilities of the hearing impaired to perceive speech is considered in the second section of the book. The research findings reported here are concerned with several approaches designed to improve the speech perception ability of children and adults with profound hearing loss.

The assessment of speech production and perception is a logical follow-up to the previous two sections. Both theoretical and practical issues are discussed in developing valid and reliable procedures to assess speech perception and production performance.

The fourth section concentrates on the phonological and phonatory aspects associated with the development of speech production and perception. Attempts are made to ascertain the nature of the relationship between these developmental concerns.

The next two sections focus on the second major division of the book, namely, speech training. The first section includes descriptions of the ways in which the Speech Spectrographic Display has been systematically employed to improve the articulatory skills of deaf adults, followed by a discussion of the current and future applications of computer technology in working with the hearing impaired.

The second section is related to the development and evaluation of several speech and auditory training programs that have been implanted for hearing-impaired children in day and public school settings. Both principles and strategies of intervention are discussed.

The final section is devoted to the third major focus of the conference—personnel preparation. Included are presentations that describe various aproaches to inservice education that have implications for evaluating preservice personnel preparation as well. The main theme underlying the papers presented was that ongoing systematic inservice training and staff development are essential for facilitating knowledge and skills on the part of practitioners to deliver more effective speech services to the hearing impaired.

The seven panel discussions and the Sensory Aids Workshop could not be included in the present volume because these would have added substantially to the length of the book, and consequently to its cost. Readers are advised, however, that all seven panel discussions as well as the proceedings of the Sensory Aids Workshop will be made available to those interested at a nominal cost. Anyone who wishes to obtain the companion volume should write to the editors at the City University Graduate School.

The proceedings of the conference as reflected in this book could not have been brought to fruition without the contributions of numerous individuals. We first would like to express our sincere appreciation to all the participants at the conference who made it the success it was, and for their sustained patience and support in bringing about its present reality. Appreciation is also extended to the members of the audience, consisting of approximately 200 professionals, for their continuing interest during the conference, and their valuable contributions during the discussion sections. We also wish to thank Linda Hoffnung for her efforts in transcribing and editing the panel discussions, and to Joanna Schmidt for her organizational and editorial skills as well as for her personal commitment to the preparation of this book. Finally, to both Lyle

Lloyd and Janet Hankin, the latter of University Park Press, our gratitude for facilitating the completion of this book.

Irving Hochberg
Harry Levitt
Mary Joe Osberger

FOREWORD

This volume is based on the conference entitled "Speech of the Hearing Impaired: Research, Training, and Personnel Preparation" held at the Graduate School, CUNY, in 1979. That was quite a special meeting with respect to the exchange between laboratory scientists, on the one hand, and practioners from school or clinic on the other. I do not mean to suggest that these different professional specialties do not normally talk to one another, but what was specal at this meeting was that they talked to one another about common phenomena. The range of subject matters was also special. Both speech production and speech perception were addressed at a very molecular level of individual speech units and were also addressed at the level of interactive speech communication. The ages of hearing-impaired children whose problems were addressed ranged from the language-acquiring infant to the language-developing school child. Furthermore, the severity of hearing loss in these children ranged from moderate to profound. Training styles and techniques of evaluation ranged from skill drills to holistic strategies of a more cognitive flavor.

We find here many new ideas and concepts still current, as well as reviews of some old persistent problems occasionally dressed up in modern labels. Under speech production, we not only learned about the results of phonetic analysis of errors made by hearing-impaired children when they speak, but we learned more global notions about their speech production systems concerning control, posture, and planning. Under speech perception, two shifts have been brought about by technological developments. First, acoustical, and electronic technology now allow us to address the impaired auditory system somewhat more successfully and thus the rehabilatative programs emphasize more auditory input and less visual and tactile inputs used since the early nineteenth century. On the other hand, a second aspect of technological development reminds us not only of improved systems for conveying information to the eye and to the skin but also of the necessity for different kinds of encoding and perhaps different learning strategies associated with different information displays.

Contributions and discussions about training, assessment, and professional preparation brought together several themes. Our teachers and clinicians seem more comfortable, perhaps by virtue of their training, with an analytic approach that leaves them to work on particular speech items and to assess their training programs with such items. On the other hand school administrators and counselors note the sometime discrepancy between apparently successful performance on smaller units and the less successful everyday communication that is demanded outside the classroom. There appear to be in contemporary fields, some useful concepts (or at least useful labels) like cognitive strategies, pragmatics, global communication, and others but, so far at least, they have not found their way to significant contributions in closing the gap between educational atomism and the demands of real-world holism.

An important problem, not entirely new, related to terminology that arose during the conference. For several years now, professionals in the field have avoided speaking about "the deaf," because of socially unacceptable connotations. Instead we created the term "hearing impaired" and gathered together under that label everyone from mild hearing loss to profound deafness. Now we talk to each other, as did the authors of papers and discussants at this conference, about the "hearing impaired," as if there were a unity to this extreme range of implied hearing levels. To be sure, some of our speakers specified "profoundly hearing impaired" or even "profoundly deaf," as opposed to "severely hearing impaired" and "moderately hearing impaired." Those are clumsy words. It seemed as if it would have been simpler to talk about the deaf, the profoundly deaf or the severely hearing-impaired. The reader must be aware of this terminological problem not as an example of lexical purity, but rather because of its effect on what we do. We already see evidence in some of the states of our country that an all-covering tent like "hearing impaired" will foster the uniform treatment of all such children, so that moderately hard of hearing children will be treated as if they were deaf.

Ira J. Hirsh
Central Institute for the Deaf
and Washington University
St. Louis, Missouri

SPEECH TRAINING THEN AND NOW: A CRITICAL REVIEW

S. Richard Silverman

CONTENTS

The title of the chapter assigned this writer requires demarcation and delineation of scope, if not precise definition. In this chapter *speech training* will refer to those activities in the home, clinic, or classroom (primarily the latter) that are directed specifically at the development, improvement, and maintenance of functional speech skills in the hearing impaired with emphasis on the severely and profoundly hearing impaired. This is not to say that a child's extramural experiences do not influence these skills; in fact, such experiences may be the critical element that determines the child's attitude toward speech or, otherwise said, the motivation to speak at all. But the intended treatment of the topic herein accommodates the theme and goals of the conference which imply the kind of specificity of target stated above.

Less easily demarcated is the "Then" of the title. Do we go back in time and develop our exposition from judicious, even occasionally biased, sampling of the available literature produced in the course of the history of the field like Bonet's *Simplification of the Letters of the Alphabet and Method of Teaching Deaf Mutes to Speak* (1620), or Holder's *Elements of Speech, Concerning Persons Deaf and Dumb* (1669), or Dalgarno's *The Deaf and Dumb Man's Tutor* including a

1

"discourse of the nature of double consonants" (1680), or van Helmont's attempt to apply Hebrew orthography to display tongue position for phoneme production (1667), or Amman's *Dissertation on Speech* (1700) "in which . . . the means are also described by which those deaf and dumb from birth may acquire speech," or Graser's *The Deaf Mute Restored to Humanity by Visible and Spoken Speech* (1829), or a fundamental German work on the development of speech of deaf mutes, Vatter's *Die Ausbildung des Taubstummen in der Lautsprache* (1875), all cited and briefly discussed by Farrar in his revision of the monumental *Arnold's Education of the Deaf* (1923)?

Certainly not to be excluded from any sampling are significant items by the Bells, father and son. Among them are A. M. Bell's effort to develop a visual symbol system that would represent articulatory features of individual sounds as presented in his *Sounds and Their Relations; Illustrated by Means of Visible Speech* (1894), his *Principles of Speech* aimed at "correction of all faults of articulation" and stammering" (1900), and A. G. Bell's collection of his lectures at the first summer meeting of the organization that bears his name, and *The Mechanism of Speech* (1907) addressed to answering questions by the assembled teachers "concerning difficulties experienced in imparting the power of articulate speech to deaf children" to which is appended a paper on vowel theories delivered to the National Academy of Science in 1879 in which vowels are stated to be "*genera* of sounds instead of individuals."

The current stress on the exploitation of residual hearing would require the inclusion in our sampling of Itard's *Traité des maladies de l'oreille et de l'audition* (1821), Urbantschitsch's classic monograph on auditory training, *Horübüngen bei Taubstummheit* (1895), and Goldstein's application of it to the American context in his *The Acoustic Method* (1939).

The Then of the title may also be elucidated in more recent literature. Schunhoff's (1957) historical review covering the period 1815–1955 dealing with the status in public residential schools of teaching speech to the deaf is particularly reflective of influential attitudes on the subject. To be noted, for example, is his inclusion of a resolution adopted in 1868 at a conference convened by E. M. Gallaudet whose invitation to heads of public residential schools indicated that the central agenda item would be "what may be termed the articulation controversy."

> Resolved, That while in our judgment it is desirable to give semi-mutes and semi-deaf children every facility for retaining and improving any power of articulate speech which they may possess, *it is not profitable*

except in very rare cases to attempt to teach congenital mutes articulation.
(italics mine)

Resolved, That to attain success in this department of instruction an added force of instructors will be necessary, and this conference hereby recommends to boards of directors of institutions for the deaf and dumb in this country that speedy measures be taken to provide the funds needed for the prosecution of this work. (Schunhoff, 1957)

Teaching methods have had their share of attention from Wright (1928), Haycock (1933), Joiner (1948), Wedenberg (1954), Ewing and Ewing (1954), Guberina (1964), Fry (1966), Clarke School (1971), Vorce (1974), van Uden (1974, 1979), Leshin, Pearce, and Funderburg (1974), Calvert and Silverman (1975), and Ling (1976). The thinking of selected workers in speech science, speech development and disorders, speech teaching, and organizational patterns is contained in a compendium edited by Connor (1971).

The above sample of literature citations points up the problem of demarcating a reasonably specific time frame in the history of the field that could be labeled *Then*. Nor would a detailed review accomplish this. On the contrary, we need but look at our references to recognize that hardly a subject treated in this volume has not been the object of past and continuing attention, some of it, for its time, impressively seminal and applicable. The historical process is continuous and resists immutable time markers for this or that trend or development. Nevertheless, for purposes of this exposition some delimitation of the period to be covered makes sense. Hence, the author shall arbitrarily confine his observations to the approximate time course of his own association with the field, which commenced in the fall of 1933. Furthermore, as requested by the editors, his presentation will be for the most part impressionistic, based on an amalgam of observation of speech training here and abroad, on his own experience in teaching hearing-impaired children, adults, and their teachers, and, of course, on continuing exchange with colleagues including practitioners and investigators. Moreover, he shall not attempt to assay the relative weights of the amalgam ingredients. Suffice to assert that it represents an integrated empirical entity.

What about the "Now" of the title? Because what shall be said on this point suggests implicitly more of a *forecast, even a hope,* than it does widespread contemporary practice as observed by the author, the arbitrary time referent for the *now* is simply this volume.

From all of this the writer will delineate what he considers to be the prominent Then influences and practices in speech training and will appose them with Now observations. In an elementary heuristic sense, this approach may be useful for teachers and clinicians, should they choose to survey their own practice.

TRANSITION FROM INTUITIVE-EMPIRICAL TO SCIENTIFIC BASE

Then   Instruction was by and large intuitively and empirically based. A substantial number of teachers were trained either in an apprentice or inservice setting in a school for the deaf or, if enrolled in a formal course of preparation, were taught by individuals whose primary qualifications consisted of experience as teachers of the hearing impaired. A popular attitude of the time, and by no means passé, is forcefully illustrated in the following comment by John Dutton Wright, Founder and then Director of the Wright Oral School in New York (1928):

> I studiously avoided technicalities as I did in the book for parents. There are enough valuable books where that form of wisdom can be found. These pages merely contain some of the plain, common sense ideas that nearly forty years of educational effort in the oral instruction of the deaf have forced to the surface of my consciousness.

Occasionally, there appeared well designed studies such as that of Hudgins and Numbers (1942) oriented to "error analysis" of deaf students' speech; but there was scant evidence in the classroom of practice resting on a carefully constructed scientific base. This is not to imply that the results were universally disappointing. We know otherwise. But it would flout experience to assert that the general results were as satisfactory as we sanguinely hoped they would or, more importantly, could be. Of course, unsatisfactory results can be attributed to something other than failure or reluctance to apply a scientific paradigm to instruction, assuming one were available. The point here is simply that such application appears generally not to have been observed. Note too, Nickerson (1975) and Ling (1976).

Now   This volume amply documents the prospect of a transition from an intuitive-empirical base to a scientific one that promises to be germane to practice. Granted that there are many open spaces between convincing experimental findings that are pertinent to training and which for the present need to be filled intuitively. The fact that this volume exists at all may enhance the probability of the transition. It represents both symbolically and substantively the felicitous deinsularization of the field and, incidentally, underlines the complexity of the problem drawing, as it does, from an imposing variety of disciplines, technologies, and professional experience.

EARLY IDENTIFICATION AND TRAINING

Then   The potential contribution to the development of speech and language of instituting a training regime at an early age has long been recognized and advocated for hearing-impaired children. As long ago as 1680, Dalgarno wrote that "successful addresses can be made to a deaf child even in the cradle." And at the start of our Then period, the White House Conference (1931) stated

> The value of preschool training for the hearing child seems now to be thoroughly established. A study of the preschool deaf and hard-of-hearing child is urgently needed, and the techniques now used for the study of hearing children should be tried out with the deaf . . . The establishment of a nursery school for deaf children where research could be carried on is urgently needed.

Despite this recommendation from a prestigious and quasi-official source and the prevalence of isolated pockets of activity in some institutions, mostly private, as shown in Miller's survey of the status of the preschool deaf child (1934) the movement toward preschool education, not to mention work with infants, was painfully slow. In this writer's opinion, this may have been due to any number or combination of causes. Lack of funds, indifference to early identification, unavailability of suitable and cost-effective tests, isolation from the mainstream of developmental and sensory psychology and the yet-to-emerge findings of psycholinguistics and neurophysiology, statutory lower age limits for admission to school, and resistance of inappropriately prepared and poorly motivated teachers are among the more prominent causes. But perhaps a more fundamental cause was the attitude of the public residential schools as revealed in Miller's survey. Representative of this point of view is the statement of Superintendent Stevenson of the California School for the Deaf, Berkeley, who is quoted by Miller as follows:

> We do not admit under five and a half. Even then beginning teachers and housemothers complain for various reasons. The preschool child should be handled as a preschool child and under special environment and for definite purposes. Then there might be some *little* (italics mine) advantage. My own experience tells me as it is now carried on it is not good.

The merits of Stevenson's argument and similar ones by his colleagues in public residential schools is not here at issue. What is important is that the large majority of deaf children were then educated in public residential schools. In 1934, for example, there were 19,627 children enrolled in schools for the deaf in the United States of whom 14,476 were in public residential schools, 4,253 in public day schools, and 898 in denominational and private schools (American Annals of the Deaf, 1934). Thus early instruction in speech was not possible for many.

Now The recognition of the potential benefits of early shaped sensory experience for a plastic maturing nervous system is a conspicuous feature of the contemporary educational scene expressed, for example, in the Head Start program (Caldwell, 1970; Kagan, 1970). The trend has encompassed very young hearing-impaired children— "even," to recall Dalgarno's 17th century phrase, "in the cradle"— and has stimulated a variety of scientific and professional activities aimed at understanding their needs and providing services for them. These include, among others, methods of early identification, developmental studies of expressive and receptive language, programs of "management," and guidance of parents. (See, e.g., Davis, 1964; Luterman, 1979; Mencher, 1976; Simmons-Martin and Calvert, 1979.) To seize the opportunity to exploit beneficially for speech development the early years of the life of a hearing-impaired child may in the long run contribute as much as any single factor to the dissipation of the lugubrious notion that intensive speech training for the profoundly deaf is a futile enterprise.

SENSORY MODALITIES AND TRAINING

Then The predominant sensory channels for the development and correction of speech were vision and touch with internal feedback cued by kinesthesia. When the commonly suggested method of development was imitation, the clear inference was that the child *watched* the teacher's model (Haycock, 1933; Joiner, 1948; Yale, 1925). Among other appeals to the eye were such visual aids as color codes for some distinctive features (New, 1942), diagrams including frontal views of visible articulatory positions and sagital sections of the head showing static tongue position for individual phonemes, orthographic systems to aid pronunciation, and symbol systems for pitch, intensity, and duration. In structured training situations, visual feedback was provided by child and teacher talking at a mirror.

The conventional classroom paradigm for the use of touch in the development and correction of speech was to have the child place his or her hand or finger tips where he or she could "sense" a sound produced by the teacher. The place could be in front of the teacher's mouth to feel the air stream or puff of air for voiceless consonants, on the teacher's nose for nasals, on the face or throat or occasionally on the sternum for voicing of consonants and vowels, and on the hyoid region for muscle tension and relaxation. For feedback the child would feel his or her own production. Suprasegmentals were conveyed by tapping patterns on a child's shoulder and by producing varying pressures with the thumb in the palm of a child's hand coincidental with speech production.

Sound sources such as the keyboard of a piano or organ, the tympanum of a drum, and a taut diaphragm stretched over the wide opening of a megaphone (Goldstein, 1939) were frequently employed. A few accounts and studies suggested the possibilities of tactile stimulation for speech training. Among them were Gault's Teletactor (1934), the Tadoma method of S. K. Alcorn used with the deaf-blind (1942), Becking's work (1953) on perception of air-borne sound on the thorax of deaf children, the Picketts' tactual vocoder (1963), and Kringelbotn's experiments combining vision and vibrotactile stimulation (1968). Yet there was little classroom evidence of application of systemtic tactile approaches. Even the placement of the child's hand on the teacher's face appeared to be more of a mindless ritualistic gesture than recognition of subtle differentiated perception related to locus of placement. Nevertheless, some children did respond favorably to teacher-produced, information-bearing tactile cues even though they were not part of any predetermined organized developmental sequence.

The full promise of the value of using residual hearing explicit in the expositions of the 19th century writers cited above and those who followed was not realized up to and including the Then period. Systematic auditory training, although enthusiastically championed by a few people, was not widely practiced in classrooms. We can only speculate about the factors and their relative influence in contributing to this situation. In this writer's opinion, the more significant among them are skepticism about the cost effectiveness of concentrated auditory training, especially for the severely and profoundly deaf; emphasis on evaluating training only on receptive skills, to the exclusion of its contribution to speech acquisition and improvement; nonreinforcing aural-oral environments; indifference to thorough audiologic assessment of auditory capacity; little early identification and consequent use of amplification; unavailability, at least in the earlier period, of convenient, durable, wearable, and acoustically effective hearing aids; failure to stress or even include aural approaches in teacher training; paucity of materials of demonstrated value for structuring the training and integrating it with speech, language, and academic instruction; and just a persistent annoyance on the part of some experienced professionals with the "exaggerated claims" advanced by ebullient advocates. The weight of these factors or combinations of them undoubtedly varied with local attitudes and circumstances.

Now The *potential* for the use of the auditory system as the method of initial choice for speech training is being increasingly recognized, discussed, and investigated if not yet widely applied. The possibilities are supported by data from the Gallaudet College Center for Demographic Studies that indicate that nearly half of hearing-impaired children have hearing levels of 84 dB or better in three speech frequencies (1971). It is reasonable to assume that, if the frequency of 250 Hz had been included in the calculation and a cut-off established at 90 dB, the numbers of children with hearing markedly significant for speech development would be much greater. A literature review is beyond the scope of this chapter. It suffices to cite some illustrative sources: Beebe, 1953; Calvert and Silverman, 1975; Ewing and Ewing, 1954; Guberina, 1964; Ling, 1976; Lowell and Stoner, 1960; Pollack, 1970; Ross and Giolas, 1978; Sanders, 1971; Simmons-Martin, 1972; Watson, 1951; Wedenberg, 1954; Whetnall and Fry, 1964. Although they may vary in details of technique and procedure, maximum emphasis on use of hearing and comprehensive intervention well beyond the traditional school setting are common to all.

The factors that have stimulated the contemporary growing interest in and activities related to auditory approaches to speech training are, in a sense, the obverse of those mentioned above as mitigating against their application in the classroom in the past. To these should be added our increasing knowledge of the temporal and spectral aspects of speech perception by the hearing impaired aided by such tools as the spectrograph and speech synthesizer. This should guide us as we take advantage of more efficient transducers and compact circuitry in the design of hearing aids. Attention to acoustic ambience in the design of new and renovated facilities is also a constructive step. Nevertheless, whether the hoped-for convergence of these encouraging factors for the use of residual hearing in speech training will be rationally and intensively applied, especially in the current pervasive institutional contexts of "total communication," remains to be seen.

As can be noted in this volume, there is a continuing interest in the coding of speech for presentation to the eye and the skin and in the role of motor activity in speech perception and production. For purposes related to speech training, computer-generated visual displays of features of speech have been investigated (Boothroyd et al., 1975), as have tactile devices (Engelmann and Rosor, 1975; Miller, Engebretson, and DeFilippo, 1976; Sparks et al., 1979). All of these are in various stages of experimentation and there is no evidence of widespread classroom use. Any appreciable use of these and other types of "sensory aids" for speech training should depend on the results of investigations of such problems as technologic design, content display, bisensory facilitation or inhibition, instructional paradigms, and, of course, rigorous "field" evaluation (see Levitt and Nye, 1971). As laboratory workers extend their efforts and interests to the field, they are likely to be confronted by many "grass roots" questions posed by teachers. For example, does the aid deliver what is intended? Will something simpler do just as well? Does the result justify the expenditure of time, energy, and money? Will apparent initial motivation wear off? Is there evidence that the training carries over to extramural situations? Viewed positively, these questions present teachers and investigators a splendid opportunity to collaborate effectively in pursuit of a common goal.

INSTRUCTIONAL APPROACHES TO SPEECH DEVELOPMENT

Then   The initial approach to speech training generally focused on articulation with emphasis on individual phonemes ("segments") as the irreducible unit of speech input to the child. Order of development of the single sounds seemed most often to be determined by their ease of production and their visibility on the face of the teacher. In the development of consonants, attention was directed to differentiating features of place, manner, and nasal-voice-voiceless distinctions communicated by vision and touch. Mouth opening with the point of tongue behind lower front teeth demonstrated vowel positions. Height of tongue was communicated by width of opening and place of arching by extraoral modeling or, on occasion, by tongue and lip manipulation. Frequently, exaggerated motor activity such as lip rounding or retraction was employed for kinesthetic feedback for "difficult" sounds. Elicited imitation by the child of exaggerated teacher models may, in part, be responsible for his or her deviant voice quality; for example, the excessively exploded stop consonant /p/ in combination with a vowel resulting in breathiness, or abnormal opening of the velar-pharyngeal port caused by excessive downward movement of the jaw resulting in hypernasality, or excessive tension felt when feeling the hyoid region resulting in harshness. The production of an individual sound was soon associated with an orthographic symbol to give the child a visual aid to pronunciation using the symbols of his culture. The Northampton symbols constitute an example of a popular system (Yale, 1925).

Development of individual sounds preceded their combination into syllables. Again, ease of production guided choice of syllabic combinations along with the knowledge that a syllable also formed a word which could be illustrated by a picture used as a stimulus to elicit speech and to show that speech communicated something, for example, /ʃu/, /θʌm/, /but/. Stored static percepts of individual sounds made accommodation to the phonetic dynamics of connected speech, including coarticulation, exceedingly difficult and may have contributed to aberrant prosody. This is not to say that the dynamics were unfamiliar to teachers or that they did not need to be taken into account in speech training, but their relative emphasis and their place in the sequence of speech training may have undervalued their basic importance.

As soon as the child could produce some vowels with ease, attention was directed to voice quality. Proper fundamental pitch and subsequent pitch control were generally more or less accomplished by the child feeling the face, larynx, or sternal area of the teacher during production of extended vowels. Eventually, intonation was communicated by written symbols for duration, intensity, and rise and fall of pitch, including phrase markers. This was then carried over to training in prosody, or as it was commonly called, rhythm. Prosodic patterns of linguistic units that occur in the language were practiced; for example, article-noun (*a ball*), article-adjective-noun (*a tall man*), and so on. Sometimes an easily produced nonsense syllable was substituted for the required phrase to avoid complication by difficulty of articulation. The attainment of mechanical skills related to stress patterns involving control of a composite of intensity, pitch, duration, rate, and phrasing led to exercises in their application to talker intent in communicating content, emotion, and purpose.

This necessarily brief review of the Then instructional approaches to speech training conveys their central features and is not intended as *the* definitive analysis of methodology. That would be presumptuous. Of course, there were variations and, in a few instances, fundamental departure from the conventional methods and the premises on which they rested.

As has been noted, in the experience of this writer, a substantial number of deaf persons educated during the period attained a high degree of functional speech ability that contributed importantly to their social, emotional, and economic self-realization. One can only speculate as to why some did well and others did not. Among the popular hypotheses accounting for success is the constant exposure to a speech-demanding and reinforcing environment in and out of school combined with consistency of method. In some institutions as a child went through school, speech training, even allowing for individual differences, was characterized by a core of common procedures and attitudes shared by the staff. Among these, for example, are an orthographic system, prosodic symbols, use of aids of one sort or another, specific drills, and, of course, the conviction that time and effort spent on speech training is worthwhile. It appears that some children respond well to this kind of situation despite theoretical objections to their training regimes.

Now The fundamental feature of the Now approach is the imposition of structure on a developmental sequence given, particularly, the early age at which an increasing number of children are identified and referred for attention. Unlike the initial emphasis on articulation, this approach rests on the recognition that phonation and prosody precede precise articulation in the developmental sequence (Lenneberg and Long, 1974). Studies of prosodic features in children's utterances suggest, for example, that children appear to learn intonation patterns before they learn segmental features (Weir, 1966). Thus, the general sequence requires the child first to vocalize, to control vocal duration and pitch, and to produce vowels and consonants in that order, as suggested by Ling (1976). This would be accomplished initially by an auditory approach as stressed by Ling and, certainly initially, as recommended by Calvert and Silverman (1975). Given the auditory sensitivity for low frequencies common to most hearing-impaired children, the rhythmic patterns that carry much information in speech are likely to be within their perceptual reach and with training are incorporated in their own speech production.

With fundamental vocalization and a semblance of prosodic patterning established and consistent with maturational status, attention is given to both the phonetic and phonologic aspects of articulation, the sequence contingent upon achievement of target behaviors. The time at which an orthographic system should be introduced or whether one should be used at all is an open question. Some workers argue that some system is helpful in communicating pronunciation and visually reinforcing production. Others contend that it orients the child too visually and fosters undesirable segmentation.

The Now approach also has its variations in application. Among them are differences in adaptation of amplification to audiologic findings, in relative emphasis on uni- and bisensory stimulation, in the integration of the approach into a context of total communication, in the use of hand cues (Cornett, 1968; Cued Speech, 1970), in manner and extent of association of speech with language and subject matter instruction, in criteria for mastery of specific skills, in responsibility for actual day-to-day implementation, in criteria for altering sequences or for shift to other emphases of approaches, in use of sensory aids, and in time devoted to formal speech training in a school or clinic schedule.

TEACHER OR SPEECH PATHOLOGIST

Then   By and large the teacher was responsible for speech training. This was probably due to the isolation of the education of the deaf from the main currents of speech therapy and pathology directed primarily toward disordered speech of those with normal hearing. Speech therapists had little or no exposure, in training or in practice, to speech problems of the severely and profoundly deaf and hence developed little, if any, interest in the subject. Even if an interest and concern were expressed, it was felt by some teachers of the deaf that speech therapists were not prepared to understand nor to address educationally the speech needs of deaf children. Furthermore, development, application to a variety of learning situations, correction, and motivation of speech had to be an all-day concern and not an isolated experience with a speech therapist detached from the rest of the day's activities. Although instructional sessions devoted exclusively to speech were usually included in the schedule of the school day, the responsibility for conducting them was the teacher's and on occasion that of a "specialist" who had a more than average interest in speech and who was trained as a teacher of the deaf. Recall that A. G. Bell's lectures were directed to teachers.

Now   There is an incipient trend, if not a major movement, to employ speech-language pathologists to teach hearing-impaired children to talk (Ross, 1976). It is argued that there is a pertinent body of knowledge from speech and psycholinguistic science and a pool of assessment methods and therapeutic procedures that can and should be profitably applied to speech development, correction, and maintenance. Furthermore, with the responsibility for instruction in language, basic skills, and subject matter, it is too much to expect the classroom teacher or even the supervisor to make the concentrated application to the child's speech needs systematically, expeditiously, and effectively. This does not mean that the teacher should have no responsibility but rather that attention to the child's speech would be influenced and guided by an appropriately qualified specialist.

How the matter should be approached is still an open question. It will probably be determined as much by local administrative organization and motivation, by availability of funds, by professional qualifications of specialists including credential requirements, by the dominant characteristics of the children to be served, by sharing experience with colleagues, by a climate of acceptance by teachers (some of whom may prefer sole responsibility for speech), as by any predetermined rigid "model."

Three salient areas of concern to the overall problem of speech training are worthy of note. They are added to those discussed in the above format and transcend attitudes toward the Then and Now points of view. They are evaluation, formulation of an oral message by severely and profoundly deaf children, and the teacher's ear.

EVALUATION

Implicit in what has been said, whether of the Then or Now period, is the pressing need for evaluation of what we do in speech training. It is a shameless and egregious bow to motherhood to state that the effectiveness of any procedure or change therein be tested by the most objective methods we can devise so that substantive grounds are established for instituting, eliminating, amending, or modifying our arrangements and practices. In many aspects of education this is devilishly difficult to accomplish. Many of the outcomes we seek may resist satisfactory measurement, and as we yield to the understandable urge and need to measure it may be a sign of our ignorance that we are more precise than a subject allows. Moreover, some anticipated results such as the ultimate social and economic usefulness of methods of training must await the passage of years before an attempt at evaluation is even appropriate. Nevertheless, the problem must be addressed.

It is helpful to clarify the purposes of evaluation. At some early stage in a child's development, decisions need to be reached about a child's demonstrated abilities and potential capacities and needs that lead to appropriate programming and, in many instances, to school placement. How much and what kind of speech training is required? Is it likely to be accessible in a special school, in a special class, in the mainstream, in a context of total communication of aural-oralism? These kinds of questions suggest evaluation that has as its purpose a combination of aptitude for learning speech and prediction about suitability of program and placement. The demand here is for establishing criteria for placement and change that are validated as best we can by measures and judgments, and which accommodate factors other than speech needs that are pertinent to the comprehensive planning for the child's education.

A purpose differing appreciably from the foregoing is that of "diagnosis." Here the purpose is to determine a child's performance of a variety of identifiable speech skills to formulate a reasonably detailed instructional plan whether immediate or long range. The basis may be an "error analysis" approach which targets for attention certain deviations in speech, or a developmental one in which a child's speech performance stands in a predetermined sequence that points to a next step in speech training. In practice, the approach is likely to be a combination of the two with relative emphasis depending, among other things, on a child's age and development. There is currently a discernable trend toward more structured diagnostic procedures than had been the case in the Then period. For example, Monsen (1975) has suggested segmental and prosodic evaluative indices of speech mechanics. The segmental indices would seek to establish coordination of laryngeal and oral articulatory gestures, accuracy of articulatory movement, and distinctiveness of phoneme images. Also included would be location of phoneme targets in phonological space, coarticulation of phonemes, and control of duration. Prosodic evaluation would consider pitch, duration, and intensity control. Ling (1976) has produced a detailed protocol that evaluates segmental and nonsegmental aspects of speech at both phonetic and phonological levels. It should be very helpful in lesson planning for speech.

Another distinctive purpose for evaluation is to assess a child's progress in speech. At a refined analytical level, diagnostic protocols may be applied to this purpose. Periodic checks of the needs therein assessed can indicate whether and to what extent specific objectives established by them have been achieved. Less easily evaluated is progress in the "carryover" from formal speech training during a particular training period. Has the intelligibility of a child's speech improved in and out of the classroom? Is speech an increasingly vital mechanism of social relations? . . . with those familiar to the child? . . . with strangers? Has the child's attitude toward requests for repetition of utterances been affected? Has it decreased or increased confidence in his or her ability to talk and consequently in the desire to do so? As we evaluate speech progress, realistic answers to these and similar questions must be sought conscientiously. They may cause us to examine aspects of speech training not revealed by conventional measures of skills and may contribute to more global decisions about such matters as mainstreaming, modes of communication, and even, ultimately, to career choice.

Formulation of the Oral Message

Another aspect of speech training, although intimately related to diagnostic assessment and evaluation, is worthy of special note. This is the process involved in a child's formulation of an oral message. Consider the task of the deaf child in so doing. First he must have something that he wishes to convey. Then he must produce the language appropriate to his purpose mindful of its syntactic, semantic, and phonological requirements. We know, too, that the phonology requires attention to segments frequently complicated by articulatory dynamics, to phonation that may be influenced by acoustic ambience, and to prosody involving proper mechanics applied to talker intent. Sensitivity to the ultimate goal of function speech demands of the teacher that a complete description of what children are doing when they speak include not only the actual forms produced and their context but the social uses of that speech—its *pragmatics*. Formulation of the oral message does indeed require coherence in satisfying the multiple demands of production.

All of this has to be taken into account by the teacher as evaluation and subsequent instructional planning are extended beyond the analysis of mechanical speech skills. In so doing, the teacher must, for example, attend to a child's revisionary behavior because it is reasonable to assume that the deaf talker will frequently be asked by a listener to repeat an utterance because it has not been understood when first spoken. The query may be in the form of a simple "What," a quizzical facial expression, or whatever. In investigation of listener uncertainty with normally hearing children it has been found that interaction between speaker and listener may contribute as much to articulatory inconsistency as to phonetic context (Weiner and Ostrowski, 1979). In language performance, revisions appear to be more frequent than repetitions in answer to the question "What?" (Gallagher, 1977).

For her speaking deaf pupil the teacher must ask what the pupil has internalized about what must be changed if he or she is not understood. Should the pupil change the language? And if so, does he or she change its structural, lexical, or phonologic features? And if the latter, does he or she change articulation, phonation, or prosody? Does this change derive from an internalized phonologic system including a catalogue of "error probabilities," as suggested by Calvert and Silverman (1975)? The answers to such questions should influence the teacher's response to revision, or lack thereof. In seeking to encourage self-monitoring and self-correction, careful judgment is required of the level of specificity of intervention. If, for example, the teacher has decided that a particular phoneme needs correction does the teacher identify the phoneme for the child? Does the teacher say a phoneme needs correction without identifying it? Or does the teacher merely say to the child, "Say that again and watch your speech"? A recent experience of this writer illustrates the significance of the problem of revisionary behavior. In the course of a lesson in a class of 6-year-olds that this writer observed, the teacher responded with "What did you say?" to the child's oral production of a sentence. The child's language was not only structurally perfect but it was impressively rich for a 6-year-old. The intent of the teacher's question was to improve the speech but in response the child changed her superb language. Perhaps, this occurred because the lesson was emphasizing language or because the child was simply not aware that revision of speech mechanics may be the response of choice to the frequently encountered "what" question.

The entire question of self-monitoring, of which revisionary behavior is an essential aspect, should command the attention of investigators and planners of speech training. As suggested by Vegeley (1964), it is the fundamental process initiated when a person compares his or her speech to certain standards of speech correctness. The deaf person can do this only by indirect comparisons based on knowledge, gained through training, that in order to be understood certain sounds have to be produced in certain ways. This is supplemented by the reinforcement received in communicating orally with normally hearing people.

THE TEACHER'S EAR

As fundamental as any factor that contributes to the effectiveness of any program or procedure of speech training is the teacher's (clinician's) ear. Obviously, responses—whether to an isolated segment or to a complex message—depend on what one thinks one has heard. This, in turn, determines whether in a particular instance and for a particular child the teacher reinforces the production by acceptance or by some form of reward, or whether and how the teacher intervenes to "fix" or to change what is being said. What one thinks one has heard influences decisions related to the reasons for intervention. Should the teacher intervene because he or she does not understand the child (despite reverse auditory training in listening to deaf talkers), or to call attention to something that is being stressed in the child's program at that time, or to make a judgment that a naive listener would not understand the speech?

Pertinent to these questions, Vegeley (1964) found that normally hearing listeners were consistently better than deaf talkers in their ability to predict the intelligibility of the speech of deaf talkers. Vegeley's results underline the fact that people with normal hearing serve as a vital part of the deaf talker's feedback loop for speech. This is so obvious that it is hardly worth mentioning. Nevertheless, the feedback, depending so heavily on the ear of the listener, may be imperfect and may on occasion actually reinforce a talker's mistakes and punish some of the better speech. Increased emphasis on ear training of all who have to do with the speech of hearing-impaired children should reduce, if not avoid, the occurrences of such situations.

SUMMARY

This review has addressed speech training of hearing-impaired children from the point of view of past and current practices, including topics importantly related to them. The title, however catchy, implies a questionable construct. It is difficult to demarcate with any degree of validity or precision what is past or current in an essentially continuous professional and scientific process. Nevertheless, faithful to this assignment and given the latitude by the editors to discourse impressionistically, the author singled out as worthy of Then and Now treatment the following topics: transition from an intuitive-empirical base to a scientific one; early identification; sense modalities in speech training; instructional approaches; and the issue of teacher or specialist responsibility for speech training. Contemporary needs for methods of evaluation in speech training, for an understanding of the complexity of the task faced by a hearing-impaired child in formulating an oral message, and for increased emphasis on ear training of teachers are discussed.

Finally, whatever one may think of the ideas and practices of those who have gone before, we should admire and be grateful to them for having undertaken to teach speech at all and for their persistent conviction that their efforts, in the face of skepticism, incredulity, and indifference, were worthwhile. In a profound sense this conference is an expression not of a sharp break with them but of a continuity that we hope is stimulating and productive.

REFERENCES

Alcorn, S, K. 1942. Development of speech by the Tadoma method. In Report of the Proceedings of the 32nd Meeting of the Convention of American Instructors of the Deaf, 1941. U.S. Government Printing Office, Washington, D.C.

American Annals of the Deaf. 1934. Schools for the deaf in the United States. Am. Ann. Deaf 79:8–31.

Amman, J. C. 1700. Dissertatio de Loquela (Dissertation on Speech). John Walters, Amsterdam.

Becking, A. G. T. 1953. Perception of airborne sound in the thorax of deaf children. In Proceedings of the International Course in Paedo-audiology. Groningen, Verenigde Drukkerijen Hoitsema, N.V.

Beebe, H. H. 1953. A Guide to Help the Severely Hard-of-Hearing Child. S. Karger, Basel.

Bell, A. G. 1907. The Mechanism of Speech. Funk & Wagnalls, New York.

Bell, A. M. 1894. Sounds and Their Relations. Volta Bureau, Washington, D.C.

Bell, A. M. 1900. Principles of Speech. Volta Bureau, Washington, D.C.

Bonet, J. P. 1890. Simplification of the Letters of the Alphabet and Method of Teaching Deaf Mutes to Speak, (1620) Translated. London, 1890.

Boothroyd, A., P. Archambault, R. E. Adams, and R. D. Storm. 1975. Use of a computer-based system of speech training aids for deaf persons. Volta Rev. 77:178–193.

Caldwell, B. M. 1970. The rational for early intervention. Except. Child. 36:717–726.

Calvert, D. R., and S. R. Silverman. 1975. Speech and Deafness. A. G. Bell Association for the Deaf, Washington, D.C.

Clarke School for the Deaf. 1971. Speech Development. Clarke School for the Deaf, Northampton, Mass.

Connor, L. E. (ed.). 1971. Speech for the Deaf Child: Knowledge and Use. A. G. Bell Association for the Deaf, Washington, D.C.

Cornett, R. O. 1968. Cued speech. In Report of Proceedings of the 43rd Meeting of the Convention of American Instructors of the Deaf. U.S. Government Printing Office, Washington, D.C.

Cued speech. 1970. Aust. Teacher Deaf 11:153–165.

Dalgarno, G. 1680. Didascalocophus, or the Deaf and Dumb Man's Tutor. Timo. Halton, Oxford.

Davis, H. 1964. The young deaf child: Identification and management. Acta Otolaryngol. Suppl. 206.

Engelmann, S., and R. Rosor. 1975. Tactual hearing experiment with deaf and hearing subjects. Except. Child. 41:243–253.

Ewing, I. R., and A. W. G. Ewing. 1954. Speech and the Deaf Child. A. G. Bell Association for the Deaf, Washington, D.C.

Farrar, A. 1923. Arnold's Education of the Deaf. 2nd Ed. Francis Carter, Derby, England.

Fry, D. B. 1966. The development of the phonological system in the normal and deaf child. In F. Smith and G. A. Miller (eds.), The Genesis of Language: A Psycholinguistic Approach. M.I.T. Press, Cambridge, Mass.

Gallagher, T. M. 1977. Revision behaviors in the speech of normal children developing language. J. Speech Hear. Res. 20:303–318.

Gallaudet College, Center for Demographic Studies. 1971. Audiological Examinations of Hearing Impaired Students. Gallaudet College, Washington, D.C.

Gault, R. H. 1934. The use of the sense of touch in developing speech. Volta Rev. 36:82–83.

Goldstein, M. A. 1939. The Acoustic Method for the Training of the Deaf and Hard-of-Hearing Child. Laryngoscope Press, St. Louis, Mo.

Graser, J. B. 1829. The Deaf Mute Restored to Humanity by Visible and Spoken Speech. Bayreuth.

Guberina, P. 1964. Verbotonal method and its application to the rehabilitation of the deaf. In Report of Proceedings of the International Congress on Education of the Deaf and the 41st Meeting of the Convention of American Instructors of the Deaf, 1963. U.S. Government Printing Office, Washington, D.C.

Haycock, G. S. 1933. The Teaching of Speech. Hill & Ainsworth, Stoke-on-Trent, England.

Holder, W. 1669. Elements of Speech. London.

Hudgins, C. V., and F. C. Numbers. 1942. An investigation of intelligibility of speech of the deaf. Genet. Psychol. Monogr. 25:289–392.

Itard, J. M. G. 1821. Traité des Maladies de l'Oreille et de l'Audition. Paris.

Joiner, E. 1948. Our speech teaching heritage. Volta Rev. 50:417–422.

Kagan, J. 1970. The determinants of attention in the infant. Am. Sci. 3:298–305.

Kringelbotn, M. 1968. Experiments with some visual and vibrotactile aids for the deaf. 113:311–317.

Lenneberg, E. H., and B. S. Long. 1974. Language development. In Psychology and the Handicapped Child (U.S. Department of Health, Education and Welfare). U.S. Government Printing Office, Washington, D.C.

Leshin, G. (ed.), M. F. Pearce, and R. S. Funderburg. 1974. Speech for the Hearing Impaired Child. University of Arizona, Tucson.

Levitt, H., and P. W. Nye. (eds.) 1971. Sensory Aids for the Hearing Impaired: Proceedings of a Conference. National Academy of Engineering, Washington, D.C.

Ling, D. 1976. Speech and the Hearing Impaired Child. A. G. Bell Association for the Deaf, Washington, D.C.

Lowell, E. L., and M. Stoner. 1960. Play It by Ear! John Tracy Clinic, Los Angeles.

Luterman, D. 1979. Counseling Parents of Hearing-Impaired Children. Little, Brown & Company, Boston.

Mencher, G. T. (ed.). 1976. Early Identification of Hearing Loss. S. Karger, New York.

Miller, J. D., A. M. Engebretson, and C. L. DeFilippo. 1976. Preliminary research with a three-channel vibrotactile speech reception aid for the deaf. In Speech and Hearing, Defects and Aids, Language Acquisition. John Wiley, New York.

Miller, M. K. 1934. The status of the preschool deaf child. Am. Ann. Deaf 79:414–427.

Monsen, R. 1975. (Personal communication). In D. R. Calvert, and S. R. Silverman (eds.), Speech and Deafness. A. G. Bell Association for the Deaf, Washington, D.C.

New, M. 1942. Color in speech teaching. Volta Rev. 44:133–138, 199–203.

Nickerson, R. S. 1975. Characteristics of the speech of deaf persons. Volta Rev. 77:342–362.

Pickett, J. M., and R. H. Pickett. 1963. Communication of speech sounds by a tactual vocoder. J. Speech Hear. Res. 6:207–222.

Pollack, D. 1970. Educational Audiology for the Limited Hearing Infant. Charles C Thomas, Publisher, Springfield, Ill.

Ross, M. 1976. Verbal communication: The state of the art. Volta Rev. 78:324–328.

Ross, M., and Giolas, T. G. 1978. Auditory Management of Hearing-Impaired Children. University Park Press, Baltimore.

Sanders, D. A. 1971. Aural Rehabilitation. Prentice-Hall, Englewood Cliffs, N.J.

Schunhoff, H. F. 1957. The Teaching of Speech and by Speech in Public Residential Schools for the Deaf in the United States, 1815–1955. West Virginia Schools for the Deaf and Blind, Romney, W.Va.

Simmons-Martin, A. 1972. The oral/aural procedure: Theoretical basis and rationale. Volta Rev. 74:541–551.

Simmons-Martin, A., and D. R. Calvert. (Eds.) 1979. Parent-Infant Intervention. Grune & Stratton, New York.

Sparks, D. W., L. A. Ardell, M. Bourgeois, B. Wiedmer, and P. K. Kuhl. 1979. Investigating the MESA (Multipoint electrotactile speech aid): The transmission of connected discourse. J. Acoust. Soc. Am. 65:810–815.

Urbantschitsch, V. 1895. Horübüngen bei Taubstummheit. Urban & Schwarzenberg, Vienna.

van Helmont, F. M. 1667. A Brief Description of the Truly Natural Hebrew Alphabet. Sulzbuch (Germany).

van Uden, A. 1974. Dove Kinderen Leren Spreken (How Children Learn to Speak). Universitaire Pers Rotterdam, Rotterdam, Holland. (Summary in English)

van Uden, A. 1979. How to converse with a speechless and languageless child. In A. Simmons-Martin and D. R. Calvert (eds.), Parent-Infant Intervention. Grune & Stratton, New York.

Vatter, J. 1875. Die Ausbildung des Taubstummen in der Lautsprache. Frankfurt A.M.

Vegeley, C. 1964. Monitoring monosyllabic words by deaf children. In Report of the Proceedings of the International Congress on Education of the Deaf and the 41st Meeting of the Convention of American Instructors of the Deaf. U.S. Government Printing Office, Washington, D.C.

Vorce, E. 1974. Teaching Speech to Deaf Children (The Lexington School for the Deaf. Education Series, Book IX). A. G. Bell Association for the Deaf, Washington, D.C.

Watson, T. J. 1951. Auditory training and the development of speech and language in children with defective hearing. Acta Otolaryngol. 40:95–103.

Wedenberg, E. 1954. Auditory training of severely hard of hearing preschool children. Acta Otolaryngol. Suppl. 110.

Weiner, F. F., and A. A. Ostrowski. 1979. Effects of listener uncertainty on articulatory inconsistency. J. Speech Hear. Disord. 44:487–493.

Weir, R. H. 1966. Some questions on the child's learning phonology. In F. Smith and G. A. Miller (eds.), The Genesis of Language. M.I.T. Press, Cambridge, Mass.

Whetnall, E., and Fry, D. B. 1964. Learning to Hear. William Heinemann, London.

White House Conference on Child Health and Protection. 1931. Special Education: The Handicapped and the Gifted. The Century Co., New York.

Wright, J. D. 1928. Speech Teaching to the Deaf. The Wright Oral School, New York.

Yale, C. A. 1925. Formation and Development of Elementary English Sounds. Gazette Printing Co., Northampton, Mass.

RECENT RESEARCH ON THE SPEECH PRODUCTION ABILITIES OF THE HEARING IMPAIRED

CHAPTER 1

GENERAL EFFECTS OF DEAFNESS ON PHONATION AND ARTICULATION

Randall B. Monsen

In contrast to the situation of the normally hearing child, the deaf child is confronted with the task of learning how to produce speech sounds by how they look on the face, how they feel through vibration, what he or she is told or shown about them, and only to some degree by their auditory qualities, as filtered and distorted by impaired hearing. Thus, to study the speech of the deaf is really to study the participation of hearing in speech acquisition and speech production. No matter how innate language may be, a child must first hear samples of it to produce it normally. To some extent, not being able to hear one's own speech as it is being uttered, at least during the period of language acquisition, may also play an important role in learning to speak normally. In this sense, the general effect of deafness on speech production is that it forces the individual to try to learn speech by an imitation that is not wholly, or even in large part, auditory.

Although deafness exerts a dominant effect on the learning of speech, it is by no means the only important factor in shaping speech production abilities. The amount and quality of speech training and the use of suitable amplification devices (among other factors) are also of obvious importance. After all, without speech training and sound amplification, the effect of deafness is quite clear, consistent, and un-avoidable: it prevents an individual from ever learning to speak. Effective teaching thus interferes with the otherwise neat correlation between not hearing and not speaking. Nevertheless, if we are going to talk about the general effects of deafness on speech, it is useful to assume that all other things are held constant, that is, the child receives competent speech training and practice in listening through a hearing aid. On the other hand, the degree of hearing impairment is a factor that varies over a wide range and must, of course, be taken into account. In general, it appears that the effects of hearing impairment on speech production are proportional to the severity of the impairment (as estimated by pure tone thresholds). This relationship is probably valid up to the point of profound deafness.

The abnormal sensory conditions under which the hearing impaired learn to speak cause their speech to have certain shared characteristics. These shared characteristics are prominent enough that they can be easily noted among hearing-impaired children speaking languages other than English. This is to say only that the speech of the hearing impaired bears the imprint of the sensory deficit which shaped it. It appears to do so according to the following general principles:

1. *If available, an incoming auditory signal will be imitated.* In cases in which the incoming auditory signal is merely distorted by the hearing impairment, but in which it nevertheless remains the most prominent sensory image of speech, the distorted speech signal will serve as a model to be imitated. Although a child may succeed in imitating this distorted signal, the resulting speech will obviously also be distorted. Examples of this phenomenon range all the way from the "shushing" articulation of /s/ in the speech of individuals with mild to moderate hearing impairments (in which a phrase like "so few" will often be pronounced as "sho few") to the speech of the severely hearing impaired, in which many of the speech sounds, though often recognizable, are nevertheless different in quality from normal. Special techniques of speech training must be developed for this type of malarticulation, because the individual must be taught to produce sounds differently from how they are perceived.

For the profoundly deaf, on the other hand, there is no real acoustic image to imitate, even when sound amplification is used. The profoundly deaf do not "hear" merely a muffled or severely filtered version of speech; instead, speech is delivered to them as a spectrally unanalyzed blur equivalent in all known respects to the vibration on the skin (Nober, 1967; Risberg, 1977). Therefore, the profoundly deaf child must learn speech by nearly total dependence on the visual and vibratory images of speech sounds.

2. *Sounds made by visible articulatory gestures are better produced than those made by concealed gestures; the more visible, the better produced.* Many, or indeed most hearing-impaired children can learn to produce labiodental or interdental fricatives, as in the words *five* or *thing*, even though they may have never heard what these phonemes sound like when produced either by themselves or by another speaker. This is so simply because vision alone can adequately guide one to learn to produce these sounds. On the other extreme, the gestures involved in the production of voice are almost entirely invisible to a deaf language learner. In normal speech, the frequency and

intensity of voice are continuously changed over the course of a sentence to conform to the syntactic pattern and to imbue it with meaning. The patterns of fundamental frequency vary from language to language and they are learned. These variations are controlled by adducting the vocal folds properly and appropriately varying the supply of subglottal air pressure, as well as the degree of vocal fold tension. Changes in vocal fold tension are particularly important in bringing about frequency changes in normal speech. For those who have been and are unable to correctly perceive the frequency variations found in normal speech, voice production must be learned primarily by proprioception and by trial and error. Learning to speak by trial and error results in a great deal of error. To merely phonate is not the problem; however, to control the change of frequency and intensity in a normal manner is a major difficulty. The most common deviations from normal are that the fundamental frequency (F_o) fails to vary sufficiently or that it varies too much, and in abnormal ways. In some cases, diplophonia may be produced (Monsen, 1979).

Some of the types of abnormal voice control are shown in the following figures. In Figure 1.1, narrowband spectrograms of two words are shown in which there is insufficient frequency variation. Vocal fold tension and air pressure apparently are maintained at a constant value, rather than allowed to decline smoothly. For such words spoken in isolation by normally hearing speakers, the frequency contour should fall smoothly. In Figure 1.2, narrowband spectrograms of monosyllables said by four different hearing-impaired speakers are shown in which the F_o contour indeed varies, but in a seemingly uncontrolled way; it rises and falls many times over the course of a single syllable. This would seem to be due to frequent changes in the degree of vocal fold tension. Another abnormality, F_o quaver, is shown in Figure 1.3. Here the changes of F_o are small but numerous. Abrupt changes in the positioning and tension of the vocal folds can also produce discontinuities of frequency, as shown in Figure 1.4. Finally, voice may be produced with greater tension in one vocal fold than in the other. This will cause the vocal folds to oscillate in an irregular fashion, wherein every second glottal period is different. When this happens, the voice contains two fundamental frequencies, and may be called diplophonic. An example of this is shown in Figure 1.5. In the narrowband spectrogram at the right, note the sudden appearance of additional harmonics. A portion of the speech waveform corresponding to the diplophonic episode is shown at the bottom. Note the alternation of high and low pitch periods.

3.   *In the absence of acoustic feedback, or under the influence of*

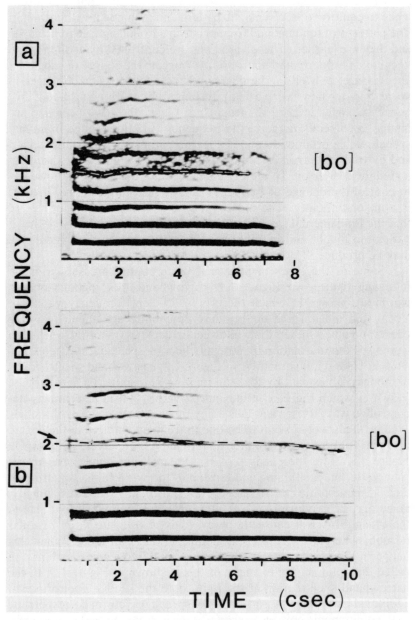

Figure 1.1.   Narrowband spectrograms of two monosyllables. Note insufficient variation of fundamental frequency as indicated by arrows and dotted lines.

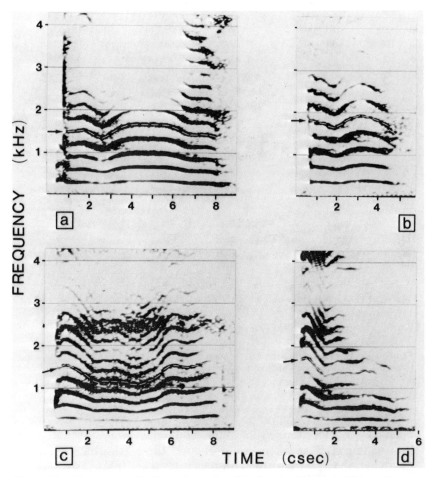

Figure 1.2.   Four monosyllabic words produced by hearing-impaired children. Excessive change of fundamental frequency, and in inappropriate directions, are indicated by arrows and dotted lines.

diminished feedback, the hearing-impaired speaker will attempt to maximize articulatory feedback.   If hearing is an insufficient guide to the articulation of a particular sound, the deaf child must rely on something else. In many cases, articulatory gestures can be produced in such a way as to maximize the feedback they provide. Two very clear examples of this are commonly encountered in the speech of the hearing impaired. The first concerns the production of fricative sounds. For nonlabial fricatives, articulators must be brought close enough together so that when air passes through, turbulence will be created. This re-

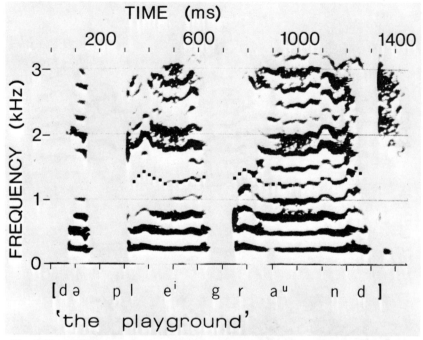

Figure 1.3.   Quavering fundamental frequency (F_o) in the utterance "the playground" as produced by a hearing-impaired female, 14 years, 7 months of age.

quires a somewhat precise positioning of the articulators—the tongue must be very close to the roof of the mouth but yet not touch it. Many hearing-impaired speakers will produce these fricative sounds by touching the two articulators. In that way, a word like "so" may be produced as [tso] or [do]. I have even observed a case in which the child produced the fricative /s/ by putting the tongue tip to the roof of the mouth and then forced air around both sides of the tongue. This creates a sound which is phonetically a voiceless /l/; that is, [ɬ]. It is a fricative sound, and it would seem to be rich in tactile feedback, but it does not sound like an /s/, or indeed like anything English.

A second clear example of maximizing articulatory feedback is to be found in the production of the stop consonants. Many deaf children learn to produce these sounds by making voiced implosives or voiceless ejectives—glottalized stop consonants. To produce voiced implosives, the larynx is momentarily depressed and phonation is begun with extremely tense laryngeal muscles. This type of production may in some measure be due to the fact that teachers often demonstrate the production of these sounds by pointing to the larynx (conveying to the child the notion that he or she should be doing something with it) or by telling the child to produce /b/, /d/, and /g/ by making voice at the same time—something which rarely is done in normal English speech. The child then says, for "boy," "day," and "go": [ɓoi̯], [ɗei̯], [ʄou̯]. In a similar manner, the voiceless stops may sometimes be produced as ejectives; that is, sounds in which the air is expelled after stop closure with a tightly closed and elevated glottis. The velar and alveolar

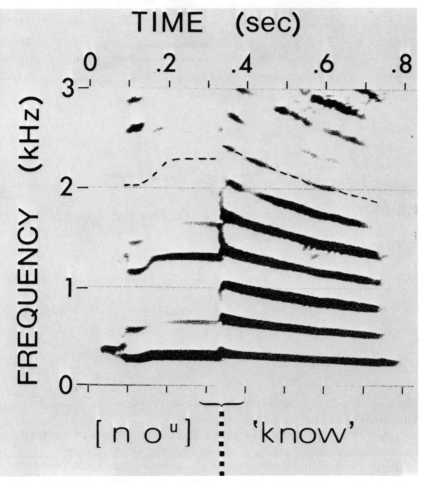

Figure 1.4.   Discontinuous change of fundamental frequency in utterances by a hearing-impaired female, 16 years, 4 months of age.

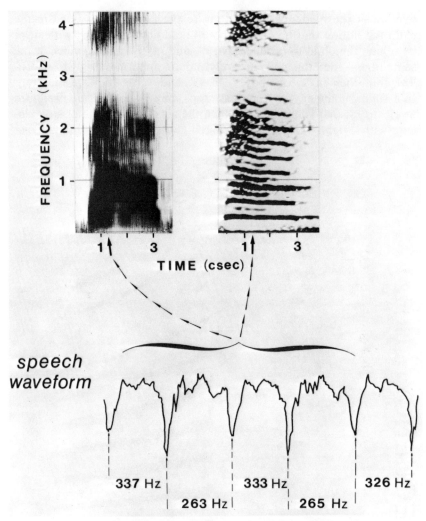

Figure 1.5.   Diplophonic phonation. (See text for discussion.)

stops are the likely candidates for this; the words "key" and "two" may sound like [k'i] and [t'u].

4.   *An inadequate visual image of articulation may predominate as a model of speech over a distorted or feeble acoustic signal.*   One of the single most noticeable acoustic facts about the speech produced by the deaf concerns the variation of the vowel formants. In normal speech, the first and second vowel formants change constantly in fre-

quency as the speaker articulates each different vowel and consonant. The movements of the vowel formants are particularly important for the listener to be able to perceive not only the intended vowel sound, but also the adjacent consonants. Among deaf speakers of low intelligibility, the second vowel formant often does not vary sufficiently in frequency, and for some speakers, the first vowel formant may also exhibit a limited range of movement. A comparison of the vowel formants in sentences said by two different speakers can be seen in Figure 1.6. Here, a sentence spoken by a highly intelligible speaker is compared with one spoken by a very unintelligible speaker. The movement in frequency of the second formant is traced by a dotted line. For the more intelligible speaker, there is considerable movement, and in an appropriate direction. For the other speaker, the second formant tends to remain nearly immobile.

It is difficult to overemphasize the importance of this characteristic of the speech of the deaf. The amount of variation of the second formant correlates highly with measured speech intelligibility (Monsen, 1978). Secondly, unlike misarticulation of just a group of sounds, the movements of the vowel formants are general features of speech, and pertain not only to all the vowels, but to the consonants as well, because the

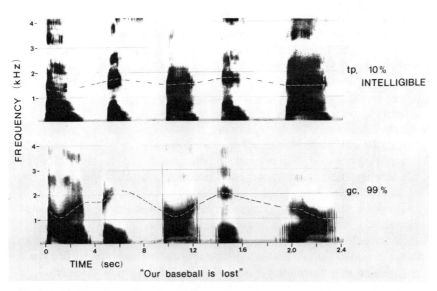

Figure 1.6.   Speech intelligibility versus movement of the second formant (dotted line). The speaker shown at the top is on the average 10% intelligible; the one at the bottom is 99% intelligible.

vowel transitions in fact convey to the listener much of the information about the identity of adjacent consonants.

Several factors may play a role in accounting for the vowel articulation of the deaf speaker. The first vowel formant lies generally below 1000 Hz, and it may be better perceived by many hearing-impaired subjects than the second vowel formant, which lies between 1000 Hz and about 2500 Hz. That is, the variation of the first vowel formant may be perceptible, whereas the variation of the second vowel formant may be only dimly perceived (if at all), because it lies in a region in which frequency discrimination is likely to be poorer. The profoundly deaf probably do not accurately locate either formant. In addition to the role of hearing, however, is the relative visibility of the different articulatory gestures that cause the vowel formants to change in frequency. Movements of the first formant can be brought about by opening and closing the mouth, which the child can see and can imitate. The changing movements of the second vowel formant, however, are brought about in large measure by the position of the tongue tip and the tongue body; these movements are difficult for a child to see or recognize as important, and they are also difficult for a teacher to describe. The profoundly deaf child may try to learn to imitate vowel sounds primarily by how they look. As a result, the articulatory gestures of lip position and mouth opening may be successfully learned, and the positions of the tongue will not. Unfortunately, it is simply not possible to achieve adequate vowel articulation without properly moving the tongue from one target to another. When the tongue is not properly moved about, the second formant tends to remain stable (between 1600 and 2000 Hz) and the listener is then unable to hear the vowel sound intended by the speaker. All vowels then tend to sound indistinct, neutralized, or schwa-like.

5. *Because speech sounds are learned by deliberate visual, vibrotactile, and auditory imitation, the coarticulation of speech sounds tends to be reduced.* In normal speech, sounds are smoothly blended into one another; this phenomenon is called coarticulation, and it appears that when sounds are smoothly blended into each other (not unlike watercolors), the recognition of sounds is enhanced rather than diminished. The normally hearing child presumably learns to coarticulate speech sounds by imitation of the acoustic image; for example, that the sound /k/ is articulated in a more front manner before front vowels and in a more back manner before back vowels. As a result of coarticulation, each phoneme of English is thus said to have allophones, that is, sound variants depending on the surrounding sounds. This contextual variation of each sound appears to be diminished in

the speech of many deaf subjects who may have learned to produce sounds in a deliberate manner as unmodified, immutable targets. For these speakers, a word is composed of individual, isolated speech sounds that are more concatenated than coarticulated.

The reduced effects of coarticulation in the speech of the deaf are easily seen. For the deaf speaker, a word is often longer simply in proportion to the number of sounds it contains. This is not true in normal speech, in which syllables tend to be produced with equal duration regardless of how many phonemes they contain. That is, when said alone, the word "so" and "sports" will both be about equal in duration, despite the fact that the first word contains two phonemes and the second contains six phonemes. The same is true of the syllables in a word. In normal speech, words tend to be said in the same amount of time whether they have one, two, three, or more syllables. This phenomenon is commonly absent in the speech of the deaf, in which longer words simply take longer to say. To a great extent, this deliberateness of articulation is primarily responsible for the slower speech of the deaf.

6. *The different sensory conditions under which deaf children learn speech tends to promote a different linguistic organization on the phonological level.* Up to now, the differences between deaf and normal speech have been discussed on a purely phonetic level. Differences may also be present in the linguistic structure of the child's phonology. For example, many deaf children appear to commit errors when trying to produce the voiced and voiceless stop consonants. For many of these subjects, the distinction between /t/ and /d/, for example, is actually collapsed into a single phoneme which is produced for both /t/ and /d/. Often this phoneme is realized as a voiceless unaspirated sound in initial position and a voiceless aspirated sound in final position. For such a person, the words "to" and "do" will both come out sounding like "do" and the words "sad" and "sat" will both come out sounding like "sat." It may appear that children are just making errors in producing these sounds, when in fact they may be realizing them in lawful phonological accordance with the rules they have learned. Bear in mind that sounds such as /t/ and /d/ appear the same from a lipreader's point of view.

There are other, more subtle examples of phonological differences between normal speech and speech produced by the deaf. For example, the distinction between two phonemes may not have collapsed, but a deaf speaker may attempt to convey it in a different way. That is, the acoustic cues used to differentiate phonemes may be rearranged or altered. The distinction between tense and lax vowels in English offers a good example. These vowels, such as /i/ and /ɪ/, are distinguished primarily by spectral differences in the formant frequencies, and only secondarily by length. However, a deaf speaker will often differentiate these vowels primarily on the basis of length and only secondarily, if at all, on the basis of their spectral properties. This may happen because vowel length may be perceptually more salient to a deaf child than vowel quality. In such a case, the speaker is distinguishing between phonemes, but on a different basis than the normal speakers of the language do.

In summary, the speech of the deaf tends to differ from normal speech because of the different sensory conditions under which it must be learned. The dependence on vision, vibration, proprioception, the feedback provided by a hearing adult, and distorted hearing in learning to speak can ultimately lead to differences in the phonological organization of speech. Because speech sounds are learned by deliberate visual, vibrotactile, and auditory imitation, the coarticulation of speech sounds tends to be reduced; speech may then be slower than normal and arythmic. Furthermore, deaf children may imitate the visual image of articulation, and in doing so ignore important movements of the tongue which they cannot see. At the same time, they may attempt to maximize articulatory feedback in producing some speech sounds. Some sounds can be adequately imitated on a visual basis, and these may be produced well. Finally, those fortunate enough to receive an auditory signal will use that signal, even when it is severely distorted, as a basis for learning to produce speech.

REFERENCES

Monsen, R. B. 1978. Toward measuring how well hearing-impaired children speak. J. Speech Hear. Res. 21:197–219.
Monsen, R. B. 1979. Acoustic qualities of phonation in young hearing-impaired children. J. Speech Hear. Res. 22:270–288.
Nober, E. H. 1967. Vibrotactile sensitivity of deaf children to high intensity sound. Laryngoscope 77:2128–2146.
Risberg, A. 1977. Hearing loss and auditory capacity. Paper presented at the Conference on Speech-Processing Aids for the Deaf, Gallaudet College, Washington, D.C.

CHAPTER 2

SUPRASEGMENTAL AND POSTURAL ASPECTS OF SPEECH PRODUCTION AND THEIR EFFECT ON ARTICULATORY SKILLS AND INTELLIGIBILITY

K. N. Stevens, R. S. Nickerson, and A. M. Rollins

CONTENTS

SEGMENTAL, SUPRASEGMENTAL, AND POSTURAL ASPECTS OF SPEECH

The characteristics of the speech stream can be described broadly in terms of segmental aspects and suprasegmental aspects. The segmental aspects describe how individual speech segments are produced. The production of individual speech sounds requires a specification of the target configurations that the articulatory structures achieve and the way in which the movements of these structures toward or away from the target configurations are actualized and are coordinated. The suprasegmental aspects of an utterance are those characteristics that span linguistic units longer than a phonetic segment. In normal speech production, these suprasegmental aspects include the contour of fundamental frequency versus time, the durations of certain of the speech events and of pauses, and the assignment of relative prominence or stress to different syllables.

An individual speaker can impose his or her own characteristics

35

on the utterances, and these characteristics also span linguistic units longer than the phonetic segment. For example, an individual may have a particular average fundamental frequency, may use a restricted or an expanded range of fundamental frequency, may impose greater-than-normal variations in durations of speech events in particular syntactic positions, or may tend to nasalize all vowels more than the average speaker. Although these personal characteristics of a speaker are also suprasegmental in the sense that they span linguistic units larger than a segment, they are more appropriately described as *postural* characteristics. They depend to some extent on the overall average posture that is assumed by the articulatory, laryngeal, and respiratory structures in preparation for speech production. These postural aspects can influence how the segmental features are produced as well as the suprasegmental attributes of the speech. We assume that the term *posture* includes not only some static state of readiness for speaking, but also the range over which the configurations or states of various structures are allowed to vary.

In describing the speech of the deaf, we often encounter deviant acoustic characteristics that span entire utterances, and that can be ascribed to improper postural characteristics of the speech production system. (See, for example, reviews in Ling, 1976; Nickerson, 1975.) One common deviation from normalcy relates to the voice quality observed in many deaf speakers—a quality often described as breathiness. This deviant voice quality is presumably a consequence of improper positioning of the vocal folds with too wide an average glottal opening during voiced sounds (Hudgins, 1937; Stevens, Nickerson, and Rollins, 1978). Another problem relating to larynx posture is an average fundamental frequency (F_o) that is too high or too low. This deviant F_o probably arises because the average vocal-fold tension is too high or too low (Angelocci, Kopp, and Holbrook, 1964; Boone, 1966). Improper adjustment of vocal-fold posture can also result in an F_o contour that is overly sensitive to adjustments of the tongue position for individual vowels (Angelocci et al., 1964; Bush, 1979; Mártony, 1968).

Deviant nasalization characteristics in the speech of a deaf individual can be the result of improper posture of the velopharyngeal structures (Hudgins, 1934; Stevens et al., 1976). The normal starting posture for speech production is a closed velopharyngeal port. For many deaf speakers, however, the velum remains lowered much of the time, with the result that many vowels are improperly nasalized. Still another deviation from normal speech is the way the tongue body is positioned in the mouth. For some deaf speakers, the tongue-body position is relatively immobile as far as front-back movement during speech production is concerned, with the result that there is a rather narrow range of variation of the frequency of the second formant (Monsen, 1976).

Problems with the sequencing of syllables and words can be ascribed to improper syllable-synchronized rhythmic activities of the laryngeal and respiratory structures. These deviations from normalcy can also be regarded as postural problems that span groups of phonetic segments. Thus, for example, some deaf speakers have a tendency to insert a glottal closure between syllables or words. That is, they tend to create a reduction in sound amplitude between two syllables by cutting off the airstream at the glottis rather than by using the supralaryngeal movements to valve the airstream and thus to cause a reduction in amplitude (Bernstein, Rollins, and Stevens, 1978). Other deaf speakers insert a pause after almost every word in an utterance. That is, they treat each word as a separate unit, and do not concatenate a sequence of words to form a larger syntactic constituent that has suprasegmental attributes spanning the entire sequence.

INTELLIGIBILITY AND THE
SUPRASEGMENTAL ASPECTS OF SPEECH PRODUCTION

In the remediation of the speech of the deaf, it is important to determine what aspects of the speech should be modified in order to achieve the greatest gains in intelligibility. To the extent that the suprasegmental and the segmental aspects can be manipulated independently, it is natural to try to determine the improvements in intelligibility that can be achieved by changing each of these dimensions separately. In particular, we shall review here some evidence for changes in intelligibility that can be ascribed to modifications in certain suprasegmental characteristics of speech.

Some qualitative evidence comes from informal observations of speech produced by normally hearing individuals but with monotone pitch, or with timing modified so that each word or each syllable is produced with about the same duration, or with a pause inserted between each word. Our experience suggests that speech modified in these ways can be highly intelligible, at least when listeners hear it in the absence of noise.

On the other hand, Huggins (1978) has shown that if the timing of the syllables is adjusted so as to introduce misleading timing cues, then there can be a rather large reduction in intelligibility. Using a speech synthesis-by-rule system, Huggins adjusted the durations of the speech sounds in sentences so that syllables that were normally assigned low stress were made longer and syllables assigned high stress were made shorter. He found that listeners' errors in transcribing the modified sentences were considerably increased.

Another approach to the study of the importance of suprasegmental cues for intelligibility of speech is to start with speech of the deaf that has degraded suprasegmental characteristics and to modify these characteristics, either through instrumental means or through training of the speakers. Osberger (1978) attempted to improve the temporal aspects of the speech of deaf children by changing the durations of vowels and pauses in recorded samples artificially. Adjustment of the relative durations of stressed and unstressed vowels produced a small increase in intelligibility, whereas correction of pause durations led to a decrease in intelligibility. John and Howarth (1965) showed that speech training that emphasized timing with a few sentences produced an improved intelligibility of the words in the sentences, whereas Houde (1973) found that the intelligibility of the speech of two deaf students decreased in spite of improvements in timing, as determined from objective measurements.

In the studies of these authors, in collaboration with colleagues at the Clarke School for the Deaf in Northampton, Massachusetts, and at the Lexington School for the Deaf in New York, two kinds of data were obtained (Nickerson, Stevens, and Rollins, 1979). Objective measurements were made on several suprasegmental characteristics of the speech of a large number of deaf children, and measures of the intelligibility of the speech of these children were obtained. Similar measurements were also obtained from a smaller group of deaf children receiving speech training (with the aid of a computer-based system of visual displays) that emphasized certain suprasegmental characteristics of their speech. Acoustic characteristics of the speech and intelligibility measures were obtained for these children both before and after training.

Examples of the relations between intelligibility and the physical measures are shown in Figures 2.1 and 2.2. The physical measures in these two scatterplots are the range of fundamental frequency F_o (the average of the values of the ratio of maximum F_o to minimum F_o for each of a number of different sentences) and the average value of the ratio of the durations of stressed and unstressed vowels in a number of sentences. Each point represents one deaf student, and the intelligibility is the percentage of sentences correctly identified by listeners, each sentence being identified from a set of alternatives. The sentences within each closed set had the same number of syllables, but there was a different pattern of stress for the syllables of each sentence. These sentences were presented to listeners in two ways in different experiments: 1) the sentences were reproduced with a high quality system,

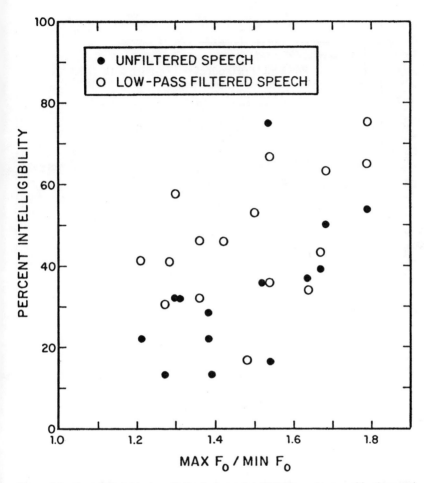

Figure 2.1   Scatterplot showing relation between intelligibility and range of fundamental frequency (F_o) in phrases and sentences for 15 deaf students. The parameters $maxF_o$ and $minF_o$ are average values of the maximum and minimum F_o in each of six different sentences. Intelligibility is obtained by presenting phrases and sentences to listeners who are required to select a response from a closed set of phrases or sentences, in which each item in the set has the same number of syllables but a different stress pattern. For the low-pass filtered speech the cut-off frequency of the filter was 200 Hz (24 dB/oct). The data for unfiltered speech in this figure and in Figure 2.2 have been reported previously by Nickerson and Stevens (1979).

and 2) they were passed through a low-pass filter with a cutoff frequency of 200 Hz (24 dB/octave), so that only the fundamental frequency contour and the temporal characteristics could be heard. We observe in each case a trend for the intelligibility, both for the wideband and the low-pass filtered speech, to increase as the physical measure

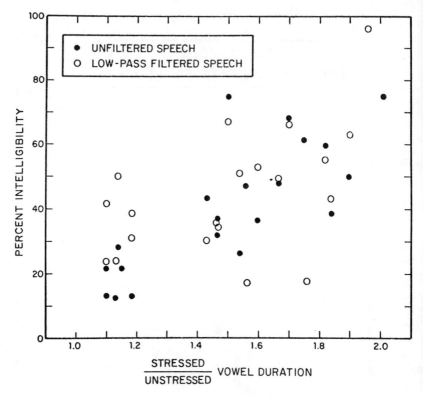

Figure 2.2.   Scatterplot showing relation between intelligibility and ratio of average durations of stressed to unstressed vowels in phrases and sentences for 20 deaf students. See legend for Figure 2.1.

approaches the same measure observed for normally hearing speakers (roughly 2.0 for each of the two measures). There is, however, a wide range of intelligibility for a given value of the physical parameter, suggesting that a number of other factors are playing a role in determining the intelligibility.

The other kind of evidence comes from observations of the speech of children who underwent a period of speech training (with the aid of a computer-based system of displays of speech parameters) on certain suprasegmental aspects of speech (Boothroyd, et al., 1975; Nickerson, Kalikow, and Stevens, 1976). The particular suprasegmental attributes that were emphasized in training sessions were different for different children. For the most part, the training resulted in improvements in the measured suprasegmental parameters of the children's speech. Examples are shown in the next three figures. These figures show that speech training resulted in a lowering of the average F_o to a value closer to the normal for the child's age (Figure 2.3), a reduction in the number of vowels (in sentences) for which the F_o value deviated significantly from the expected F_o contour for the sentence (Figure 2.4), and a reduction in the incidence of pauses between words in sentences (Figure 2.5). Data on the intelligibility of the speech of these children, measured before and after training, did not show a significant improvement in intelligibility, on the average.

A possible reason for this lack of improvement in intelligibility is that the children who were selected for training in this project tended to be those with rather severe speech problems that had persisted over several years. A more likely reason is that improvement in the suprasegmental attributes alone is not sufficient to result in an immediate

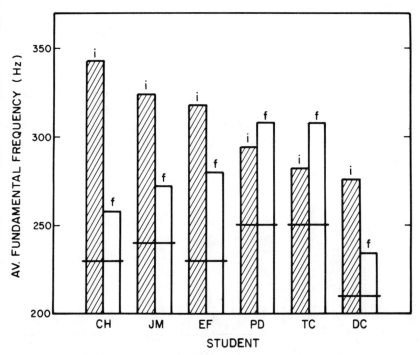

Figure 2.3.   Data on average fundamental frequency (F_o) before (i) and after (f) speech training for six students whose average F_o was considerably higher than the average F_o for normally hearing children of the same age. The students are organized with the highest initial F_o at the left. The horizontal lines for each student represent the average F_o for a normally hearing child of the same age.

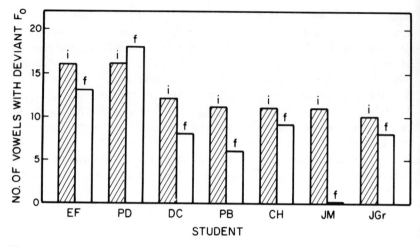

Figure 2.4.   Data indicating number of vowels (out of a total of 36 in six 6-syllable sentences) for which the F_o showed significant deviation (more than 50 Hz) from an hypothesized ideal contour. Data are given for initial (*i*) and final (*f*) recordings for students who showed such a significant F_o deviation for a substantial number of their vowels.

gain in intelligibility, although it may be accompanied by an improvement in the naturalness or overall quality of the speech. Reduction of errors in the articulatory or segmental aspects of the speech is probably necessary before a significant improvement in intelligibility can be achieved.

We shall argue in the following section that inadequacies in the

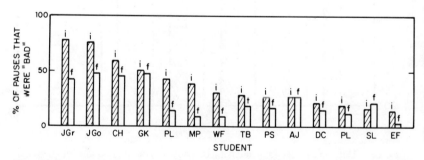

Figure 2.5.   Percentage of syllable concatenations for which there was an inappropriate pause in excess of 200 msec. Data are based on 42 concatenations in 18 phrases in sentences. Data for initial (*i*) and final (*f*) recordings are shown for 14 students who exhibited the greatest number of pauses in their speech before training was initiated.

postural attributes of speech have consequences not only for the suprasegmental parameters but also for realization of the articulatory or
segmental aspects. Thus, although improving the suprasegmental properties may be one step toward gaining more appropriate speech posture,
this gain must be accompanied by training in the utilization of this
revised posture to produce vowels and consonants with proper place
and manner of articulation and voicing characteristics. Unless careful
attention is paid to these postural effects at the segmental level and to
articulation while training proceeds on the suprasegmental aspects,
there is a danger that improved suprasegmental characteristics may be
achieved *at the expense of* precision in the articulatory maneuvers.

POSTURAL INADEQUACIES AND THEIR
RELATION TO PROBLEMS WITH SPEECH PRODUCTION

At first glance it might seem that errors or inadequacies in posture are
most likely to create problems with the suprasegmental characteristics
of speech. Thus, as noted earlier, a deaf speaker might have too high
an average fundamental frequency, or nasalize entire utterances. However, improper posture can also interfere with the correct realization
of a number of the segmental aspects of speech production. That is,
postural inadequacies can create conditions that make it extremely
difficult to produce certain speech sounds with the appropriate characteristics. We can illustrate this relation between improper posture
and poor segmental characteristics with several examples.

Figure 2.6 shows spectra sampled at the middle of vowels spoken
in words by four different children—one with normal hearing, and the
other three with profound hearing impairment. The spectra are sampled
with a time window of about 25 msec, and the frequency resolution is
sufficient to resolve the individual harmonics of the fundamental frequency. For the vowel /æ/ produced by the normally hearing child
(panel AS of the figure) we see well-defined peaks in the spectrum
envelope corresponding to the vocal tract resonances or formants. The
curve above the spectrum represents a smoothed (all-pole) spectrum
for this vowel. The spectra of the vowels produced by the three deaf
children in the other panels of the figure do not show such well-defined
peaks corresponding to the formants. For example, the vowel /ɑ/ (produced by BC) has a broad peak in the spectrum envelope between
about 800 Hz and 2700 Hz, with only minor fluctuations in the amplitudes of individual harmonics that would give some evidence of formant
locations. Similar lack of clear peaks for at least some of the formants
is evident in the other two spectra. Apparently, for these hearing-

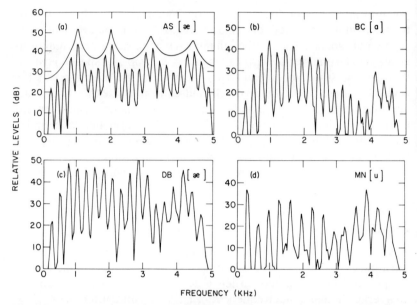

FREQUENCY (KHz)

Figure 2.6.   Short-time spectra (time window 26 msec) sampled in vowels produced in words by a normally hearing child (AS, panel a), and by three deaf children (panels b, c, d). Individual harmonics for each spectrum are resolved, as shown. The smooth curve in panel a is derived by a calculation procedure that represents the spectrum by a series of formants (a linear prediction procedure).

impaired children a representation of vowel production by a glottal source with a smooth spectrum that is filtered by the vocal tract is not adequate.

There are at least three possible reasons for this deviation from the normal vowel-production mode for the deaf children:

1.   Because the vocal folds are in a posture that is somewhat abducted, there is acoustic coupling to the subglottal acoustic system, introducing additional resonances or spectral peaks into the output spectrum that tend to fill in the spectral valleys in the normal vowel spectrum and hence to make the formant peaks less distinct.

2.   The spectrum of the sound from the glottis is not smooth but contains irregularities not normally seen in the speech of hearing individuals.

3.   Inadvertent acoustic coupling to the nasal cavities through a partially open velopharyngeal port can result in the presence of additional resonances that give rise to a spectrum with less distinct peaks and valleys.

Any of these possibilities is the consequence of improper posture either in the laryngeal or in the velopharyngeal region; and this improper posture makes it difficult for the child to achieve a wide range of vowels with distinctive spectral characteristics. There is evidence from data we have gathered that there are children that exhibit each of the problems represented by these three possibilities.

A related problem concerned with laryngeal posture is illustrated in Figure 2.7. This figure shows spectra of the vowel [ɑ] produced by a normally hearing child and by two deaf children who were judged to have breathy voices (Stevens et al., 1978). The spectra were obtained from a filter bank with rather broad filters, and hence the individual harmonics are not resolved as they are in Figure 2.6. In the case of the deaf children, the spectrum is dominated by a large amplitude at

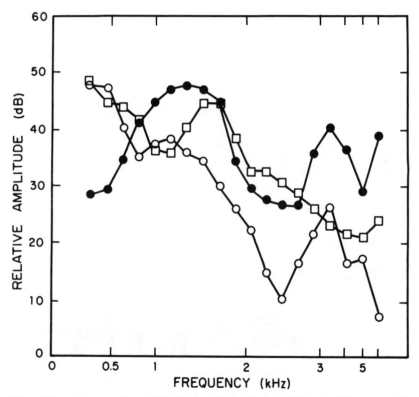

Figure 2.7.   Spectrum of vowel [ɑ] (obtained from a 19-channel filter bank) for a normally hearing child (closed circles) and two deaf children who were judged to have breathy voices (open circles and open squares).

low frequencies, presumably representing the amplitude of the fundamental component of the periodic glottal waveform. The vocal folds are probably in a somewhat abducted configuration for these two children, and this posture leads to a glottal output that has a strong first harmonic in relation to the higher harmonics (Fischer-Jorgensen, 1967; Stevens, 1977), as well as to possible acoustic coupling to the subglottal system, as noted above. The strong low-frequency energy in the spectrum would again make it difficult for the children to generate vowels with distinctive acoustic characteristics, particularly with good definition of the first formant.

This aspect of the glottal spectrum resulting from improper laryngeal configuration is highlighted in Figure 2.8, which shows spectrograms of the utterance "caught the ball" produced by the same deaf child on two occasions during a speech training session in which an effort was being made to improve the voice quality with the aid of a

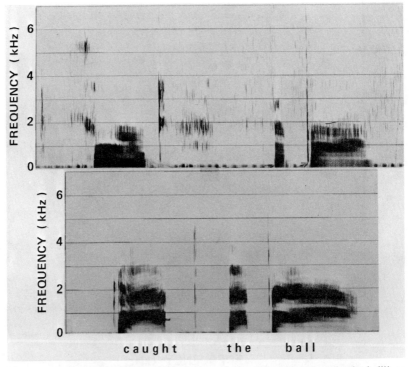

Figure 2.8.   Spectrograms of a deaf child producing the phrase "caught the ball" on two different occasions. The child used her habitual breathy voice for the utterance in the upper spectrogram, which shows enhanced spectral energy at low frequencies, below the first formant. In a speech training session, the child was able to change her voice quality to remove the breathiness, resulting in the spectrogram at the bottom of the figure.

computer-based system of displays. The upper spectrogram depicts the utterance produced with the child's habitual voice quality, and the strong low-frequency energy in each of the vowels is evident close to the base line of the spectrogram. When the child managed to switch to a more clear voice quality, the change was obvious to listeners, and the strong low-frequency spectral energy in the vowels disappeared, as the lower spectrogram shows.

Another example of a situation in which improper speech posture leads to an interaction between an articulatory configuration and the behavior of the larynx is the shift in fundamental frequency that is observed for some deaf children when they produce certain vowels. This observation has been made by teachers of the deaf, and has been documented in more quantitative terms by Bush (1979). Figure 2.9 shows that there is a group of deaf children for whom the average fundamental frequency is considerably higher when they produce the high vowels [iɪʊu] than when they produce the other vowels. Furthermore, Bush has shown that the children who show less variation in F_o from one vowel to another also tend to produce a smaller range of variation in vowel formant frequencies. Thus, at least for some children, the control of F_o is not independent of the adjustment of the vocal tract to produce different vowel configurations.

A characteristic that is observed in the speech of a number of deaf children is the tendency to produce a glottal closure between words in an utterance. An example of an utterance produced by such a child is shown in Figure 2.10. Evidence for glottalization is seen in the irregular vocal fold vibrations occurring at the onsets of some of the vowels (e.g., at the beginning of *Bill*, *played*, *in*, and both syllables of *water*). Deaf speakers with these characteristics seem to utilize a glottal closure or constriction to create a reduced amplitude for the sound during the consonantal region between adjacent syllabic nuclei. A consequence of the glottal closure is elimination of the airflow above the glottis, and hence no sound is generated to indicate the place or manner of articulation for the consonant. Thus, a deaf speaker who has the "postural" problem of glottalizing regularly between syllables is severely impaired in his or her ability to produce acoustic attributes that indicate manner and place of articulation for consonants (Bernstein et al., 1978). Production of correct place of articulation is of no avail unless there is proper control of airflow to generate the proper sound source.

Still another postural problem is related to the positioning of the tongue. There are some deaf speakers who maintain the tongue body in a relatively backed position, and who seem to be unable to cause the tongue body to undergo much displacement in a front-back direction during speech production. Apparently, the muscles that maintain

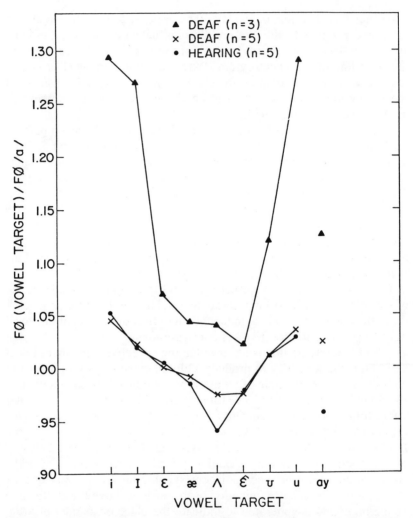

Figure 2.9.   Data on average fundamental frequency for different vowels in words produced by 5 normally hearing boys and two groups of deaf boys, as shown. The ordinate is the ratio of the fundamental frequency used to produce the indicated vowel and the fundamental frequency used to produce vowel /ɑ/. The deviant group of 3 deaf children produce several vowels with a fundamental frequency that is considerably higher than for the vowel /ɑ/. (From Bush, 1979)

the rather static tongue-body position remain tensed as part of an overall deviant speech posture. A consequence of this problem is a narrow range of movement of the second formant from one vowel to another, so that a limited range of vowel qualities is generated (Monsen, 1976). The spectogram in Figure 2.10 is an example of an utterance with a

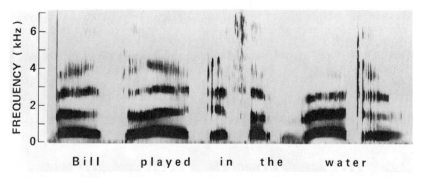

B i l l   p l a y e d   i n   t h e   w a t e r

Figure 2.10.   Spectrogram of a sentence produced by a deaf child who glottalized at many syllable boundaries. This child also shows a relatively restricted range of variation in the second formant frequency.

narrow range in the frequency of the second formant, presumably because of this somewhat rigid tongue-body positioning. This relative immobility of the tongue body would presumably also have consequences for correct tongue placement and shaping for consonants as well as vowels.

CONCLUDING REMARK

In speech training of deaf children it is important that the correct postural aspects of speech production be developed, inasmuch as these aspects are prerequisites for developing proper articulatory skills as well as proper speech quality and prosodic aspects of speech. Because inadequacies in the postural aspects of speech have consequences for both the articulatory and the suprasegmental aspects of speech production, we believe that speech training activities should be structured so that articulatory skills are developed at the same time as the suprasegmental aspects. Improvement in postural skills should facilitate improvement in articulation and the production of selected speech sound sequences with the correct acoustic characteristics. Training on suprasegmental aspects of speech without specific attention to articulatory skills, however, probably is not an appropriate strategy, because it will not lead directly to improvements in intelligibility, and it could lead to a regression in articulatory ability.

REFERENCES

Angelocci, A. A., G. A., Kopp, and A. Holbrook. 1964. The vowel formants of deaf and normal hearing 11- to 14-year-old boys. J. Speech Hear. Disord. 29:156–170.

50   Stevens, Nickerson, and Rollins

Bernstein, J., A. M. Rollins, and K. N. Stevens. 1978. Word and syllable concatenation in the speech of the deaf. Paper presented at the meeting of the A. G. Bell Association for the Deaf, June 25, St. Louis.
Boone, D. R. 1966. Modification of the voices of deaf children. Volta Rev. 68:686–694.
Boothroyd, A., P. Archambault, R. E. Adams, and R. D. Storm. 1975. Use of a computer-based system of speech analysis and display in a remedial speech program for deaf children. Volta Rev. 77:178–193.
Bush, M. 1979. Articulatory proficiency and F_o control by profoundly deaf speakers. Paper presented at the meeting of the American Speech-Language-Hearing Association, November 16, Atlanta.
Fischer-Jorgensen, E. 1967. Phonetic analysis of breathy (murmured) vowels in Gujarati. Annual Report of the Institute of Phonetics, University of Copenhagen 2:35–85.
Houde, R. A. 1973. Instantaneous visual feedback in speech training for the deaf. Paper presented at the meeting of the American Speech and Hearing Association, November, Detroit.
Hudgins, C. V. 1934. A comparative study of the speech coordination of deaf and normal subjects. J. Genet. Psychol. 54:3.
Hudgins, C. V. 1937. Voice production and breath control in the speech of the deaf. Am. Ann. Deaf 82:338–363.
Huggins, A. W. F. 1978. Speech timing and intelligibility. In J. Requin (ed.), Attention and Performance. VII. Lawrence Erlbaum Associates, Hillsdale, N.J.
John, J. E. J., and Howarth, J. M. 1965. The effect of time distortions on the intelligibility of deaf children's speech. Lang. Speech 8:127–134.
Ling, D. 1976. Speech and the Hearing-Impaired Child: Theory and Practice. A. G. Bell Association for the Deaf, Washington, D.C.
Mártony, J. 1968. On the correction of the voice pitch level for severely hard of hearing subjects. Am. Ann. Deaf 113:195–202.
Monsen, R. B. 1976. Normal and reduced phonological space: The production of English vowels by deaf adolescents. J. Phonet. 4:189–198.
Nickerson, R. S. 1975. Characteristics of the speech of deaf persons. Volta Rev. 77:342–362.
Nickerson, R. S., D. N. Kalikow, and K. N. Stevens. 1976. Computer-aided speech training for the deaf. J. Speech Hear. Disord. 41:120–132.
Nickerson, R. S., and K. N. Stevens. 1979. Approaches to the study of the relationship between intelligibility and physical properties of speech. Paper presented at the Institute on Speech Assessment and Speech Improvement for the Hearing Impaired, National Technical Institute for the Deaf, June 20–23, Rochester, N.Y.
Nickerson, R. S., K. N. Stevens, and A. M. Rollins. 1979. Research on computer based speech diagnosis and speech training aids for the deaf. Final Report on Contract No. 300-76-0116 with the U.S. Office of Education; BBN Report No. 4029, March.
Osberger, M. J. 1978. The effect of timing errors on the intelligibility of deaf children's speech. Doctoral dissertation, City University of New York.
Stevens, K. N. 1977. Physics of laryngeal behavior and larynx modes. Phonetica 34:264–279.
Stevens, K. N., R. S. Nickerson, A. Boothroyd, and A. M. Rollins. 1976.

Assessment of nasalization in the speech of deaf children. J. Speech Hear. Res. 19:393–416.

Stevens, K. N., R. S. Nickerson, and A. M. Rollins. 1978. On describing the suprasegmental properties of the speech of deaf children. Bolt Beranek and Newman Report No. 3955, November.

CHAPTER 3

SEGMENTAL CHARACTERISTICS OF THE SPEECH OF HEARING-IMPAIRED CHILDREN: FACTORS AFFECTING INTELLIGIBILITY

Harry Levitt and Harvey Stromberg

CONTENTS

> Errors, errors, everywhere,
> nor any one to correct.
> (With apologies to Coleridge)

Most teachers of the hearing impaired are cast adrift in a sea of speech errors. Which errors should be corrected first? Which aspects of speech development are most important? Should the teacher work on only one problem at a time? These are important questions that are faced daily by every teacher of the hearing impaired. Unfortunately, there are no simple solutions. The overall objective of our research is to determine the underlying causes of the speech problems exhibited by the hearing impaired, and in so doing, to provide a framework for developing more effective speech training procedures.

The purpose of this paper is to examine the organization of errors, or more generally, characteristic abnormal patterns in the speech of the hearing impaired. Abnormal speech patterns do not develop at random. There are reasons why hearing-impaired persons speak the way they do. Previous studies on the speech of the hearing impaired (e.g.,

---

Water, water, everywhere,
nor any drop to drink.
The Rime of the Ancient Mariner, Coleridge

Hudgins and Numbers, 1942; Markides, 1970; Nober, 1967; Smith, 1975) show remarkable similarities in the types of errors and inadequacies that are reported, although the subjects in these studies came from different geographic regions with significant dialectal differences and were exposed to different methods of speech training. Despite the similarities in the types of speech problems exhibited by hearing-impaired speakers, there are nevertheless vast differences in the intelligibility and overall quality of the speech produced by individual hearing-impaired persons. How does one take into account the differences in the speech problems exhibited by individual hearing-impaired persons without losing sight of the general structure of these problems and their likely causes? This chapter presents an approach to this quandary, together with the results obtained for an important segment of the hearing-impaired population, severely to profoundly hearing-impaired children at schools for the deaf or at regular schools with special programs for the hearing impaired.

PATTERNS IN THE SPEECH OF THE HEARING IMPAIRED

Methods of Analysis

There are many different ways in which the sounds of speech can be classified and, consequently, many different ways of specifying the differences between the speech of the hearing impaired and that of normally hearing persons. Because we are particularly interested in those differences that are likely to affect intelligibility, we have chosen to use as the basis of our classification system the smallest self-contained unit of speech that affects meaning, that is, the phoneme.

The reasons for choosing a classification system that is directly linked to meaning are both obvious and subtle. It is obvious that a classification system in which each category boundary corresponds to a change in meaning is likely to show up deviant speech patterns that affect meaning adversely and hence reduce intelligibility. A more subtle but eminently practical reason is that the normal ear is a remarkably sensitive instrument for categorizing sounds according to meaning. Although the use of modern instrumentation in the analysis of the speech of the hearing impaired is strongly encouraged, the limitations of such measurements are recognized. Whereas instrumental methods are particularly good for measuring many of the suprasegmental aspects of speech (e.g., fundamental frequency contours, syllabic duration) and certain important articulatory characteristics (e.g., formants, formant transitions, voice-onset time, degree of nasalization), the ear is, as yet, unmatched in identifying the sounds of speech. If this were not the case, machines for reliable, automatic speech recognition would have been developed long ago.

Given the limitations of instrumental methods and the many difficulties encountered with subjective judgments, we believe that the most effective way of analyzing the speech of the hearing impaired is to combine the best of both approaches, but to move in a direction that will allow for the further development of objective methods of measurement; that is, to systematically reduce the unreliability of subjective judgment by extending the range of applicability of objective instrumental techniques. In this regard, we feel it is important to find out first how the speech of the hearing impaired differs from that of the normally hearing using subjective judgments as needed (but geared to the most reliable types of subjective judgments), and then to find out the acoustic and other physically measurable correlates of these speech characteristics. The data reported in this chapter, derived primarily from phonetic transcriptions, represent the first stage in our ongoing research effort. Acoustic and other instrumental analyses of the most significant speech problems identified by this analysis are currently in progress.

It is convenient to label the differences between the speech of the hearing impaired and that of normally hearing persons as "errors," but it is important to recognize that this label may be misleading for those hearing-impaired persons whose speech is produced according to a different but consistent set of phonological rules. This is particularly true of young hearing-impaired children whose phonological systems may be at a different stage of development than their normally hearing peers. The data reported in this study are for older hearing-impaired children who showed an awareness of and attempted to produce the intended phonological forms, although they were not always successful. For these children the use of the term *error* for the difference between the targeted sound and that actually produced appears reasonable. An alternative view of the use of the term *error* is provided by Fisher et al. (Chapter 11, this volume). For those circumstances under which the term *error* is misleading, the term *difference,* or some other appropriate descriptor, should be used.

It is hypothesized that the errors or other inadequacies in the speech of the hearing impaired can be subdivided into three groups:

1. Errors or inadequacies that are common to the vast majority of hearing-impaired speakers
2. Errors or inadequacies that are common to specific subgroups of

hearing-impaired speakers—Such subgroups may include children who, for better or worse, have been exposed to uniquely different methods of speech training, subgroups that differ in terms of the type and amount of hearing impairment (e.g., conductive versus sensorineural impairment, mild versus profound, whether or not there is some residual hearing at high frequencies), and most importantly, subgroups that differ in terms of the age of onset of the hearing impairment (e.g., prelingually versus postlingually acquired hearing impairment).

3. Errors or inadequacies that are unique to the speech of individual hearing-impaired persons

Of the data we have gathered thus far, which deals primarily with the speech of prelingually deafened children with severe to profound hearing impairments, the segmental errors show a preponderance toward the first of these three categories. That is, there appears to be a significant number of segmental errors that are common to the majority of severely to profoundly hearing-impaired children. This chapter is concerned with the segmental characteristics of the speech of the hearing impaired. Given detailed information on the errors produced by a reasonably large number of children, it is possible to develop a quantitative description of these characteristic errors and their underlying patterns. For reasons given earlier, the errors are specified in terms of a phonemically based classification system. An analogous model for specifying suprasegmental error patterns is under development and is not reported in this chapter. Aspects of the suprasegmental characteristics of the speech of these and other hearing-impaired children may be found in the work of Levitt, Smith, and Stromberg (1974), Levitt et al. (1976), Osberger and Levitt (1979), and Reilly-Peterson (1979).

Data obtained by Smith (1975) and Gold (1978, 1980) for four groups of children were analyzed. The four groups were: 1) 20 children, between 8 and 10 years of age attending an oral school for the deaf (hearing levels poorer than 80 dB); 2) 20 children, as above, but between 12 and 14 years of age attending an oral school for the deaf (hearing levels poorer than 80 dB); 3) 19 children between 10 and 11 years of age with hearing levels poorer than 80 dB, mainstreamed into the regular school system; and 4) 18 children between 10 and 11 years of age with hearing levels better than 80 dB, mainstreamed into the regular school system. All of the children studied were attending schools in New York City, and in each case deafness was acquired prelingually. Speech intelligibility scores for the children ranged from 0% to just under 100%. Recordings were obtained of each child reading a set of 20 sentences developed by Smith (1975). Each sentence was read twice in order to eliminate reading errors as far as possible, and the better of the two utterances was used for subsequent analysis.

The recorded utterances were transcribed by skilled listeners, referred to as *raters*. These raters were provided with copies of the test sentences, and knowing what the children were attempting to say, they provided broad phonetic transcriptions of the recorded utterances. In addition, the suprasegmental characteristics of the speech were analyzed by a second group of raters (these data are not reported here). The intelligibility of each child's speech was measured by having normally hearing listeners, not familiar with the speech of the deaf, listen to randomized sets of these recorded utterances. The listeners wrote down what they heard, and the percentage of content words correctly identified was used as the measure of intelligibility. In order to minimize learning effects, no listener heard the same sentence more than once. A balanced experimental design was used such that each listener heard utterances provided by several children and each utterance was heard by three listeners.

The reliability of the phonetic transcriptions was reasonably high. The raters were in agreement on more than 70% of their judgments, and when they disagreed the differences were confined to a few relatively subtle judgments.

The broad phonetic transcriptions provided a basis for classifying the segmental characteristics of each child's speech. The phonemes produced were divided into the following categories: 1) target phoneme identifiable; 2) target phoneme substituted by another recognizable phoneme (including, as a special case, the glottal stop); 3) target phoneme distorted beyond recognition; 4) target phoneme omitted. In addition, two special categories were used for vowels and diphthongs: 5) vowel diphthongized excessively; and 6) intended diphthong fails. From a data-analysis point of view, each of the above categories represents a possible substitution for the target phoneme. For example, category 4 may be viewed as the substitution of an "omission" for the target phoneme. Using the above classification system, a *substitution matrix* was derived for each child, the rows of the matrix showing the target phonemes and the columns showing the substitutions. The entries along the diagonal of the matrix represent the correct or adequate productions of the target phonemes. The substitution matrices obtained for each of the children were subjected to an analysis similar to that used in the analysis of variance (Brownlee, 1965). From this analysis a common substitution matrix was obtained for all of the children as well as average matrices showing how the four groups of children differed from each other (as groups). In addition, individual difference matrices were obtained showing how each child differed from his or her group matrix. Details of this analysis may be found in Levitt et al. (1980).

A striking finding that emerged from the above analysis was that the major difference between the matrices obtained for the different children was the relative frequency of occurrence of the error substitutions and that there were only relatively small differences in the pattern of substitutions between children. Furthermore, the differences between substitution patterns that were observed were more closely related to the child's relative speech intelligibility rather than to between-group differences, although certain between-group differences were also observed. The two variables are not independent of each other in that children with hearing levels better than 80 dB and attending a regular school usually had better speech intelligibility.

The differences in error patterns that were observed were greatest between children with very good intelligibility (measured intelligibility greater than 95%) and those with very poor intelligibility (measured intelligibility less than 5%). Children with very poor speech intelligibility not only showed a higher rate of certain errors (i.e., omissions, substitutions, or unrecognizable distortions) than the highly intelligible children, but also produced errors of a kind that never occurred with the intelligible children. Even so, the relative frequency of these differences in error type was small compared to the very large differences observed in the frequency of occurrence of those errors that were common to all children. In other words, there were highly significant differences between children and between the above-mentioned groups of children in terms of the overall frequency of error substitutions, but once this factor was extracted, the pattern of errors (i.e., the *relative* frequency of substitutions of each type, given that a substitution has occurred) is very similar across children within groups and also, to a lesser extent, across experimental groups. The major exceptions to this trend occurred with those few children whose speech intelligibility scores lay at the extremes of the range (i.e., 0% or 100%).

Of particular interest in this chapter is the structure of this common pattern of errors. Because the errors observed by the raters seldom involved the substitution of a vowel for a consonant, or vice versa, it is convenient to analyze the error patterns for vowels and consonants separately. The next two sections provide such an analysis.

Patterns in the Production of Vowels

We have chosen to show in the diagrams that follow the error patterns obtained for the two groups of children at a school for the deaf. The error patterns for these two groups of children are virtually identical, within the limits of statistical testing. These data have been selected for illustration because more detail can be extracted from the substitution matrices of the groups showing a high error rate. The hearing-impaired children attending regular school show similar error patterns; but because of their lower frequency of errors it was difficult to establish, for the less common error types, whether or not the observed error rates were significantly different from zero. In order to develop a concise description of the most common error types, only error rates in excess of 0.5% were included in the analysis of error patterns.

In order to provide an explicit yet concise description of the prevalent error patterns, Figure 3.1 shows the errors grouped according to vowel type and error type. Error types have been subdivided according to the articulatory maneuvers involved. These are identified along the top row of the diagram. The vowel types showing these errors are identified in the first vertical column of the diagram. Thus, each row of the diagram corresponds to a specific vowel type (front, central, back, and schwa-like vowel) and each column of the diagram corresponds to a different error type. Ten basic error types are shown: 1) tense-lax substitutions; 2) substitution of the intended vowel by neighboring vowel in the vowel quadrilateral (near-neighbor); 3) substitu-

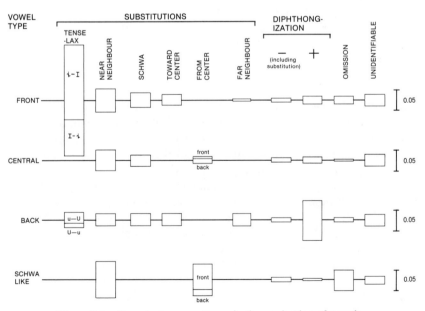

Figure 3.1.   Prevalent error patterns in the production of vowels.

tion by a schwa or schwa-like vowel; 4) substitution by a vowel (other than a near neighbor) that is closer to the center of the vowel quadrilateral; 5) substitution by a vowel that is further away from the center of the vowel quadrilateral; 6) substitution by a vowel on the opposite side of the vowel quadrilateral (far-neighbor substitution); 7) substitution of a diphthong by a vowel (usually by the major component of the diphthong or a near neighbor of the major component), identified as *diphthongization* − in the diagram; 8) substitution of a vowel by a diphthong or excessive diphthongization of the vowel, identified as *diphthongization* + in the diagram; 9) omission of the intended vowel or diphthong; and 10) unidentifiable distortion. Note that there is some overlap between error types, but that no error is counted more than once. For example, error type 4, substitution of a more central vowel, does not include substitutions by a near neighbor (2), but it should be borne in mind that a greater proportion of near-neighbor substitutions will be toward rather than away from the center of the vowel quadrilateral. Similarly, substitutions by a schwa or schwa-like vowel (3) are separate from, but similar to, error type 4.

Each box in the diagram corresponds to a specific error type occurring with a specific vowel type. The height of each box represents the average frequency of occurrence of that error type for that vowel type. These frequencies were derived from the average substitution matrix. Scale markers showing relative frequency per unit height appear at the end of each row. Unless otherwise indicated, all substitutions represented by a given box occur with roughly equal frequency, that is, within ±2.5 percentage points of their average frequency of occurrence.

The following is an example illustrating how to interpret the diagram. Consider the top left-hand box, representing tense-lax substitutions for the front vowels. Because /i/ and /ɪ/ are the only front vowels subject to this substitution, they are identified specifically in the figure. Furthermore, the box is made up of two smaller boxes, one corresponding to the substitution /i/ to /ɪ/ and the other to the substitution /ɪ/ to /i/. Two boxes are shown because the two versions of this error type have significantly different frequencies of occurrence. The height of the box corresponding to the /i/-to-/ɪ/ substitution is greater than that of any other box in the diagram, indicating that this substitution was observed more frequently than any other vowel substitution.

The average frequency of occurrence of the /i/-to-/ɪ/ substitution may be obtained by comparing the height of the box representing this substitution to the scale marker shown on the right-hand side. The height of the box is roughly four times the height of the scale marker which, in turn, corresponds to an average frequency of substitution of 0.05. The average frequency of occurrence of /i/-to-/ɪ/ substitutions is, therefore, (4 × 0.05) = 0.20, or 20%. The height of both boxes (representing the sum of both the /ɪ/-to-/i/ and /i/-to-/ɪ/ substitutions) is 5.6, corresponding to an average frequency of occurrence of (5.6 × 0.05) = 0.28, or 28%. That is, the average frequency of occurrence of the tense-lax substitution involving the front vowels (either /ɪ/-to-/i/ or /i/-to-/ɪ/) is 28%.

The frequencies calculated above represent average values and correspond to the mean rates of these substitutions obtained for the two groups of children at a school for the deaf. Individual children will show very different rates of substitution. To a first approximation, however, the pattern of substitutions will be very similar across children (excluding those children whose intelligibility scores are close to either 100% or 0%). A good estimate of the frequency of a specific substitution for any one child (within the population studied) is obtained by multiplying the average frequency of the substitution by an adjustment factor which takes into account the overall rate of substitutions for that child. For example, the overall rate of phoneme substitutions for the children represented by the diagram was roughly 48%; that is, on average, 48 out of every 100 phonemes was either substituted by another phoneme, omitted, or distorted beyond recognition. A child with better than average speech would have a smaller overall error rate, say 19% for purposes of illustration. This error rate is about 2/5 of the average error rate (i.e., 19/48 is approximately equal to 0.4, or 2/5). Thus, to a first approximation, the frequency of tense-lax substitutions involving the front vowel for this child is approximately 0.4 × 0.28 = 0.112, or roughly 11%. Expressed another way, for this child, roughly one out of nine occurrences of the front vowels /i/ or /ɪ/ (in the context of read sentences) will be heard as its tense-lax cognate, /ɪ/ or /i/, respectively.

The next column in the diagram shows near-neighbor substitutions. These are substitutions in which the target vowel is substituted by a neighboring vowel in the vowel quadrilateral, for example, /ɪ/ and /ɛ/, /ɛ/ and /æ/ confusions. The use of a single box to represent all of the near-neighbor substitutions implies that each substitution occurs with roughly the same frequency and that the height of the box corresponds to average frequency of substitution. The criterion used for grouping substitutions within a single box was that the observed frequency of occurrence of each substitution within the group be within ±2.5 percentage points of the average frequency of substitution for the entire group.

Viewed as a whole, Figure 3.1 shows that by far the most common error involving the vowels is that of substituting one vowel for another and that, of these, the tense-lax substitution involving the front vowels /i/ and /ı/ is the most frequent. The next most frequent type of substitution is that involving near neighbors, followed by substitutions to more central or to a schwa-like vowel. The trend toward substituting a more central vowel also occurs within near-neighbor and tense-lax substitutions. Substitutions away from the center occur relatively infrequently except when the intended vowel is a schwa or a schwa-like vowel. Similarly, omissions occurred relatively infrequently except for this vowel group. Errors of diphthongization showed moderate frequencies of occurrence except for the back vowels which are often diphthongized. Unidentifiable substitutions occurred with moderate frequency and were roughly equally frequent for all vowel types.

Patterns in the Production of Consonants

Figure 3.2 shows the error patterns obtained for the consonants. The format of the diagram is the same as that of Figure 3.1. The rows of the diagram indicate consonant types (stops, fricatives, affricates, nasals, glides, and laterals). The columns indicate error types. These have been divided into six basic groups (omissions, asynchrony, constriction errors, placement errors, glottal substitutions, and unidentifiable distortions). The first three of these groups have been further subdivided into two parts, resulting in a total of nine error categories:

1. *Omission of target phoneme (Omissions, all).* This error type is subdivided according to the place of articulation of the target phoneme (front, middle, and back, represented by the symbols f, m, and b in the figure), and position in the word of the target phoneme (initial, medial, and final, represented by the symbols I, M, and F in the figure).

2. *Omission of part of the intended phoneme (Omissions, part).* This error type occurs with only the affricate. Three specific forms of this error type are identified: that in which the first component (i.e., the stop component) of the sound is omitted; that in which the second component (i.e., the fricative component) is omitted; and that in which the remaining component is subject to a voiced-voiceless substitution (shown by the dotted box).

3. *Lack of synchrony in the control of voicing (Asynchrony, voicing).* This error has two basic forms, that in which the target phoneme is voiced and is replaced by its voiceless cognate (represented by the symbol V-V̄) and that in which the target phoneme is voiceless and is replaced by its voiced cognate (represented by the symbol V̄-V).

4. *Lack of synchrony in control of the velum (Asynchrony,*

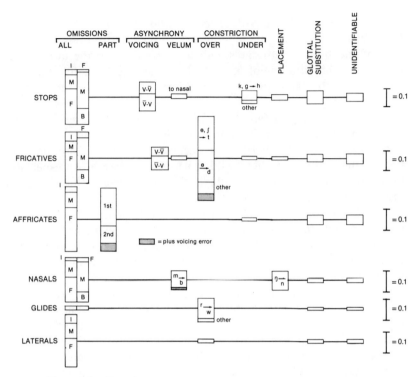

Figure 3.2.   Prevalent error patterns in the production of consonants.

velum).   Improper control of the velum, usually in conjunction with other articulatory events, will result in a nasal consonant being substituted for a stop or vice versa. The substitution of /m/ by /b/ is particularly frequent and is shown by a separate box. The small dotted box shows nasal to stop substitutions in which the stop is also subjected to a voiced-to-voiceless substitution.

   5.   *Vocal tract constriction too great (Constriction, over).*   If the constriction in the vocal tract is too great, fricatives will be substituted by a stop. The substitutions of /θ/ or /ʃ/ by /t/ and /θ/ by /d/ are especially frequent and are shown by separate boxes.[1] Another form of over constriction is that in which the oral opening for a glide is reduced. A specific form of this substitution, which occurs relatively frequently, is that from glide /r/ to /w/ and is represented by a separate box.

---

[1] By far the most common substitution of this type was that of /ð/ to /d/. This substitution is not treated as an error because of its common occurrence in the speech of normally hearing children of the same dialect.

6. *Insufficient vocal-tract constriction (Constriction, under).* Insufficient closure results in stop-to-fricative substitutions, or in the case of fricatives or affricates, substitution of /h/ for the target phoneme. The substitutions of /k/ or /g/ by /h/ are significantly more frequent than other substitutions of this form and are represented by a separate box.

7. *Incorrect placement of the articulators (Placement).* This error type involves substitutions in place of articulation with no accompanying problem other than an occasional voicing substitution. As before, the dotted box shows additional voicing errors. An especially frequent place-of-articulation substitution is that from /ŋ/ to /n/ and is represented by a separate box.

8. *Substitution of glottal stop (Glottal substitution).* In this case, a glottal stop was substituted for the target phoneme.

9. *Unidentifiable distortion (Unidentifiable).* This error type covers those cases in which the target phoneme is substituted by an unidentifiable sound.

The above categorization of error types is based on the articulatory features associated with the target and substituted phonemes, respectively. It is important to bear in mind that these error categories are relatively broad and their articulatory descriptions are inferred; that is, they are not the result of direct articulatory measurements.

Viewed as a whole, Figure 3.2 shows that by far the most common type of consonant error is that of omission. Note that the scale in Figure 3.2 is different from that of Figure 3.1. In this case, the height of the scale marker corresponds to an error rate of 0.1, which is twice that used in the vowel diagram. Because of the high frequency of occurrence of omission errors, this error type has been further subdivided according to two additional factors, position of the consonant in the word and place of articulation. Two separate, adjacent columns are used to show this subdivision of omission errors.

Omissions occur primarily in the word-final position, less frequently in word-medial position, and relatively infrequently in word-initial position. The subdivision of errors according to place of articulation shows a low rate of omissions for consonants produced at or near the front of the mouth, a moderately high omission rate for the velar consonants, and a high rate of omissions for consonants produced in the middle region of the mouth.

The factors of position in the word and place of articulation are shown for the case of omissions only because of the relatively high frequency of occurrence of these errors. A three-way analysis of variance of omission errors for the factors of consonant type (stops, fricatives, affricates, nasals, glides, and laterals), word position (initial, medial, final), and place of articulation (front, middle, back) shows not only that each of these three factors is highly significant, but that there are also important interactions. For example, although the ordering of omission rates by word position is the same for each consonant type (that is, frequency of omissions greater for word-final position than for word-medial position, which in turn is greater than for word-initial position), the relative frequency of omission as a function of word position differs between consonant types. For example, consonant omissions in the word-initial position are slightly less frequent for the stops than for the fricatives, but omissions in the word-medial and word-final position are relatively more frequent for the stops. Similarly, omission of stops produced at the front of the mouth is less frequent than omission of fricatives with the same place of articulation; for other places of articulation, the stops show a higher average rate of omissions than the fricatives. These subtleties are evident in Figure 3.2 when the relative heights of the corresponding boxes under the omissions column are compared.

After omission errors, the next most common error type is that of overconstriction. Unlike omission errors, which occurred frequently with all consonant types, errors of overconstriction occurred only with fricatives and glides. Furthermore, the bulk of these errors involved a small subset of substitutions of /θ/ or /ʃ/ by /t/, /θ/ by /d/, and /r/ by /w/. Of these, the voiceless-fricative-for-stop substitutions involve similar articulatory mechanisms, a factor to be taken into account in developing more effective speech training procedures to reduce the high frequency of occurrence of this specific error type.

A particularly important error category is that classified as *asynchrony*. The most common form of this error is that of the voiced-voiceless substitution. For the stops, the substitution of the voiced for the voiceless cognate (shown by the symbol V̄-V in the diagram) occurred more frequently than the voiced to voiceless form (V-V̄). The relative frequency of these substitutions was more nearly equal for the fricatives.

Voicing substitutions also occurred frequently in combination with other error forms, as shown by the dotted boxes in Figure 3-2. The most common cases in which a voicing substitution occurred jointly with another error type were those of partial omission in affricates, asynchrony or improper velum control, overconstriction in fricatives resulting in fricative-to-stop substitutions (a particularly frequent substitution is that of /θ/ by /d/), and substitutions in place of articulation.

Although it is reasonable to conclude that voicing errors in stops are a result of asynchronous timing in the sequence of articulatory events constituting a stop, the reasons for classifying voicing errors in fricatives as errors of asynchrony are more subtle. Experiments in the development and evaluation of speech training strategies for the fricative sounds (Guttman, Levitt, and Bellefleur, 1970; Levitt, 1973; and Levitt and Nye, 1971) have shown that hearing-impaired children have relatively little difficulty in learning the voiced-voiceless distinction for fricatives produced in isolation but that difficulties occur when the sounds are produced in context. It is believed that, for the most part, voicing errors for fricatives in context occur because of an inability to control the onset and termination of voicing during the flow of speech rather than an inability to produce voicing, per se, hence the designation of this error type as one of *asynchrony*. It is important to remember that the timing problems underlying voicing errors in stops are quite different from those involving fricatives. As a reminder of this difference, the boxes showing voiced-voiceless substitutions for stops and for fricatives are not aligned immediately below each other in Figure 3.2.

Another common set of errors classified under the general heading of *asynchrony* result from improper velar control. As noted earlier, if the target sound is a stop and the velum is not raised fully at the appropriate time, a nasal consonant will be substituted. Conversely, if the target is a nasal consonant and the velum is not lowered at the appropriate time, then a stop may be substituted. This error can take several forms. For example, the velum may be raised throughout, leading to a simple substitution of the form /b/ for /m/, or the velum may be raised too late, leading to a substitution of the form /mb/ for /b/. The stop component may also be produced by implosion. The substitution of /m/ for /b/, as judged at a phonemic level, is especially frequent for substitutions of this type and the various causes of this substitution must be studied in greater detail.

Errors of placement were relatively infrequent. The most common of these errors was the substitution of /n/ for /ŋ/. Because these two nasal consonants sound very similar, it is likely that a fair proportion of the reported substitutions were a result of perceptual confusions rather than errors in production. Aside from this substitution, which may involve a substantial perceptual component, errors involving place of articulation were, on average, the least frequent of all the error types.

Glottal substitutions occurred with all consonant types, but showed a greater frequency of occurrence with the stops and affricates. The stop component in the affricate may have been the contributing factor in increasing the frequency of glottal substitutions for this consonant type. Similarly, unidentifiable distortions occurred with all sound types, with a slightly smaller frequency of occurrence for the vowel-like consonants (nasals, glides, and laterals). Some caution should be exercised in interpreting the relative frequencies of these two error types. Whereas most of the error types showed a frequency of occurrence in direct proportion to the overall error rate, the relative proportion of glottal substitutions and unidentifiable distortions increased at a greater than average rate. That is, the less intelligible children showed a greater relative proportion of glottal substitutions and unidentifiable substitutions than the more intelligible children, many of whom did not exhibit these errors.

DISCUSSION

In view of the complexity and diversity of the problems in analyzing the speech of the hearing impaired, it is not surprising that, despite decades of research, there still does not exist a comprehensive, quantitative description of the speech of the hearing impaired. This paper represents a limited attack of this problem in that a reasonably comprehensive description of segmental errors has been derived for a specific population of hearing-impaired children. The results of this analysis not only allow for limited but reasonably accurate predictions to be made of the speech problems of individual children within the population studied, but more importantly, well defined trends have been observed which we believe are generalizable to other populations of hearing-impaired persons and which may provide new insights for the development of more effective speech-training and speech-assessment procedures.

Before embarking on a discussion of the error patterns observed and their implications for speech training, it is important to recognize the limitations (and strengths) of the procedures used in this study.

A major drawback of a phonetic analysis approach is that of variability between judgments. Even the most highly trained, experienced raters will exhibit some variability in their phonetic evaluations. Of greater concern are the relatively large differences between raters. In order to combat this problem, two or more evaluations were obtained independently from different raters. This strategy does not eliminate the problem but it does reduce the effects of inter-rater variability while providing information on the reliability of the various types of phonetic judgments. For an analysis of inter-rater differences on phonetic judgments of the type used in this paper, see Gold (1978).

Another important limitation that is closely linked to the problem of rater reliability is that of confounding between perceptual and articulatory cues. For example, the raters reported a fairly high rate of substitutions between the nasal consonants /n/ and /ŋ/, particularly when the target sound was /ŋ/. Since /n/ and /ŋ/ are perceptually very similar, many of the reported substitutions may have been the result of judgmental errors on the part of the raters. Unfortunately, the acoustic characteristics of /n/ and /ŋ/ are also very similar, thereby making it difficult to resolve this ambiguity using simple acoustical analyses. It is possible using sophisticated instrumentation to measure the articulatory movements involved, but this would be a major study in itself.

Although confusions between perceptually similar sounds occur in the speech of normally hearing persons, they occur far more frequently in the speech of the hearing impaired. It is difficult to separate the degree to which articulatory and perceptual factors contribute to misidentifications in speech, but the fact that such misidentifications are much more frequent in the speech of the hearing impaired suggests that production problems play a prominent role. Speech problems that result in misidentification of phonemes will typically have an adverse effect on intelligibility. Certain errors, however, will have a greater effect than others in reducing intelligibility. The effect of different error types on intelligibility has been a subject of interest for some time, but discussion of this research is beyond the scope of this paper.

Having placed the problems of analysis in perspective, let us now examine the major findings of this study. A key observation was that although there are vast differences between hearing-impaired children in terms of overall speech intelligibility, there are marked similarities between children with respect to the types and relative frequencies of the most common segmental errors. As a result it has been possible to summarize the main findings on the underlying patterns of segmental errors in terms of two relatively simple diagrams for vowels and consonants, shown in Figures 3.1 and 3.2, respectively.

Errors of the type shown in these two diagrams have been reported by many different researchers, although not always in the same terms (Hudgins and Numbers, 1942; Markides, 1970; Nober, 1967; Smith, 1975). In view of the vast differences between the populations studied (i.e., children attending schools with different educational philosophies, in different countries, and at different periods in time), the similarities in the error patterns that have been reported are quite striking. These similarities between the error types further support the notion that there is a common body of speech problems that are exhibited by a majority of persons with severe to profound hearing impairment. The contribution of this chapter lies not so much in providing a detailed summary of the most common error types, but in placing these error patterns in perspective.

The method used in deriving Figures 3.1 and 3.2 is based on the analysis of variance, which provides a quantitative assessment of the extent to which various errors differ between the four groups of children and which errors are common to all of the children. The largest difference between children was found to be the overall frequency of occurrence of segmental errors. Once this variable is taken into account, there are relatively small differences in the segmental error patterns exhibited by the four groups of children.

It is important to recognize that there are exceptions to the above trend. The major exceptions were found to occur with children whose speech was either very intelligible or virtually unintelligible (i.e., children with intelligibility scores in excess of 95% or less than 5%, respectively). As a result, it is possible to predict, with a precision that is comparable to the precision of measurement, the error patterns exhibited by individual children within each of the four groups studied (for mathematical details of the method of prediction, see Levitt et al., 1980). Less precise predictions are to be expected for other groups of children with similar hearing impairments, but preliminary estimates of the accuracy of predictions indicate that at least the ranking of most common errors will be essentially the same. Note also that the anticipated error patterns for children with markedly different forms of hearing loss, such as those with significant amounts of high-frequency residual hearing, or for children with postlingually acquired impairments will be quite different.

More important than the ability to predict the frequency of occurrence of specific error types is that of identifying underlying trends in the pattern of errors. One of the criteria used in constructing the vowel and consonant diagrams is that the errors be subdivided into relatively homogeneous groups according to both the articulatory mechanisms involved and the sound type.

It is revealing to note that, in order to obtain relatively homogeneous groupings of the vowel errors, it was necessary to subdivide the vowels into four basic types, front, back, central, and schwa-like (i.e., /ə/, /ɚ/, /ɝ/). This grouping is somewhat different from that usually encountered in phonetic textbooks. The vowels are not only subdivided according to differences in the placement of the articulators, but also according to differences in the function of the vowel in context. Note, for example, how different the error patterns are for the central and schwa-like vowels, despite the similarities in vowel tract shape for these two vowel types.

One explanation for the relatively high rate of omission errors for the schwa-like vowels is that when a vowel omission occurs (which is seldom), it typically involves an unstressed syllable, particularly an unstressed syllable at the end of a word or phrase. The vowel in these syllables is often the schwa or schwa-like vowel such as /ə/ or /ɝ/. In this case, the omission error is primarily a result of contextual factors rather than articulatory difficulties.

The consonants also show strong contextual effects. Omissions, which affect all consonants, are heavily dependent on word position. Omission errors are relatively infrequent for phonemes in word-initial position, more frequent for the word-medial position, and very frequent for the word-final position. The same trend, but less marked, also occurs with other consonant error types. The reasons for this trend appear to be quite complex and involve not only differences in the way consonants in word-final position are produced but also dialectal variations and problems of improper speech planning (McGarr and Harris, this volume). It is important to know under what conditions these problems are least likely to occur because these are the conditions under which new contrasts or phoneme types are most easily learned.

A comparison between the vowel and consonant diagrams shows several striking differences. The vowel diagram shows that the most common errors involve incorrect placement of the articulators, as manifested by the high incidence of near-neighbor and other vowel-for-vowel substitutions. Furthermore, there is a marked bias toward more neutral vowel positions, as shown by the high rate of substitutions toward either a schwa or more central vowel. Dynamic factors also play a part, as in errors of diphthongization, but these are markedly less frequent, and errors of omission seldom occur. In contrast, the most frequent consonant error is that of omission. Errors involving dynamic characteristics of speech (asynchrony or lack of movement) are the next most frequent; errors of articulatory placement are relatively infrequent. When comparing the two diagrams, remember that the scale of the consonant diagram is half that of the vowel diagram (as shown by the scale markers on the right-hand side of each diagram). An exception to this overall trend for consonant errors is exhibited by the glides. These consonants (often referred to as semi-vowels) have an error pattern more closely associated with that of the vowels, that is, a low rate of omission errors and a relatively high rate of placement errors[2] as compared to other consonants.

The vowels and consonants (semi-vowels excluded) involve very

---

[2] The substitution of /w/ for /r/, which is relatively frequent, may be viewed as a placement error and not only as an error of overconstriction (see Figure 3.2).

different articulatory mechanisms and hence it is not surprising that basically different error patterns have been observed for these two sound types. From a teaching point of view, it is significant to note that the vowels are acquired earlier and are easier to produce than the consonants. Secondly, the vowels are more closely associated with and affected by the prosody of an utterance than the consonants. Thirdly, the articulatory differences between vowels in normal speech are not well defined. Both the production and perception of vowels are affected substantially by a variety of factors, including contextual, dialectal, perceptual, and cognitive variables. In contrast, the articulatory differences between consonants are more sharply defined and misarticulations are both easier to define and easier to perceive.

It is not coincidental that the sounds that are easier to produce are also the ones that are acquired earlier. Most speech training programs introduce the teaching of vowels at an early stage; for example, just after the elements of prosody have been taught and before the teaching of consonants (Ling, 1976). At the same time, because the articulatory distinctions between vowels are not absolutely firm (i.e., they are influenced substantially by context and a host of interactive variables) it is to be expected that subtle errors, such as tense-lax, near-neighbor, and centralization substitutions, will abound but that gross errors, such as omissions, will occur infrequently. An important practical question is: what degree of precision in vowel production is to be expected from a hearing-impaired child before moving on to the teaching of consonants? This is an important question, as is the analogous question relating to the teaching of prosody as a base for the teaching of segmental characteristics. Research addressing these issues and on the objective evaluation of speech-training strategies, such as that reported by Osberger (this volume), is much needed.

A major concern in any good speech-training program is that of assessment. Effective assessment protocols are needed for a variety of purposes, to measure progress (or lack of progress), to identify special problem areas, to provide the basic information needed in planning individualized speech training curricula, and, on a broader scale, to evaluate the effectiveness of different teaching methods or instrumental aids to speech training, as well as answering basic research questions of the type cited above. Conventional methods of speech testing, however, are laborious, time-consuming, and, as a result, seldom used. There is a need for the development of more efficient, practical speech tests. The vowel and consonant diagrams shown here provide useful guidelines for the development of more efficient tests. As a rule, test efficiency is improved if there is some prior knowledge of the quantities to be measured. Thus, for example, if one knew which speech characteristics or speech errors are most revealing regarding a hearing-impaired child's speech production skills, then test items that elicit examples of these characteristics or errors will provide the needed information speedily and efficiently.

In conclusion, it is the hope of the authors that the consonant and vowel diagrams shown in Figures 3.1 and 3.2 are of a temporary nature. As noted earlier, the error patterns shown in these diagrams are made up of three major components: errors common to the vast majority of hearing-impaired persons; errors common to specific subgroups of the hearing impaired, such as those educated according to a specific system; and idiosyncratic errors that are specific to each individual. For those fortunate few hearing-impaired children who have received and benefited from truly effective speech training that began at an early age, many of the error types shown in these diagrams either do not exist or occur only rarely. Hopefully, as a result of improved teaching, the majority of hearing-impaired children will be classified in this category.

REFERENCES

Brownlee, K. A. 1965. Statistical Theory and Methodology in Science and Engineering. John Wiley & Sons, Inc., New York.

Gold, T. 1978. Speech and hearing skills: A comparison between hard-of-hearing and deaf children. Doctoral dissertation, City University of New York.

Gold, T. 1980. Speech production in hearing-impaired children. J. Commun. Disord. 13:397–418.

Guttman, N., H. Levitt, and P. A. Bellefleur. 1970. Articulatory training of the deaf using low-frequency surrogate fricatives. J. Speech Hear. Res. 13:19–29.

Hudgins, C. V., and F. C. Numbers. 1942. An investigation of the intelligibility of the speech of the deaf. Genet. Psychol. Monogr. 26:293–392.

Levitt, H. 1973. Speech processing aids for the deaf: An overview. IEEE Trans. Audio Electroacoust. AU-21:269–273.

Levitt, H., and P. W. Nye. 1971. Sensory Training Aids for the Hearing Impaired. National Academy of Engineering, Washington, D.C.

Levitt, H., C. R. Smith, and H. Stromberg. 1974. Acoustical, articulatory and perceptual characteristics of the speech of deaf children. In G. Fant (ed.), Speech Communication: Proceedings of the Speech Communication Seminar, Stockholm. Halsted Press, New York.

Levitt, H., R. E. Stark, N. McGarr, et al. 1976. Language communication skills of deaf children, 1973–75. Paper presented at the Institute on Language Assessment for the Hearing Impaired, May, Rome, N.Y.

Levitt, H., H. Stromberg, C. Smith, and T. Gold. 1980. The structure of segmental errors in the speech of deaf children. J. Commun. Disord. 13:419–441.

Ling, D. 1976. Speech and the Hearing-Impaired Child: Theory and Practice. A. G. Bell Association for the Deaf, Washington, D.C.

Markides, A. 1970. The speech of deaf and partially hearing children with special reference to factors affecting intelligibility. Br. J. Disord. Commun. 5:126–140.

Nober, E. H. 1967. Articulation of the deaf. Except. Child. 33:611–621.

Osberger, M. J., and H. Levitt. 1979. The effect of timing errors on the intelligibility of deaf children's speech. J. Acoust. Soc. Am. 66:1316–1324.

Reilly-Peterson, A. 1979. Syllable nucleus duration in the speech of hearing and deaf children. Doctoral dissertation, City University of New York.

Smith, C. R. 1975. Residual hearing and speech production in deaf children. J. Speech Hear. Res. 18:795–811.

CHAPTER 4

ARTICULATORY CONTROL IN A DEAF SPEAKER

Nancy S. McGarr and Katherine S. Harris

CONTENTS

Although some children who are born severely or profoundly hearing impaired or become hearing impaired in infancy achieve intelligible speech, the vast majority do not. Speech intelligibility is fairly well correlated with residual hearing (Boothroyd, 1970; Smith, 1972), at least until 90 dB, and overall intelligibility is well correlated with the percentage of segmental errors, and to a lesser extent with supraseg-mental deviancy (Levitt, Smith, and Stromberg, 1974). Although many educators of the hearing impaired would claim that their students' characteristic unintelligibility is a consequence of faulty teaching practices (Haycock, 1933; Ling, 1976), independent investigations have been remarkably consistent in showing similar patterns of segmental and suprasegmental errors in the speech of hearing-impaired talkers trained in a wide variety of programs (Hudgins and Numbers, 1942; Johnson, 1975; Levitt et al., 1976; Smith, 1972). Furthermore, teachers experienced with the group can discriminate between these speakers and others in production of disyllables (Calvert, 1961) and are better at decoding their speech (McGarr, 1978). If we accept the point of view

---

The acoustic measurements were described in a paper presented at the meeting of the Acoustical Society of America, Atlanta, Georgia, April 1980. The work described in this chapter was supported by Grants NS-13617, NS-13870, and RR-05596 to Haskins Laboratories.

that there is a generic "deaf speech"[1] pattern, not dependent at least on the fine-grained details of the training procedure, we may ask: what are its characteristics?

One hypothesis, primarily concerned with consonant articulation, is that deaf speakers place their articulators fairly accurately—especially for those places of articulation that are highly visible—but fail to normally coordinate the movements of several articulators (Huntington, Harris, and Sholes, 1968; Levitt et al., 1974). Thus, we may suggest that the errors in deaf speech are the consequences of incorrect motor planning in time.

A second hypothesis, primarily concerned with vowel articulation, is that deaf speakers move their articulators through a relatively restricted range, thereby "neutralizing" vowels (Angelocci, Kopp, and Holbrook, 1964; Monsen, 1976). However, this hypothesis fails to account for the great variability in the speech production of deaf talkers, a point we will discuss in further detail later.

A third hypothesis is that the inability of deaf speakers to control the suprasegmental characteristics of their speech makes both segmental and suprasegmental characteristics more difficult for listeners to decode (Harris and McGarr, 1980). Suprasegmental aspects of speech may be so abnormal as to mislead the listener. Deaf speakers may not preserve phonological contrasts or may produce them in a way that makes information about the intended contrast unavailable to the listeners, and perhaps blocks information about other contrasts. That fundamental frequency (McGarr and Osberger, 1978) and overall duration levels (e.g., Osberger and Levitt, 1979) are often deviant in deaf speakers is well known. These deviations alone might interfere with a listener's ability to decode a speech signal, even if other suprasegmental contrasts were preserved in either a normal or an abnormal way.

On an entirely different level, poor control of the speech source function may simply provide inadequate support for the acoustic realization of upper articulator movement. Deaf speakers characteristically take in less air in speech respiration (Forner and Hixon, 1977; Whitehead, this volume) and may, in addition, convert air into acoustic energy inefficiently due to poor control of the larynx.

---

[1] For convenience in the ensuing discussion, we will call the speech characteristic of the group *deaf speech* and for the purposes of the paper, speakers of deaf speech will be called *deaf*. By making this identification, we wish to acknowledge the fact that persons who are severely to profoundly hearing impaired do not necessarily produce this characteristic speech.

This chapter presents a preliminary attempt to assess these hypotheses by examining a number of productions of some very simple utterances by a single deaf talker using listeners to judge production accuracy utterance by utterance. Although it is obvious that more subjects must be studied in order to reach firm conclusions, the authors believe that the general technique of examining interarticulator programming in depth with combined perceptual, acoustic, and physiological techniques is a promising avenue.

METHODS AND PROCEDURES

The prelingually deaf speaker in this study was a woman in her mid-40s who graduated from an oral school for the deaf, and has received remedial speech classes as an adult. Her pure tone average is 105 dB. Informal ratings of spontaneous speech samples suggest that her productions would be characterized as fairly typical of her group. For purposes of comparison, productions of a hearing speaker who has frequently served as an experimental subject were also examined.

Each subject produced approximately 20 repetitions of each of six utterance types. These utterances were nonsense words of the type /əpipɑp/, /əpipip/, and /əpɑpip/ with stress on either the /i/ or the /ɑ/. For this paper, data are presented primarily for the first and third utterance types. Paint-on surface electrodes were used to record from the orbicularis oris muscle (Allen, Lubker, and Harrison, 1972); conventional hooked-wire electrodes were inserted into the genioglossus muscle. The electrode preparation and insertion techniques for the genioglossus muscle electrodes have been reported in detail elsewhere (Hirose, 1971). Conventional acoustic recordings were made at the same time as the electromyography.

The acoustic and electromyographic (EMG) data obtained from the two speakers were analyzed in several ways. First, for the deaf speaker, the acoustic recordings of six utterance types were randomized and presented to listeners inexperienced in hearing deaf speech. The listeners were required to select one of the six utterance types presented on an answer sheet for each item they heard. Confusion matrices were obtained. The hearing subject's productions were not checked perceptually, but informal listening suggested that perceptual errors would not be made. Second, acoustic measurements were made on the interactive computer system at the Haskins Laboratories and with conventional sound spectrography. Third, the EMG signals were rectified, integrated, and then further analyzed, as described below.

RESULTS

Listener Judgments

First, examining the results of the listening test, the authors found that the deaf speaker was judged to be fairly intelligible (at least as measured by a closed-response listening task). Table 4.1 shows the confusion matrix obtained from the listeners' scores. An item was considered to be correct if 9 out of 10 listeners identified it as the originally intended utterance. The average percentage correct for all utterance types was 75%. Overall, there were more errors of stress than of the segment type (e.g., a vowel identity error). In fact, only for the utterance /əpɑˈpip/ was there a significant number of vowel errors. In this case, the listeners perceived the utterance as /əpiˈpip/ 32% of the time.

Using these listener judgments, all tokens (repetitions) of an item were divided into two categories: "perceived correct" utterances and "stress error" utterances. Only for the intended utterance /əpɑˈpip/ was there an additional category (that of a vowel error).

Acoustic Measurements

The acoustic cues used to convey contrastive stress in normal speech production have been extensively studied (Fry, 1958, 1964; Harris, 1978). In general, speakers convey changes in contrastive stress to listeners by differences in acoustic cues such as vowel duration, fundamental frequency, amplitude, and formant frequency. For the deaf speaker, two questions are of interest. First, what acoustic cues does a deaf speaker use to convey contrastive stress to the listener and how do these cues compare to those used by the normal speaker? Second, can productions perceived as being incorrect in the speech of the deaf be explained as differing systematically from those utterances perceived as being correct?

If stress may be conveyed at least in part by differences in vowel duration, we might expect that for perceived correct utterances in the

Table 4.1. Confusion matrix of listeners' judgments for the deaf speakers

	1	2	3	4	5	6
1. əˈpi pɑp	88	08				
2. əpiˈpɑp	25	75				
3. əˈpi pip			83	17		
4. əpiˈpip			07	91		
5. əˈpɑ pip					67	29
6. əpɑˈpip				32	16	51

speech of the deaf, the stressed vowel would be longer than the unstressed vowel. Conversely, stress error utterances may be due, in part, to an inappropriate vowel duration ratio.

The measurements of vowel duration show that the deaf speaker was like the hearing speaker in some ways, but not in others. Figure 4.1 shows the measurements of vowel duration for the hearing speaker (FBB) and the deaf speaker's "perceived correct" utterances (MH ↑) and "stress error" utterances (MH ↓). Dark bars represent stressed vowels; open bars represent unstressed vowels. As expected, overall duration of the vowels produced by the deaf speaker was considerably longer than those of the hearing speaker.

For the hearing speaker, there is always a shift toward longer relative duration for a vowel when it is stressed than when it is not, although this pattern is apparently complicated by differences in intrinsic vowel duration in that productions of /ɑ/ are in general longer than productions of /i/ in the same phonetic environment. An acoustic analysis of a second hearing speaker shows less effect of intrinsic vowel duration. The deaf speaker did not, however, show consistent differences in intrinsic vowel duration between /i/ and /ɑ/ within the same phonetic context.

On average, the deaf speaker appears to be conveying contrastive stress by varying vowel duration in the sense that intended stressed

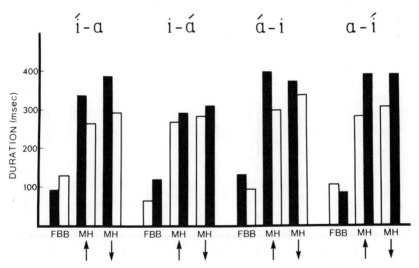

Figure 4.1.   Mean duration of vowels for the hearing speaker (FBB) and the deaf speaker (MH). *Arrows* indicate perceived correct (↑) and stress error (↓) utterances.

vowels were always longer than unstressed vowels in the same utterance, and across utterances. For example, in the utterance /'i-ɑ/, when perceived as intended, the average duration of /i/ was 334 msec; in the contrastive pair /i-'ɑ/, when /i/ was not stressed, its duration was 267 msec. The same pattern—stressed vowels longer than unstressed—holds for all vowels perceived as correct. However, we find nearly the same pattern for stress error utterances. That is, when an unstressed /i/ was perceived in the first contrast /'i-ɑ/, the duration of the /i/ was 380 msec. When a stressed /i/ was perceived in the contrastive pair /i-'ɑ/, the /i/ was 285 msec. Thus, the same pattern of vowel durations were found in both perceived correct and stress error utterances.

In Figure 4.2, the data show the mean vowel durations and their standard deviations. The durations of the hearing speaker's utterances show very little variability, as reflected in the small standard deviations. In contrast, the deaf speaker was exceedingly variable. Standard deviations were fairly large for the deaf speaker and vowel durations for correct and incorrect utterances often fell within the same range.

The data in Figures 4.1 and 4.2 suggest that the deaf speaker is not conveying stress contrasts primarily by differences in vowel duration and also that perceived stress errors are not due simply to a consistently used incorrect pattern of duration. It would seem, however, that the deaf speaker learned the stress rules of relative vowel

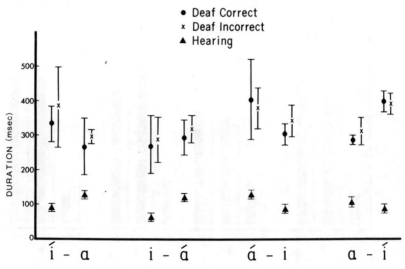

Figure 4.2.   Means and standard deviations of vowel duration for the hearing and deaf speaker.

duration but is unable to use them to produce an acoustically constant output.

Figure 4.3 shows measurements of fundamental frequency (F_o) obtained from extracting individual pitch periods from the middle portion of each vowel and calculating the frequency from the period. In making these measurements, we noted frequent abnormalities of the waveform. For the hearing speaker, F_o is higher for stressed than for unstressed vowels, as expected. For the deaf speaker, F_o is higher for the intended stressed vowel in three of the four utterance types, but for /'ɑ-i/, F_o is slightly lower for the intended stressed vowel in both perceived correct and stress error utterances. Again, as with duration, patterns are the same for perceived correct and stress error utterances.

In Figure 4.4, the data show mean F_o and its standard deviation. For the hearing speaker, the standard deviations are small, again reflecting little variability. Obviously, the standard deviations for the deaf speaker are large, indicating that the utterances were quite variable. Again, these data suggest that perceived errors are not due simply to a consistently used incorrect pattern of F_o.

Figure 4.5 shows measurements of the amplitudes of the vowels relative to a standard, the first production of an unstressed /ɑ/ in the utterance /ə'pipɑp/. For the hearing speaker, not surprisingly, stressed /ɑ/ had greater amplitude than stressed /i/ and the amplitude of a given

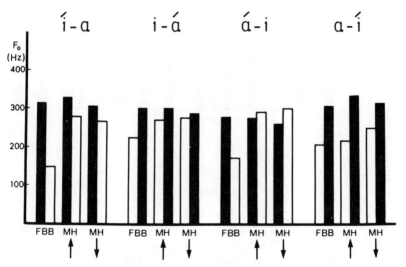

Figure 4.3.   Mean fundamental frequency (F_o) for the hearing and deaf speaker.

82   McGarr and Harris

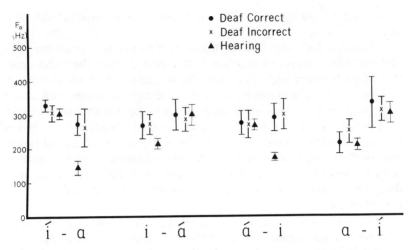

Figure 4.4.   Means and standard deviations of F_o for hearing and deaf speakers.

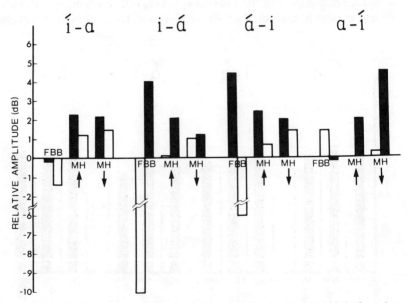

Figure 4.5.   Mean relative amplitude of the vowels for the hearing and deaf speakers.
The standard was the first production of an unstressed /ɑ/ in the utterance /əˈpipɑp/.

vowel increased with stress. For the deaf speaker, the stressed vowel always had a higher amplitude than the unstressed vowel. But again, it is clear that this deaf speaker is not conveying contrastive stress to the listener by differences in relative amplitude because "correct" and "incorrect" productions show the same pattern.

Another way in which stress change may be conveyed acoustically is by differences in vowel color. Fry (1964) has shown that listeners are more likely to perceive a syllable as unstressed if the formant values are less extreme, or more like the neutral schwa. Physiological explanations for the effect have been proposed by Lindblom (1963), and by Harris (1978). Without going into the details, it should be noted that the Harris study included measurements of productions of the same disyllables by the same speaker (FBB). Therefore, the values for the deaf speaker were measured and are presented in Table 4.2. The results show neither a consistent pattern overall, nor a systematic difference between correct and incorrect utterances. It should be noted, however, that measurements were extremely difficult to make, apparently because of the mismatch between spectrograph filter and fundamental frequency (cf. Huggins, 1980), or because of source function abnormalities.

This deaf speaker appears, at least on average, to have learned

Table 4.2.   Mean values for F_2 and F_3 for the deaf speaker's utterances perceived correct or perceived incorrect

	F_2	F_3	F_2	F_3
1. ə'pi pɑp	i		ɑ	
Correct	2170	2990	1546	2369
Incorrect	2060	2940	1500	2330
2. əpi'pɑp				
Correct	2162	2950	1625	2475
Incorrect	2170	2880	1670	2370
3. ə'pi pip	i		i	
Correct	2188	3055	2066	2766
Incorrect	2190	3060	2110	2950
4. əpi'pip				
Correct	2246	2980	2280	3100
Incorrect	2200	2900	2166	3100
5. ə'pɑ pip	ɑ		i	
Correct	1620	2600	2040	2880
Incorrect	1550	2592	2150	2875
6. əpɑ'pip				
Correct	1733	2600	2100	2966
Incorrect	1650	2320	2100	2970

some rules for conveying stress increase: vowel duration longer; F_o higher; and amplitude higher. Furthermore, it is not likely that these were specifically included in this deaf speaker's training program, because theoretical discussions of suprasegmental production at this level are relatively recent in the literature on training deaf speakers. More likely, this speaker has extracted this information from her low-frequency residual hearing and then generalized it to abstract rules. However, the variability in her production suggests an inability to coordinate the production mechanism so as to achieve these stress contrasts in a consistent acoustic manner, and although she communicates the information that should allow listeners to judge stress, they evidently cannot use it.

EMG Results

The EMG results were examined to see if they revealed any systematic differences between normal and deaf interarticulator programming, or between correctly and incorrectly perceived utterances. In these utterances, orbicularis oris (OO) activity is associated with pursing and closing the lips as for the /p/. For the vowel /i/, the genioglossus (GG) bunches the tongue and brings it forward in the mouth (Raphael and Bell-Berti, 1975; Raphael et al., 1979).

Figure 4.6 shows data for the hearing speaker producing the utterance type /ə'pɑpip/. At the top of each column is the ensemble average of the EMG wave forms. This was obtained by rectifying and integrating the EMG potentials for each repetition and aligning them with respect to an acoustic event. The signals were digitized and the ensemble average calculated by averaging each sample for each repetition of an utterance type (Kewley-Port, 1973). A sample of four of the 20 repetitions are seen in the columns below the average. For this utterance type, the line-up point for averaging the EMG and acoustic events, indicated by the vertical line at 0 msec, is the release burst of the second /p/.

The data for orbicularis oris show three well-defined peaks of activity corresponding to the lip gestures for the three /p/ closures in /ə'pɑpip/. The line-up point falls between peaks 2 and 3. The duration of the interval between peaks 1 and 2 is greater than between peaks 2 and 3 reflecting stress on the /ɑ/, and the consequently longer vowel. One notable feature of these data is the striking similarity of the EMG patterns for all tokens. For the genioglossus, there is a peak of activity for the /i/ and no activity for the /ɑ/ as expected, because the genioglossus is active in raising and bunching the tongue. Indeed, peak genioglossus activity (for the vowel) occurs approximately at the time of

[ə'pɑpip]

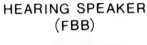

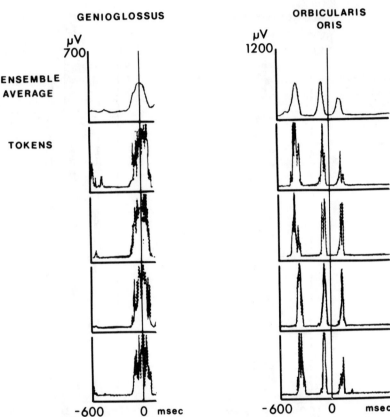

Figure 4.6. /ə'pɑpip/ as produced by a hearing speaker. Data plots at the top show the EMG averaged for about 20 tokens for the genioglossus and orbicularis oris muscles. Four individual tokens are shown below. The vertical line indicates the acoustic release of the /p/ closure.

the acoustic line-up event—the /p/ burst-release. This is not surprising because EMG activity precedes the articulatory event to which it is related by about 50 to 100 msec.

Figure 4.7 shows data for the utterance /əpɑ'pip/, again for the hearing speaker. The interval between the second and third peaks of orbicularis oris activity is greater than that between the first and second

[əpɑˈpip]

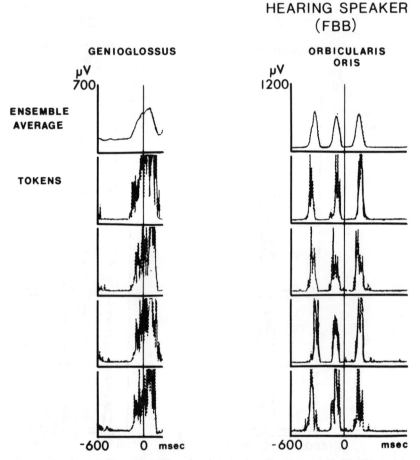

Figure 4.7.   /əpɑˈpip/ as produced by a hearing speaker. Data presented as in Figure 4.6.

peaks because stress occurs on the final syllable. Also, the duration of genioglossus activity is longer in this utterance type because /i/ is stressed. Note, however, that peak activity for the genioglossus still occurs at the release of the second /p/, between peaks 2 and 3. Once again, the patterns of activity for all these tokens look remarkably similar.

Figure 4.8 shows parallel data for several of the deaf subject's productions of /əˈpɑpip/. Each of these tokens was a perceived correct utterance. Examining the EMG activity for orbicularis oris we see that, as for the hearing subject, there are three well-defined peaks of activity and the interval between the second and third peaks is greater than that between the first and second peaks. However, the duration of each peak is prolonged. The /p/ release falls between the second and third peaks as for the hearing speaker.

Turning to the genioglossus EMG, peak activity is less well defined and occurs later than for the hearing speaker; it follows /p/ release. Furthermore, there is considerable variability from token to token in the duration of genioglossus activity. In some instances, this activity starts fairly early (token 3) and at other times, later (token 4).

Figure 4.9 shows the data for the deaf speaker's production of /əpɑ'pip/. Here again, the overall duration of EMG activity is prolonged for both muscles, but the pattern more closely resembles that of the hearing speaker for orbicularis oris than for genioglossus. The variability and "lateness" of the genioglossus are again observed. These data show that the deaf speaker was somewhat like the hearing speaker

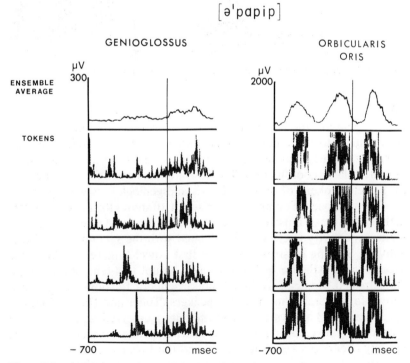

Figure 4.8. /ə'ɑpip/ as produced by a deaf speaker. Data presented as in Figure 4.6.

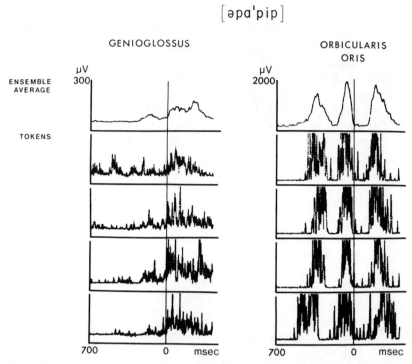

Figure 4.9.   /əpɑ'pip/ as produced by a deaf speaker. Data presented as in Figure 4.6.

with respect to "the visible aspects of articulation," but quite variable with respect to the timing of lingual control. This variability appears to be particularly manifested in what we would describe as abnormal interarticulator coordination. To illustrate this notion further, the data for selected tokens of orbicularis oris and genioglossus were plotted.

For purposes of comparison, Figure 4.10 shows the averaged EMG activity for these muscles for the hearing speaker. Onset of the genioglossus activity is closely coordinated with the second peak of oris activity. Shifting of stress from the first vowel (Figure 4.10A) to the second vowel (Figure 4.10B) does not disrupt this temporal relationship. Indeed, this closely timed interarticulator relationship has been shown for several other hearing speakers (Tuller and Harris, 1980).

Figure 4.11 shows one of the tokens, perceived as correct, that most closely resembles those of the hearing speaker. Peak genioglossus activity occurs between the second and third peaks of orbicularis oris activity, but the peak is late relative to acoustic event. Timing between the articulators differs from the hearing speaker in that genioglossus activity begins after the second orbicularis oris peak occurs, and continues well into the third burst of orbicularis oris activity.

Figure 4.11B shows a token perceived as a stress error. Genioglossus activity begins quite late relative to orbicularis oris activity,

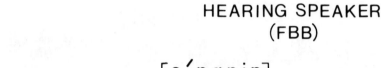

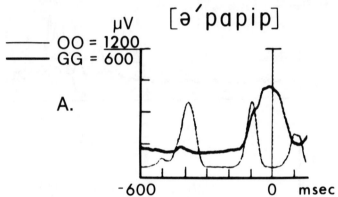

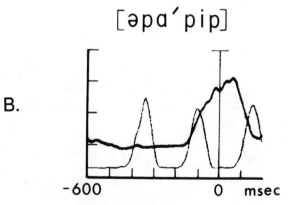

Figure 4.10.   Ensemble average of the EMG potentials for genioglossus and orbicularis oris for the utterance type /əpɑpip/ produced by the hearing speaker. The vertical line indicates the acoustic release of the /p/ closure.

and in fact, it peaks simultaneously with the third oribularis oris peak. This pattern was never seen for the hearing speaker.

Figure 4.11C shows another token perceived as a stress error. Genioglossus activity begins too soon in this case, although a peak occurs between the second and third peaks of orbicularis oris activity.

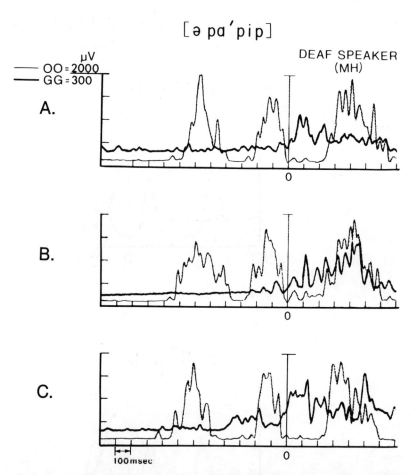

Figure 4.11. A, A single selected token of the EMG potential from the genioglossus and orbicularis oris muscles as produced by the deaf speaker. The vertical line indicates the acoustic release of the /p/ closure. In Figure 4.11A, peak genioglossus activity occurs between the second and third oris peaks, but is late relative to the acoustic event. This pattern was most like normal. In Figure 4.11B and C, the single tokens show that genioglossus activity was either too late or too early, respectively. (Single tokens filtered with settings used for the average in Figure 4.8.)

[əpɑ'pip]

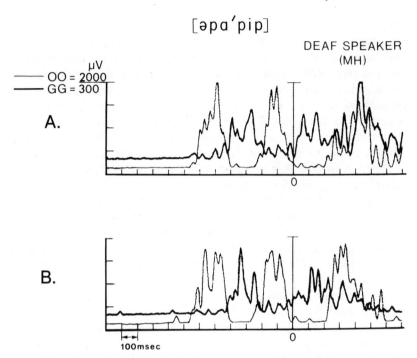

Figure 4.12.   A shows an example of a perceived vowel error, with genioglossus activity occurring between the first and second oris peaks. This token was perceived as /əpi'pip/. Figure 4.12B shows an example of an utterance perceived as correct although genioglossus activity clearly occurs between the first and second oris peaks as seen above. Data after Figure 4.11.

However, the genioglossus activity continues beyond the final burst of orbicularis oris activity.

Figures 4.12A and B show respective examples of a perceived vowel error, and an instance in which there was inappropriate genioglossus activity for the /ɑ/, but listeners perceived the vowel as correct. These two final examples were quite unusual with respect to the normal. It should be emphasized that although there was substantial token-to-token variation in the deaf speaker, the type of physiological patterns do not differ systematically from "correct" to "incorrect" tokens.

DISCUSSION

Although this study obviously does not allow definitive answers to questions about other deaf speakers, it does suggest some further directions for research. First, these results give ample evidence of the instability of deaf production. The speaker does not produce a "wrong" pattern in a stereotyped way; rather, production is variable in all acoustic and physiological measurements examined. If the results for this speaker are replicated in further work, one cannot assume the deaf speaker simply operates in a reduced or deviant phonological space whether the distortion of phonology is produced by explicit teaching or some other aspect of the speaker's experience. Although the instability can be noted in transcription studies (Oller and Eilers, 1982), it is better documented in studies that go beyond traditional transcriptions (Fisher et al., this volume).

At a segmental level, there is an apparent failure of consistent interarticulator programming. Overall, a tight temporal coupling of activity in articulatory muscles is lacking. In the normally hearing speaker producing a stop consonant-vowel syllable, activity of the tongue muscles for the vowel is well underway when acoustic release for the stop takes place—this may not be so in this deaf speaker. The more important difference between deaf and normal subjects, however, is that the relationship between lip and tongue activity varies from token-to-token in the deaf speaker. However, the variability of the relationship arises from the lingual rather than the labial component; that is, it is the invisible rather than the visible aspect of articulation which varies.

The second hypothesis about deaf speech described above is that the tongue is relatively immobile in this group, as inferred from acoustic measures of formant positions, and this contributes to the unintelligibility of the speech. The present speaker shows some neutralization of formant values, as we can infer by comparing her values in the present context with those of Peterson and Barney (1960). That the tongue is, on average, more centralized than that of the normal speaker may be inferred from the fact that the normal speaker shows about the same values for /i/ as Peterson and Barney, in spite of the context difference.

The present EMG technique cannot, of course, be used to ascertain tongue position. Furthermore, the absolute level of EMG activity is not interpretable, because the amplitude of the recorded EMG activity reflects the distance of the active electrode from the firing muscle fibers, as well as the distance between the electrode tips, variables which are uncontrolled in all such techniques. Genioglossus fibers for our speaker are active, however, and the relationship between activity for the nonspeech and speech gestures was not different for deaf and normal speakers. Therefore, the rather low activity level of genioglossus activity reflects, at least in part, a rather weak insertion, rather than a relatively inactive tongue. Apparently, the deaf talker is at least capable of contracting an appropriate muscle for /i/, and leaving it relatively inactive for /ɑ/.

A third hypothesis about deaf speech is that source function control is a substantial source of unintelligibility. The present speaker apparently knew the rules for conveying stress by varying F_o, duration, and intensity, even though she showed the characteristic overall durational lengthening of deaf speech. What is puzzling is that listeners were not able to extract this information from the signal, as shown by the similarity of "correct" and "incorrect" tokens in acoustic measures. We examined the possibility that incorrect tokens were those in which conflicting cues were presented, but no such readily apparent pattern emerged. It is possible that the contours of intensity and F_o were abnormal, although the syllable center values were in appropriate ratio.

A question we could not answer within the framework of the present study is what contribution source function irregularities may make to even segmental unintelligibility. The present experiment suggests an articulatory variable, interarticulator timing, which deserves greater attention. However, it would be interesting to know how much a deviant and inadequate source in and of itself prevents the listener from interpreting the segmental cues he or she receives, however inadequate they may be. The authors intend to pursue this topic further by examining simple nonsense syllables within a wider range of structures, attempting to use various instrumental techniques to manipulate the source function.

ACKNOWLEDGMENTS

We are grateful to our colleagues Fredericka Bell-Berti and Carole E. Gelfer for their helpful comments and assistance.

REFERENCES

Allen, G. D., J. F. Lubker, and E. Harrison. 1972. New paint-on electrodes for surface electromyography. J. Acoust. Soc. Am. 52:124(A).

Angelocci, A. A., G. A. Kopp, and A. Holbrook. 1964. The vowel formants of deaf and normal-hearing eleven- to fourteen-year-old boys. J. Speech Hear. Disord. 29:156–170.

Boothroyd, A. 1970, Distribution of hearing levels in the student population of Clarke School for the Deaf. S.A.R.P. Report #3. Clarke School for the Deaf, Northampton, Mass.

Calvert, D. R. 1961. Some acoustic characteristics of the speech of profoundly deaf individuals. Doctoral dissertation, Stanford University.

Forner, L. L., and T. J. Hixon. 1977. Respiratory kinematics in profoundly hearing impaired speakers. J. Speech Hear. Res. 20:373–497.

Fry, D. B. 1958. Experiments in the perception of stress. Lang. Speech 1:126–152.

Fry, D. B. 1964. The dependence of stress judgments on vowel formant structure. In Proceedings of the Fifth International Congress on Phonetic Sciences. S. Karger, Basel.

Harris, K. S. 1978. Vowel duration change and its underlying physiological mechanisms. Lang. Speech 21:354–361.

Harris, K. S., and N. S. McGarr. 1980. Relationships between speech perception and speech production in normal hearing and hearing-impaired subjects. In J. Subtelny (ed.), Speech Assessment and Speech Improvement for the Hearing Impaired, pp. 316–337. A. G. Bell Association for the Deaf, Washington, D.C.

Haycock, G. S. 1933. The Teaching of Speech. A. G. Bell Association for the Deaf, Washington, D.C.

Hirose, H. 1971. Electromyography of the articulatory muscles: Current instrumentation and techniques. Haskins Lab. Status Rep. Speech Res. SR-25/26:73–86.

Hudgins, C. V., and F. C. Numbers. 1942. An investigation of the intelligibility of the speech of the deaf. Genet. Psychol. Monogr. 25:289–392.

Huggins, A. W. F. 1980. Better spectrograms from children's speech. J. Speech Hear. Res. 23:19–27.

Huntington, D. A., K. S. Harris, and G. Sholes. 1968. An electromyographic study of consonant articulation in hearing impaired and normal speech. J. Speech Hear. Res. 11:147–158.

Johnson, D. D. 1975. Communication characteristics of NTID students. J. Acad. Rehab. Audiol. 8:17–32.

Kewley-Port, D. 1973. Computer processing of EMG signals at Haskins Laboratories. Haskins Lab. Status Rep. Speech Res. SR-33:173–183.

Levitt, H., C. R. Smith, and H. Stromberg. 1974. Acoustic, articulatory, and perceptual characteristics of the speech of deaf children. In G. Fant (ed.), Proceedings of the Speech Communication Seminar (Stockholm). John Wiley & Sons, New York.

Levitt, H., R. E. Stark, N. S. McGarr, et al. 1976. Language and communication skills of deaf children 1973–1975. Unpublished report, City University of New York.

Lindblom, B. E. F. 1963. Spectrographic study of vowel reduction. J. Acoust. Soc. Am. 35:1773–1781.

Ling, D. 1976. Speech and the Hearing-Impaired Child: Theory and Practice. A. G. Bell Association for the Deaf, Washington, D.C.

McGarr, N. S. 1978. The differences between experienced and inexperienced listeners in understanding the speech of the deaf. Doctoral dissertation, City University of New York.

McGarr, N. S., and M. J. Osberger. 1978. Pitch deviancy and intelligibility of deaf speech. J. Commun. Disord. 11:237–247.

Monsen, R. B. 1976. Second formant transitions of selected consonant-vowel combinations in the speech of deaf and normal hearing children. J. Speech Hear. Res. 19:279–289.

Oller, D. K., and R. E. Eilers. 1982. A pragmatic approach to phonological systems of deaf speakers. In N. Lass (ed.), Speech and language: Advances in basic research and practice, Vol. 6. Academic Press, Inc., New York.

Osberger, M. J., and H. Levitt. 1979. The effect of timing errors on the intelligibility of deaf children's speech. J. Acoust. Soc. Am. 66:1316–1324.

Peterson, G. E., and H. L. Barney. 1960. Control methods used in a study of the identification of vowels. J. Acoust. Soc. Am. 32:693–703.

Raphael, L. J., and F. Bell-Berti. 1975. Tongue musculature and the feature of tension in English vowels. Phonetica 32:61–73.

Raphael, L. J., F. Bell-Berti, R. Collier, and T. Baer. 1979. Tongue position in rounded and unrounded front vowel pairs. Lang. Speech 22:37–48.

Smith, C. R. 1972. Residual hearing and speech production of deaf children. Doctoral dissertation, City University of New York.

Tuller, B., and K. S. Harris. 1980. Temporal models of interarticulator programming. J. Acoust. Soc. Am. 67:S64.

CHAPTER 5

SOME RESPIRATORY AND AERODYNAMIC PATTERNS IN THE SPEECH OF THE HEARING IMPAIRED

Robert L. Whitehead

CONTENTS

The study of the respiratory and aerodynamic components of speech are important in understanding the speech production process in the hearing-impaired population. In the past, a number of aberrant respiratory characteristics have been observed during speech produced by hearing-impaired individuals (Hudgins, 1934; Hudgins and Numbers, 1942). More recently, Forner and Hixon (1977) investigated respiratory patterning during speech for hearing-impaired speakers who demonstrated difficulties in controlling respiration for speech. Using magnetometers, which measured changes in the antero-posterior diameter of the chest wall, they found, in general, that the hearing-impaired subjects spoke on lower lung volumes and used higher volumes of air during syllable production when compared with normally hearing subjects.

The aerodynamic aspects of speech produced by the hearing im-

This study was conducted in the course of an agreement with the U.S. Department of Education.

97

paired has been studied by several investigators (Gilbert, 1974; Hutchinson and Smith, 1976) who agree on the existence of at least two prominent characteristics. First, during consonant production there is often inappropriate glottal activity in the form of a blurring of the voiced/voiceless distinction. Secondly, there appears to be inefficient valving of the air stream during consonant production. This may take the form of high volume velocities in which low flow rates normally occur, or low flow rates in which higher ones would usually be expected to occur.

There seems to be limited information regarding the possible relationships between respiratory patterning for speech and overall speech intelligibility for hearing-impaired individuals. Such information would be beneficial if a complete understanding of the factors that affect speech intelligibility in the hearing impaired is to be obtained. In addition, data relative to the coordination of the respiratory, phonatory, and aerodynamic aspects of speech in the hearing impaired is somewhat limited. Because of the unique interactive aspects of respiration and upper airway dynamics in speech production, such data would provide additional information pertaining to speech production in the hearing impaired and thus further aid in clarifying the factors affecting speech intelligibility.

The present study was therefore undertaken to describe and quantify the respiratory characteristics of hearing-impaired young adults who varied in degree of speech intelligibility. In addition, this study was designed to investigate selected simultaneous respiratory, phonatory, and aerodynamic measures that may affect speech intelligibility in the hearing-impaired speaker.

PROCEDURES

Subjects

Subjects for this study included five normally hearing adult males; five hearing-impaired adult males with intelligible speech (as measured by the NTID rating scales), and 15 hearing-impaired adult males with speech intelligibility ranging from semi-intelligible to unintelligible. The age range for all the subjects was from 19 years to 34 years. Each of the hearing-impaired subjects had a bilateral, congenital, sensorineural hearing loss. The mean pure tone average (three frequency) for the five hearing-impaired subjects with intelligible speech was 89.5 dB hearing level (HL), whereas for the 15 hearing-impaired subjects with semi-intelligible or unintelligible speech, the mean pure tone average was 102.5 dB HL.

This investigation was divided into two components, the first being the analysis of respiratory patterns only, and the second, the analysis of simultaneous respiratory, phonatory, and aerodynamic patterns. All subjects participated in the respiratory-only portion of the study. For the simultaneous portion, all the normally hearing and hearing-impaired subjects with intelligible speech participated, whereas only eight of the hearing-impaired subjects with semi-intelligible speech participated.

Instrumentation

Respiration   To collect the respiratory data, antero-posterior diameter changes of the rib cage and abdomen were sensed with paired magnetometer coils (Mead et al., 1967). Signals from the magnetometers were fed simultaneously through an amplifier (Lexington Instruments A122RB) to separate channels of a Honeywell 5600CC instrumentation recorder and to a Tektronix two-channel storage oscilloscope. During analysis, signals were played back from the FM recorder into the oscilloscope from which the displays could be traced onto translucent paper. The utterances were picked up by two microphones, fed into separate amplifiers, and recorded on the FM recorder and an Ampex AG440 AM tape recorder.

Each magnetometer coil was attached to the chest wall with double-sided adhesive tape. The generating coils were positioned at the midline on the anterior surface of the chest wall, one for the rib cage and one for the abdomen, whereas the sensing coils were positioned posteriorly at the same axial level as their generator mates.

The tasks were performed with the subjects in an upright position leaning back on a foam pad against the wall. Subjects were instructed to avoid unnecessary movement such as raising their arms, using sign language or fingerspelling, or shifting their positions during recordings.

Recordings were made during two nonspeech activities: resting tidal breathing and isovolume maneuvers. The isovolume maneuvers occurred at tidal end-expiration level, that is, functional residual capacity (FRC), and 1 liter above FRC. For each of the two levels, the subjects closed the glottis and slowly displaced volumes back and forth between the rib cage and abdomen. For a more detailed description of this procedure, see Forner and Hixon (1977).

Phonatory   To obtain an estimate of glottal activity, an FJ Electronics electroglottograph was used. Two surface electrodes were attached on each side of the larynx slightly below the thyroid cartilage.

The electrodes monitored impedance changes across the vocal folds. These changes were then amplified and recorded onto a third channel of the Honeywell FM recorder. For playback, the glottographic channel of the FM recorder was connected to a Honeywell visicorder (1858 CRT).

Aerodynamic   Air flow, in terms of volume velocity, was measured using a face mask and Honeywell pneumotach. The pressure changes associated with the air flow through the pneumotach were picked up by a Statham pressure transducer (PM15E) and fed to a Honeywell bridge amplifier (Acudata 113) which was connected to a fourth channel on the Honeywell FM recorder. An audio microphone was placed directly in front of the face mask/pneumotach system and was connected to both the FM and Ampex AM tape recorders.

Figure 5.1 presents the equipment for collection and analysis of the phonatory, aerodynamic, and acoustic data.

Speech Samples

For the respiratory-only portion of the investigation, all subjects read the first paragraph of the Rainbow Passage. In the simultaneous portion of the study, the subjects uttered CV syllables comprised of the vowel /ɑ/ and the vowel /i/ and the consonants /t/, /d/, /k/, and /g/. Each syllable

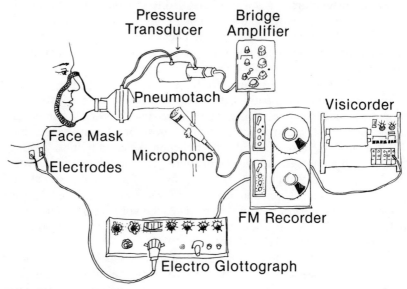

Figure 5.1.   The equipment used for collection and analysis of the phonatory, aerodynamic, and acoustic data.

was produced three times in succession. The normally hearing and hearing-impaired subjects with intelligible speech correctly articulated all the syllables. The hearing-impaired subjects with semi-intelligible speech perceptually misarticulated the consonants in the syllable task, as judged by the investigator, but did approximate a plosive production as seen on the visicorder tracing of air flow. Thus, although there were misarticulations, the manner of articulation was either correct or an accurate approximation.

Data Analysis

Figure 5.2 illustrates the relative motion display used to analyze the respiratory data. The isovolume lines trace the relative motion pathway during the shifting of volume between rib cage and abdomen at the two fixed lung volumes. Both lines have slopes of − 1, meaning that for

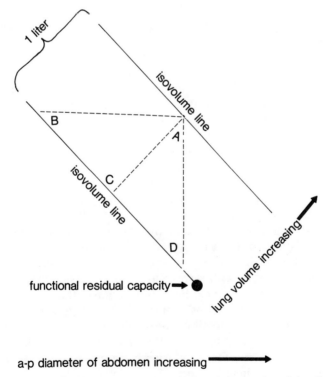

Figure 5.2.   Diagram of the display used for analysis of the relative motion of the rib cage and abdomen during speech production (reproduced with permission from Forner and Hixon, 1977).

any shift in volume between the rib cage and abdomen, equal diameter changes occur. Thus, the diagram provides: 1) a display of change in lung volume; 2) the relative volume contributions of the rib cage and abdomen to changes in lung volume (slope); and, 3) the separate volume displacements of the rib cage and abdomen (chest wall configuration).

The change in lung volume between any two points is a function of the distance between the two points measured perpendicular to the isovolume lines (AC). Increasing volume is upward and to the right, whereas decreasing volume is downward and to the left. The pathways AB and AD in Figure 5.2 reflect 1 liter change in lung volume as indicated by the perpendicular measurement line AC. The pathways such as AB and AD are identified as respiratory limbs for purpose of analysis.

The relative contributions of the rib cage and abdomen to lung volume change are indicated by the slope of the line between any two points. For the pathway AB in Figure 5.2, total volume change is accomplished by displacement of the abdomen, whereas AD shows the rig cage alone accounting for total volume change. Pathway AC shows equal rib cage and abdominal contribution.

The volume displacement of the rib cage is indicated by position along the vertical axis of the diagram, with upward movement indicating increased lung volume. Abdominal volume displacement is along the horizontal axis, with increasing volume extending toward the right. Every point on the diagram defines a different chest wall configuration and any series of points provides a descriptor of the changing shape of the moving chest wall. A detailed explanation of the data collection and analysis procedures can be found in Hixon, Goldman, and Mead (1973) and Forner and Hixon (1977).

In the present study, the respiratory display was used to investigate only lung volume and number of syllables per respiratory limb. Discussion of the slope of the respiratory limbs and the chest wall configuration is not presented in this chapter.

For each subject, the average lung volume per respiratory limb was calculated with respect to volume at initiation, volume at termination, and volume per limb. In addition, although there was variation across subjects in terms of lung volumes during speech, group averages were determined to allow for a more general analysis of the findings.

With respect to the air flow measures, for each subject the peak volume velocity for the plosive consonants in the two vowel environments was calculated in cubic centimeters/second. Measurement was made only in the first consonant-vowel (CV) monosyllable of the three-succession CVs uttered by each subject. The glottographic trace was used to obtain an estimate of the onset of voicing for the plosive consonants.

RESULTS

Respiratory-Only

Figure 5.3 presents a typical display of the respiratory limbs during the reading of the first paragraph of the Rainbow Passage for a normally hearing subject. Each limb starts at a minimum of 700 cc above FRC and is terminated at or slightly above FRC. The length of each limb is dependent, in part, on the linguistic components of the speaking task, that is, timing, stress, phrasing, and number of syllables. Although not analyzed, the limbs for this subject demonstrate an almost equal contribution of the rib cage and abdomen for lung volume change. As the speaker approached FRC, however, several of the limbs indicated that volume change was accomplished mainly by the displacement of the abdomen.

Figure 5.4 presents a typical plot of the respiratory limbs during the reading task for a hearing-impaired subject with intelligible speech. The initiation of the limbs, that is, the volume of air in the lungs at the beginning of an utterance, is slightly less than that seen for a normally hearing subject. Thus, even though the hearing-impaired speaker has completely intelligible speech, he does not appear to take in as much air for speech as his normally hearing counterpart. It is also noted that several of the limbs extended below FRC, something which seldom occurs in normally hearing speakers.

Figure 5.5 presents a typical plot of the respiratory limbs during the reading task for the hearing-impaired subjects with semi-intelligible or unintelligible speech. For this subject, only a few of the limbs are initiated above FRC and even those began with a lung volume of less than 500 cc. The majority of limbs began below FRC and, of course, continued further below FRC until the completion of the utterance. As the subject continued below FRC, the lung volume change was accomplished almost solely by abdominal displacement.

The mean averages of lung volume at initiation of the respiratory limbs, lung volume at termination of the limbs, and lung volume per limb were calculated for the subjects in each of the three groups and are presented in Figure 5.6. Also included in this figure is the amount of variation in the average lung volumes across subjects. As noted, the mean volume at initiation of the limbs was 900cc for the normally hearing subjects, 750 cc for the hearing-impaired subjects with intelligible

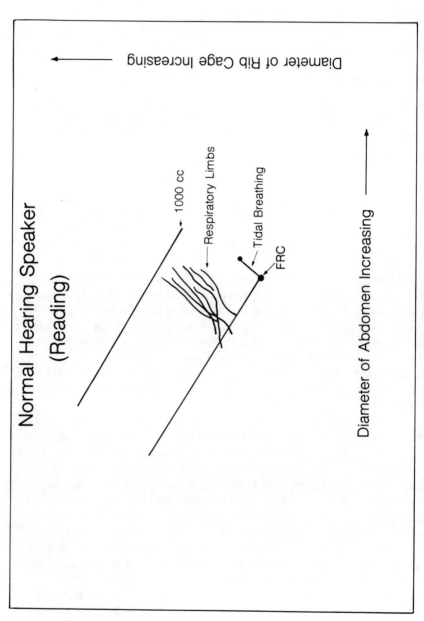

Figure 5.3.   A typical display of the respiratory limbs during reading of the first paragraph of the Rainbow Passage for normally hearing subjects.

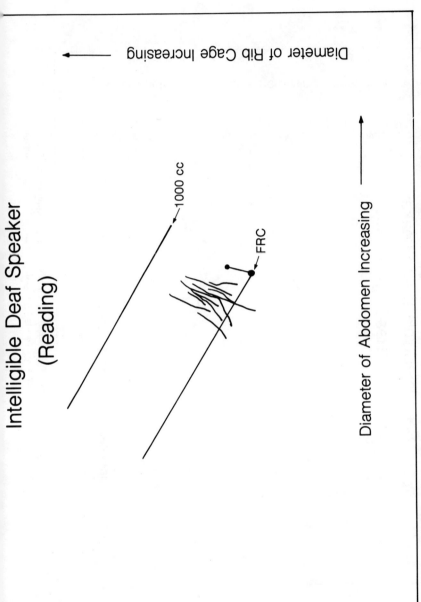

Figure 5.4. A typical display of the respiratory limbs during reading of the first paragraph of the Rainbow Passage for hearing-impaired subjects with intelligible speech.

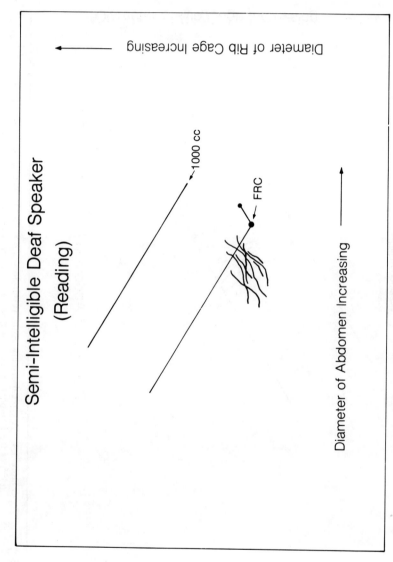

Figure 5.5.   A typical display of the respiratory limbs during reading of the first paragraph of the Rainbow Passage for hearing-impaired subjects with semi-intelligible or unintelligible speech.

speech and 125 cc for the hearing-impaired subjects with semi-intelligible or unintelligible speech. With respect to lung volume at termination, the normally hearing and intelligible hearing-impaired subjects, for the most part, terminated at or about FRC. A few of the intelligible hearing-impaired speakers went below FRC before their limb was terminated. The hearing-impaired subjects with semi-intelligible and unintelligible speech, however, all terminated well below FRC, at an approximate average lung volume of −500 cc. Figure 5.6 also presents the mean of the average volume per limb for the three groups of subjects. Again, the normally hearing and intelligible hearing-impaired subjects both used approximately the same volume of air per limb, 825 cc. The semi-intelligible and unintelligible hearing-impaired subjects had a mean average of about 550 cc of air per limb.

The average number of syllables per respiratory limb were calculated for each of the subjects. The means and standard deviations of these averages are presented in Figure 5.7. The normally hearing subjects, who had an average lung volume per limb of 825 cc, produced a mean average of 14 syllables per limb, whereas the intelligible hearing-impaired subjects, who also had approximately 825 cc of air per limb, produced a mean average of 10 syllables per limb. The semi-intelligible and unintelligible hearing-impaired subjects, who demonstrated an average lung volume per limb of 550 cc, however, produced a mean average of 3 syllables per respiratory limb. Thus, the average lung volume per limb per syllable was 180 cc for the semi-intelligible and unintelligible hearing impaired subjects, 82 cc for the intelligible hearing-impaired subjects, and 55 cc for the normally hearing speakers.

Simultaneous

Figure 5.8 presents the means and standard deviations of peak volume velocity in cubic centimeters/second for the plosive consonants produced in the CV environment with the vowel /ɑ/ for the three groups of subjects. For the normally hearing and intelligible hearing-impaired subjects, the peak volume velocities are quite consistent. In addition, there is a clear voiced/voiceless distinction in peak air flow for these two groups. That is, a voiceless plosive was produced with approximately twice as much peak air flow as the voiced cognate. With respect to the semi-intelligible hearing-impaired subjects, however, there was a consistent pattern in which the voiced consonants were produced with greater air flow and the voiceless consonants with less air flow when compared with the normally hearing and intelligible hearing-impaired subjects. Thus, the voiced/voiceless distinction was not clearly

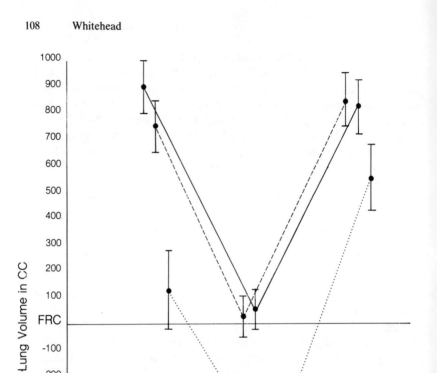

Figure 5.6.   The means and standard deviations of the averages of lung volume at initiation of respiratory limbs, lung volume at termination of respiratory limbs, and lung volume per limb, during the reading task for normally hearing, intelligible hearing-impaired, and semi-intelligible hearing-impaired speakers.

evident for the hearing-impaired subjects with semi-intelligible speech. Similar results were found for the positive consonants in the CV contexts with the vowel /i/ and are presented in Figure 5.9.

Each glottographic trace, which was a part of the visicorder readout of the air flow, was measured with respect to the onset of voicing in comparison with the peak volume velocity. For the voiceless plosives produced by the normally hearing and intelligible hearing-impaired subjects, there was an average delay of approximately 40 msec between peak air flow and onset of voicing. The voiced plosives produced by these subjects were characterized by a voicing onset pattern which occurred at an average of 9.5 msec before peak air flow. The semi-intelligible hearing-impaired subjects, however, demonstrated a glottographic pattern for the voiceless consonants that was very similar to that which occurred for their voiced consonants. That

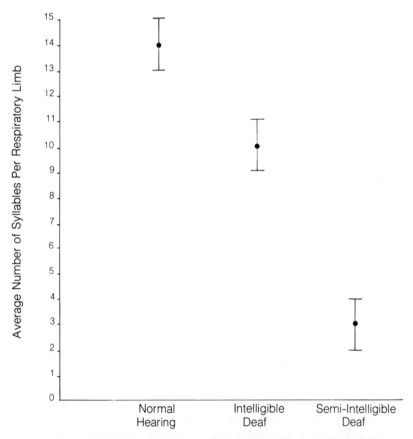

Figure 5.7.   The means and standard deviations of the average number of syllables per respiratory limb for normally hearing, intelligible hearing-impaired, and semi-intelligible hearing-impaired speakers.

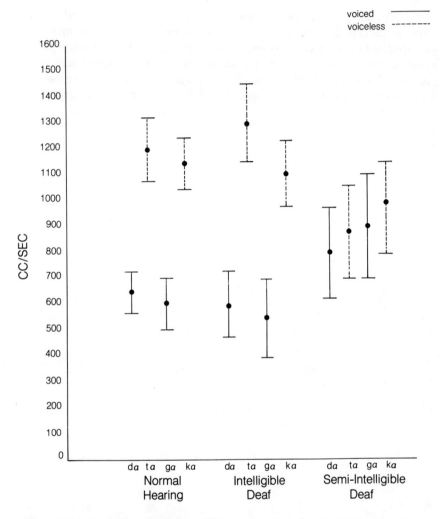

Figure 5.8.   The means and standard deviations of peak air flow for plosive consonants in the CV environment with the vowel /ɑ/ produced by normally hearing, intelligible hearing-impaired, and semi-intelligible hearing-impaired speakers.

is, for both voiced and voiceless plosives, the onset of voicing occurred an average of 6 msec before peak volume velocity.

As a measure of respiratory activity during production of the CV syllables, the average lung volume, as measured by the respiratory limbs, at the initiation of the CV sequence was calculated. Figure 5.10 presents the means and standard deviations of the lung volumes at initiation of the CVs (vowels pooled) for the three groups of subjects. As may be seen, the normally hearing and intelligible hearing-impaired subjects tended to initiate their CVs with approximately the same amount of air in their lungs. The semi-intelligible hearing-impaired speakers, however, attempted production of the CVs with substantially less air in their lungs when compared with the other two groups.

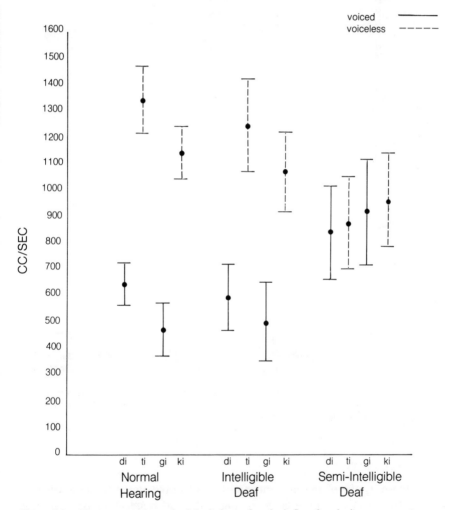

Figure 5.9.   The means and standard deviations of peak air flow for plosive consonants in the CV environment with the vowel /i/ produced by normally hearing, intelligible hearing-impaired, and semi-intelligible hearing-impaired speakers.

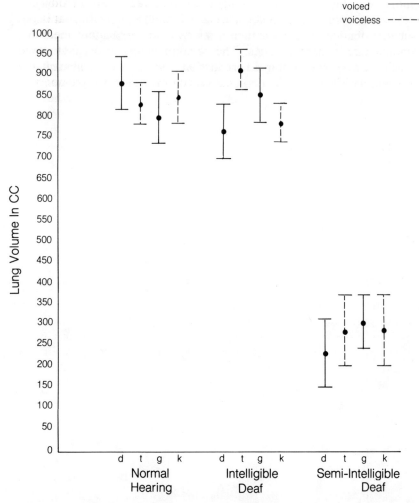

Figure 5.10.   The means and standard deviations of the lung volumes at initiation of the CV syllables (vowels pooled) for normally hearing, intelligible hearing-impaired, and semi-intelligible hearing-impaired speakers.

DISCUSSION

One purpose of the present study was to investigate the relationships between degree of speech intelligibility and respiratory patterning in hearing-impaired individuals. In addition, an attempt was made to quantify the respiratory characteristics for the groups of subjects in the study. The normally hearing subjects in the present study performed much the same as reported by Hixon et al. (1973). That is, the amount of air inhaled per phrase of utterance in continuous speech was about twice the depth for tidal breathing. It is interesting that almost all the hearing-impaired speakers with intelligible speech initiated their respiratory limbs at levels less than was characteristic for the normally hearing speakers. It appears, therefore, that even though some hearing-impaired speakers have intelligible speech, they have not learned to initiate speech with as much air in their lungs as normally hearing speakers. In general, it was also found that as the degree of speech intelligibility decreased for the hearing-impaired speakers, the point at which respiratory limbs were initiated in connected speech, that is, the volume of air in the lungs, also decreased. Thus, it was not uncommon for subjects with semi-intelligible or unintelligible speech to attempt the continuous speech task with the volume of air in their lungs equal to or slightly above/below FRC.

In view of the above findings, one question which may be raised for hearing-impaired speakers with good speech intelligibility is, what effect does the reduced lung volume at initiation of speech, small though it may be in some instances, have on selected speech production skills, particularly as the speaker approaches the end of an utterance? If there is very little effect, then it is possible that the semi-intelligible hearing-impaired speaker may not need to be taught to achieve the identical lung volumes that occur at the initiation of speech by the normally hearing speaker.

During the continuous speech task, the normally hearing speakers, depending on the linguistic components of the utterance, would usually terminate their respiratory limbs above or at FRC, whereas the intelligible hearing-impaired speakers would, at times, terminate their limbs below FRC. In contrast, the semi-intelligible and unintelligible hearing-impaired speakers almost always terminated their limbs well below FRC. As noted by Forner and Hixon (1977), when speaking at levels below FRC, the speaker must use higher than average muscular pressure to achieve speech and must also work against inspiratory recoil forces. The consistent pattern of speaking at or below FRC for the hearing-impaired subjects, particularly those with semi-intelligible and unintelligible speech, indicates that the lack of sufficient air and the resultant unusually heavy demands put on the respiratory system may be a significant contributor to their speech problems, which, in turn, would have an effect on overall speech intelligibility.

The data from this investigation suggest that part of the difficulties in speech production for the hearing impaired may be due to an inability to coordinate respiratory patterning during speech with the valving of the vocal tract at the laryngeal and articulatory levels. The results of this study indicated that this incoordination may be demonstrated in several ways. First, the semi-intelligible and unintelligible hearing-impaired speakers had very high volumes of air expended per syllable in continuous speech. They averaged approximately 180 cc per syllable, which was several times greater than what occurred for the normally hearing speakers. It appears, therefore, that these hearing-impaired subjects were exhibiting a reduced resistance in the vocal and articulatory tracts and were thus inefficiently valving the air stream during speech production. Similar results regarding inefficient valving have been reported by other investigators (Forner and Hixon, 1977; Hutchinson and Smith, 1976). Furthermore, for the subjects in the present study, speech was undertaken with reduced lung volumes, thus creating an obvious mismanagement and incoordination of the mechanisms for speech production.

A second indicator of a coordination problem may be demonstrated by the glottographic and air flow data. These data indicated that the semi-intelligible hearing-impaired speakers, when compared with the normally hearing and intelligible hearing-impaired speakers, had: 1) intrusive voicing in voiceless plosive consonant production; 2) produced voiced plosives with greater air flow; 3) produced voiceless consonants with less air flow; and 4) initiated the CV utterances at substantially lower lung volumes. The picture of disordered laryngeal and aerodynamic functioning presented by these findings adds further support to the suggestion that many of the speech problems demonstrated by the hearing impaired may be the result of air stream mismanagement through inappropriate and inefficient vocal tract valving.

One finding of this study that must be considered when discussing the respiratory characteristics of hearing-impaired speakers was the linguistic patterning used during continuous speech. The normally hearing speakers, and, for the most part, the intelligible hearing-impaired speakers, took inspirations of air at appropriate sentence or phrase boundaries, thereby creating an acceptable flow of speech that undoubtedly contributed to intelligibility. The semi-intelligible and unintelligible hearing-impaired subjects, however, would inhale at inappropriate times, thus not appearing to follow any logical linguistic pattern. This may have been due, in part, to the fact that as a group they initiated speech at low lung volumes, as well as wasted a great deal of air as demonstrated by the very high rates of air expenditure per syllable. The linguistically inappropriate inspirations of air probably were a major contributor to reduced intelligibility.

In general, it appears from the data in this investigation that some of the patterns that semi-intelligible and unintelligible hearing-impaired individuals exhibit when attempting speech are: 1) initiation of speech at low lung volumes; 2) continuing speech well beyond FRC; 3) inefficient valving of the air stream by intrusive voicing and air wastage; and 4) respiratory inspirations occurring without regard for linguistic boundaries.

With respect to the clinical implications of these findings, a number of factors must be considered. It is obvious that if intelligible speech is to be obtained by hearing-impaired individuals, one must not forget the respiratory and upper airway dynamics requisite for intelligible speech. The clinician should be aware of the fact that many hearing-impaired individuals with poor intelligibility may be attempting speech with reduced lung volumes, and should be prepared to assess this behavior pattern in a client. It must also be remembered that speech involves more than respiration. Thus, the clinician should be able to determine the existence of inefficient and/or inappropriate vocal tract valving during speech production and how the deficiencies may or may not contribute to the speech problems. Also, based upon information from this and other studies, the linguistic programming used by the speaker and its relation to the respiratory and vocal tract valving patterns should be assessed. It appears that a speech correction program that focuses on the fundamentals of speech production, that is, respiration, upper airway dynamics, and linguistic programming may be necessary to improve the intelligibility of some hearing-impaired speakers.

The data from the present investigation have shown some general trends with respect to the relationships between selected measures of speech physiology and degree of perceived speech intelligibility. Additional research into the exact effect of such physiological measures on speech intelligibility is needed. These data would then be helpful in obtaining a complete understanding of the factors that contribute to speech intelligibility in hearing-impaired individuals.

REFERENCES

Forner, L., and T. Hixon. 1977. Respiratory kinematics in profoundly hearing-impaired speakers. J. Speech Hear. Res. 20:373–408.

Gilbert, H. R. 1974. Simultaneous oral and nasal airflow during stop consonant production by hearing impaired speakers. Folia Phoniatr. 27:423–437.

Hixon, T., M. Goldman, and J. Mead. 1973. Kinematics of the chest wall during speech production: Volume displacements of the rib cage, abdomen, and lung. J. Speech Hear. Res. 16:78–115.

Hudgins, C. V. 1934. A comparative study of the speech coordinations of deaf and normal hearing subjects. J. Genet. Psychol. 44:3–48.

Hudgins, C. V., and F. C. Numbers. 1942. An investigation of the intelligibility of the speech of the deaf. Genet. Psychol. Monogr. 25:289–392.

Hutchinson, J., and Smith, L. 1976. Aerodynamic functioning in consonant production by hearing impaired adults. Audiol. Hear. Educ. 2:16-19, 22-25, 34.

Mead, J., N. Peterson, C. Gimby, and J. Mead. 1967. Pulmonary ventilation measured from body surface movements. Science 156:1383–1384.

RECENT RESEARCH ON THE SPEECH PERCEPTION ABILITIES OF THE HEARING IMPAIRED

CHAPTER 6

A SPEECH PRODUCTION APPROACH TO SPEECH PERCEPTION BY DEAF PERSONS

J. M. Pickett, Sally G. Revoile, and Lisa D. Holden

CONTENTS

This chapter considers auditory research on the perception of speech by the hearing impaired in terms of speech production. Our aims are to relate the normally perceived acoustic cues of speech to specific features of production, then to describe some research results about impaired auditory discrimination for some acoustic cue corollates of speech production, and finally to interpret this knowledge in relation to the speech teaching task. In addition to summarizing which aspects of speech one might be able to teach through residual hearing, this approach can indicate what further research on impaired hearing might contribute to our knowledge of the relations between speaking and hearing.

SPEECH CUES AND SPEECH PRODUCTION

How do speech cues function in speech communication? Essentially they are the basic sound patterns that encode a speaker's meaning.

This study was supported by the Gallaudet Research Institute and the U.S. Public Health Service through Grant NS-05464 from the National Institute of Neurological and Communicative Disorders and Stroke.

119

They arise as the result of coordinated movements of sound production by the speech organs. Some of these movements produce and control the sources of speech sounds: the turbulence of the breath stream and phonation. We will call these sound-producing movements *phonatory*. Other movements cause modulation of the source sounds (*articulatory*). Both the phonatory and articulatory movements are organized in consistent patterns of different kinds that follow language coding rules. In other words, the consistent movements of speaking produce consistent sound patterns; these patterns contain the cues that form the core fabric of speech communication.

Our task is to train the severely to profoundly deaf child to make phonatory and articulatory movements that are correctly coordinated and consistently organized according to the language coding rules. Knowledge of the hearing of speech acoustic cues can contribute a great deal to this task because there is now considerable evidence that in perceiving speech for understanding the listener interprets the sound patterns in a special way: as if they were being produced by movements of the speech organs. This recently accumulated evidence has reactivated a 50-year-old theory of speech perception called the *motor theory*. In an early extreme form of the theory, Stetson (1928) speculated that what we hear in speech is not "a mere acoustic pattern but a series of movements" being performed by the speaker. Studdert-Kennedy (1979) summarized the last 30 years of research on the acoustic cues in speech perception. Almost as extreme as Stetson, but considering the results of much auditory research on speech cues, Studdert-Kennedy said that, in effect, the listener hears the movements of the speaker.

Thus, for a better understanding of the process of learning to speak, we should profit by considering the motor theory of speech perception to be essentially correct. Then we would need to describe the features of speech movements that must be perceived for communication to take place via speech. Obviously, the perceived features would have to be those that make up the consistent phonatory and articulatory patterns of the language code. These patterns might largely be formed by characteristics of movements per se, that is, by very general features that are common to all movements of body members. Thus, for a general start we can say that the features should tell what parts of the speech mechanism are moving, where the movement is taking place, and how the parts are moving, that is, in what direction and with what speed. The speech movements are those of the chest-abdomen, the larynx, the vocal folds, the velum, and the oral shape movements and constricting movements of the tongue and lips. The location of the movement varies significantly only for the oral movements; the other movements take place in a more or less fixed region of the system of speech organs.

The features of the phonatory and articulatory modulating movements of speech are shown in Tables 6.1 and 6.2.

Movement Features

The constriction and transition movement features of Table 6.2 must be highly redundant of each other because of the fluent, "coarticulated" performance of constrictions and transitions between the constrictions and the more open vowel shapes. In other words, the vowel shape movements are determined to a very large extent by the constriction features.

It is interesting to ask whether the shape movement features of Table 6.2 are capable of generating a plausible number of syllables when combined with the nonshaping movement states of the vocal folds and frication-source production of Table 6.1. It was calculated that the tongue and lips can generate 128 different shape movements (from five two-state movement features). Assuming that the 128 shape movements themselves contain all the shape information for both consonants and a vowel, then, with two movement states each for the vocal folds, velum, and friction production, there would be 768 ($2 \times 2 \times 2$) $\times$ 128 consonant-vowel combinations and 4,608 (6×768) possible syllables with two consonants each. Lateral and retroflex tongue shapes would then give 9216 such syllables.

Finally, each constricted (consonantal) phase of a syllable may consist of significantly different subintervals characterized by combinations of the movement features. These are called *compound consonants* or, in current phonetics, *consonant clusters*. They are generated by the movement features of the velum, friction production,

Table 6.1.   Features of phonatory/sound-producing movements and corresponding variables in speech

Movement	Acoustic mechanism	Acoustic variables
Chest-Abdomen	Tracheal air pressure on closed vocal folds	Voice pitch (F_0) and relative amplitude of upper vowel spectrum
Thyroid-Cricoid	Vocal fold tension	Voice pitch
Vocal Folds		
Closed	Vibration	Periodic sound
Open	No vibration, high potential air-flow	Aperiodic friction sound or silence

Table 6.2.   Features of articulatory/spectrum-modulating movements and corresponding acoustic variables in speech

Movement	Acoustic mechanism	Acoustic variables
Velum		
Closed	Pharyngeal-oral tract resonance pattern	'Normal' F_1 in vowels 'Normal' consonants
Open	Shunted oral tract: resonances and antiresonances	Weak F_1 in vowels Low murmur in voiced consonants
Oral tract shaping (movements producing vowels) Tongue bunching Tongue hump location Tongue hump movement direction Lip rounding	Tract resonance patterns	F_1, F_2, F_3 locations and general prominence of low, middle, or upper vowel spectrum
Oral tract constricting (movements producing consonants) Fast/slow Ballistic/controlled Direction of constricting movement	Tract resonance patterns	Transitional changes in vowel F_1, F_2, F_3 locations Spectra of constriction sounds

and some of the shape movements, employed in close conjunction with the main syllable-initiating or -terminating constriction movements, compounding these into more complex movement patterns. The combinations of these as factors could generate about 27,648 (3 × 9216) syllables.

It is estimated that there are only about 4000 different syllables in English; thus it is apparent that not all of the possible combinations of movement features are employed.

CUE LEARNING AND SPEECH LEARNING

It can be assumed that a child learns to speak properly by associating each of the heard speech cues with its successful production in his or her own speech. Variant examples of a given cue are provided to the child by adult males and females, by siblings, and by himself or herself; these all become associated with the child's own speech movement patterns in producing a successful version of each cue. Thus, in terms of movement features, if the child can hear and discriminate the acoustic cues of the speech movement features, he or she can learn to produce movements with the proper features through a process of attempted imitations and communicative reinforcements (Mol, 1979; Stetson, 1951).

What acoustic cues does the child need to learn to associate with which movements? Tables 6.1 and 6.2 show the movements and related cues. Some of those movement cues may be lacking for the hearing-impaired child.

If the child cannot discriminate changes in F_o (fundamental frequency), he or she will not be able to hear the effects of the changes in the movements of the larynx and the chest and abdominal system that produce the F_o changes. These movements carry the prosodic information of the language code.

If a child cannot hear the presence or absence of a nasal murmur and its low-frequency spectrum versus the wider spectrum of the glides, laterals, liquids, and vowel sounds, he or she will not be able to hear the status of the velum during consonant production.

If a child cannot hear the differences in the general patterns of the formants, he or she will not be able to hear the vocal tract shapes formed by the tongue and lips.

If a child cannot hear differences in transitions in the formants, and also their speed of transition, he or she cannot hear the different features of the vocal tract constricting movements, and, what may be even more important, he or she cannot hear the continuities of movement between the more open shapes and the constrictions.

AUDITORY RESEARCH ON
IMPAIRED PERCEPTION OF SPEECH CUES

Recently there has been considerable research on the acoustic cues of speech to try to determine which cues the hearing-impaired person can discriminate (Pickett, 1979). Some of this research was conducted with children (see Risberg, 1977, 1979).

Let us take a few of the auditory cues to movement and determine from studies in the research literature whether they are perceived by the severely hearing-impaired listener.

Pitch Perception

One important set of movements affects the fundamental frequency, that is, the pitch, of voicing phonation. The patterns of pitch are important because they serve to indicate the stressed syllables; pitch also helps to mark the beginnings and endings of the larger units of speech, such as phrases and sentences. The patterns of pitch are produced by the coordination of two subsystems, the chest-abdomen and the larynx. Stressed syllables are spoken with a momentary increase in the subglottal pressure produced by the chest-abdomen; this causes the voice pitch to rise and the upper spectrum amplitude in vowels to increase. The laryngeal movements are used to control intonation patterns of pitch which, together with the durations of syllables, convey the prosodic information that is responsible for the blocking-out of the stream of speech into words, phrases, and sentences.

In the normal learning of speech by the child, the pitch patterns and rhythms are learned first. If the hearing-impaired child has viable pitch discrimination in the low frequencies, he or she may be able, under proper amplification, to learn to produce these basic patterns naturally, without special training.

Risberg (1977, 1979) measured low-frequency pitch discrimination of severely and profoundly deaf children. Figure 6.1 shows results for five subjects, three of which had good discrimination. At 125 Hz, two of the subjects could discriminate a pitch change of 1% to 3% difference limen (DL). These children probably could hear the pitch patterns of their parents' and their own voices. The two children with poor pitch discrimination probably would not hear voice pitch changes reliably. Their discrimination of pitch was very gross and probably came through the tactile sense.

Researchers have studied the use of tactile versions of the speech signal for partial speech perception (Erber, this volume). Tactile sensing of the speech wave can contribute the "hearing" of the timing of speech movements, particularly the occurrence of the vowel open movements. A pitch DL of 20%, as in Risberg's poor cases, however, is probably tactual and would be marginal for perceiving pitch intonation; only the most extreme changes would be felt, about half the time, as different in pitch from the average ongoing patterns of pitch of the surrounding vowels.

Formant Transition Perception

The perception of voice pitch and rhythm by the hearing-impaired child does not guarantee that he or she can also hear the articulatory movements. Articulations of the lips and tongue produce two types of changes in the spectrum of sounds: 1) changes in the general prominence of the low-, mid-, and high-frequency portions of the vowel spectrum, for vowel identification; and 2) rapid spectrum changes, that is,

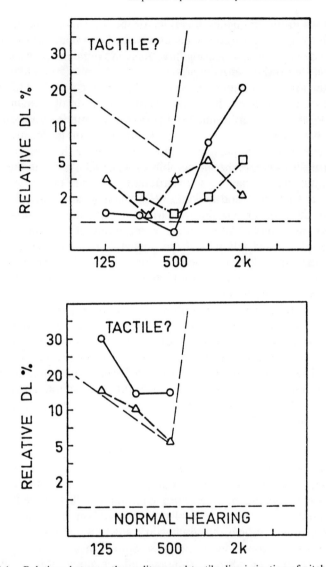

Figure 6.1.   Relations between the auditory and tactile discrimination of pitch in deaf children. The percentage of frequency change, that is, the difference limen (DL), necessary, to hear a pitch change was measured for five deaf children who listened in separate tests to pure tones at reference frequencies of 125, 375, 500, 1500, or 2000 Hz (plotted horizontally). Three of the children (results plotted in upper graph) have low-frequency pitch discrimination of ½% to 4% DL, which is nearly normal (DL = ½% in frequency) and quite adequate to hear the voice pitch variations that occur in the range 100–300 Hz. The other two children (lower graph), however, have poor pitch discrimination (DL = 10% to 30%), with frequency differences so large that they can be felt through the tactile sense. (From Risberg, 1977)

transitions in the frequency locations of the formants. The perception of these formant transitions is necessary for hearing the movements of the tongue and lips and hearing how these movements are coordinated with the "prosodic" movements.

How are transitions perceived by the hearing impaired? Some recent research by the authors has tested perception of formant transitions by severely hearing-impaired persons. Discrimination was tested for the presence of a transition versus no transition in the second formant. The results implied that among listeners with similar amounts of hearing loss some should be able to hear whether it is the lips or the tongue that is making a constriction, whereas others would not (Danaher, Osberger, and Pickett, 1973; Danaher and Pickett, 1975).

The duration of formant transitions is related to the speed of articulation movement, which varies with the rate of utterance, the type of consonant constriction, and the vowel shapes that occur between the constrictions of the consonants. For example, the transition movements of stops require only about 50 msec, glides about 75 msec, and diphthongs about 150 msec.

Recently studies by the authors tested the perception of duration of transition by hearing-impaired listeners. In these studies a brief constant-duration transition was set in a formant stimulus representing the type of transition occurring in a vowel formant after a stop consonant. The sound stimulus had a single formant that went through an upward transition of 100 Hz for 30 msec and then maintained a constant frequency of 500 Hz for 270 msec (see the "constant transition stimulus" at the top of Figure 6.2).

In the listening task, amplification was used to make the stimuli comfortably audible. Then, longer transitions were compared with the constant short-transition stimulus used as a reference. The duration of the longer transition was reduced until the listener could just hear the difference between it and the reference transition 70% of the time. The longer duration at this threshold point was taken as an index of the listener's ability to hear differences in transition duration. If the transition at threshold was very long, discrimination was poor.

The results for normal listeners, and for moderately to severely impaired listeners with either flat or sloping audiograms are shown in Figure 6.2. The results are given in mean threshold duration and this mean duration transition is diagrammed for comparisons among groups. It can be seen that the threshold for normal subjects would enable them to discriminate the formant transition of a fast stop release, which is 30 to 50 msec in duration, from that of a slower glide-consonant release, which is 75 to 100 msec in duration. For the hearing impaired, the slopes, with a mean threshold of 106 msec duration of transition,

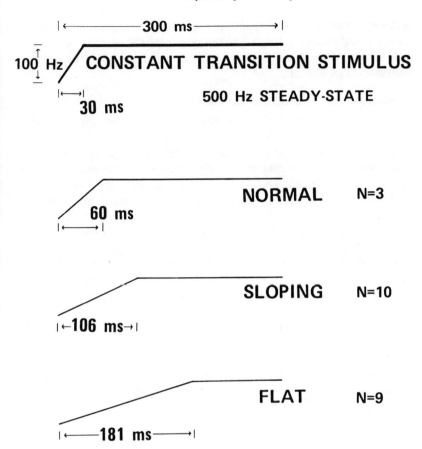

TRANSITION DURATION DISCRIMINATION

Figure 6.2.   Some results on the discrimination of duration of a formant transition by two groups of hearing-impaired listeners, with sloping, and flat audiometric contours, as compared with normal discrimination. The flat group had more hearing loss in the frequency region of the transition (always 400–500 Hz) than did the sloping group, and required a longer transition (mean of 181 msec versus 106 msec for the flat group) to be able to discriminate the transition from a very brief one of 30 msec, which was the reference "constant" transition. Further details of the experiment are given in the text.

would be expected to have some difficulty hearing stop versus glide movements. Diphthongs usually involve even slower formant movements than glides. The listeners with flat impairments might not be able to hear even this long duration movement in comparison with transitions associated with stops. (It should be noted that the listeners with a flat loss had more hearing loss in the frequency region of transition.) These results indicate that some hearing-impaired listeners will not be able to discriminate the differing rates or durations of the articulatory movements of speech.

Applications of Acoustic Cue Research

Detailed research studies of the basic auditory reception of acoustic cues can be applied to designing individual programs of speech training. The authors have found large individual differences in speech cue discrimination. The existence of such differences suggests that the parent, teacher, and clinician should have available structured programs of auditory "test" stimuli but be encouraged to remain flexible. When it is evident that an important type of movement discrimination by the model speakers is already available through hearing, it might better be left to develop naturally. The motor perception approach implies that certain types of hearing capacity should naturally result in development of certain types of correct speech articulation without training.

In another application, the motor perception approach suggests that the speech movements of deaf speakers might be studied through the reactions of normally hearing persons listening to deaf speech. To a certain extent, data on this can be found in the study of Smith (1973). She derived a phoneme confusion matrix from the responses of phoneticians listening to the speech of deaf children. The most common single defect heard was the omission of consonant phonemes when they were medial or final in the word spoken. In motor perception terms this might mean that, frequently, the deaf child makes no consonant gesture at all, where one should have been made. Smith's further analysis of her data showed that the defective consonants were frequently the less visible ones. In other words, if a deaf child cannot see the consonant articulation gesture, he or she is less likely to learn to make it. In some cases, however, invisible consonants and invisible features were heard as correctly performed. This study, or future ones of this type, might be especially designed and analyzed to shed more light on the transmission of movement features to the listeners (see Levitt and Stromberg, this volume).

Some new response tasks may be useful for investigating the transmission of movement features to listeners. For example, it has been shown in some reaction-time studies by Kozhevnikov and Chistovich in 1965 that the time delay and type of response of a listener to identify a spoken consonant reflect the motor conditions of production of the consonant (for details see Pickett, 1980, pp. 196–198). This type of test could be applied to the study of abnormal articulation and the results checked by x-ray studies of the articulations. This approach suggests that a great deal might be learned about speaking and about hearing speech through listening experiments on abnormal articulation.

REFERENCES

Danaher, E. M., M. J. Osberger, and J. M. Pickett. 1973. Discrimination of formant frequency transitions in synthetic vowels. J. Speech Hear. Res. 16:439–451.
Danaher, E. M., and J. M. Pickett. 1975. Some masking effects produced by low-frequency vowel formants in persons with sensorineural hearing loss. J. Speech Hear. Res. 18:261–271.
Mol, H. 1979. The writing on the wall for phoneticians. Proc. Inst. Phonet. Sci. (Amsterdam University) 5:1–12.
Pickett, J. M. 1979. Perception of speech features by persons with hearing impairment. In H. Hollien and P. Hollien (eds.), Current Issues in the Phonetic Sciences. John Benjamins, Amsterdam.
Pickett, J. M. 1980. The Sounds of Speech Communication. University Park Press, Baltimore.
Risberg, A. 1977. Hearing loss and auditory capacity. Paper presented at the Research Conference on Speech-Processing Aids for the Deaf, Research Institute, Gallaudet College, Washington, D.C.
Risberg, A. 1979. Bestämning av Hörkapacitet och Talperceptionsförmåga vid Svåra Hörselskador (Defining hearing capacity and speech perception ability under severe hearing impairment). A collection of articles in English, presented for the doctorate, Department of Speech Communication, Royal Institute of Technology, Stockholm.
Smith, C. R. 1973. Residual Hearing and Speech Production in Deaf Children. CSL Research Report #4. City University of New York, Communication Sciences Laboratory, New York.
Stetson, R. H. 1928. Motor phonetics. Archives Néerlandaises de Phonétique Expérimentale, 3:1–216.
Stetson, R. H. 1951. Motor Phonetics 2nd Ed. North-Holland, Amsterdam.
Studdert-Kennedy, M. 1979. Speech perception. Proceedings of the Ninth International Congress of Phonetic Sciences 1:59–81.

CHAPTER 7

SPEECH PERCEPTION AND SPEECH DEVELOPMENT IN HEARING-IMPAIRED CHILDREN

Norman P. Erber

CONTENTS

The purpose of this chapter is to survey speech perception ability in hearing-impaired children and how it relates to the ease with which they develop speech and oral language. The author will review the capacities and limitations of the various senses for speech perception and will briefly consider various speech feedback systems, including visual displays, hearing aids, and vibratory devices, that can be used to help a hearing-impaired child compensate for perceptual limitations. A teaching technique that relies on a sequence of demonstration, perception, and imitation will be discussed with regard to its use in speech development and correction.

Figure 7.1 illustrates a general relation between the speech intelligibility of hearing-impaired children and their hearing threshold levels for pure tones (Boothroyd, 1976). Speech intelligibility tends to be generally high (nearly 100% to the experienced listeners in this study) for

Preparation of this chapter was supported by Program Project Grant NS-03856 from the National Institute of Neurological and Communicative Disorders and Stroke to Central Institute for the Deaf.

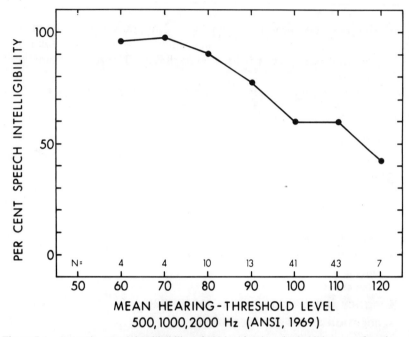

Figure 7.1   Acoustic speech intelligibility of 122 hearing-impaired children as a function of mean hearing level for 500, 1000, and 2000 Hz (dB re ANSI, 1969; better ear). Scores represent percentage of syllables correctly recognized by normally hearing listeners from a set of tape-recorded sentences (Reproduced with permission from Boothroyd, 1976).

children with hearing levels better than about 70 dB, but becomes progressively lower for children with poorer pure tone thresholds. These lower levels of performance for severely and profoundly hearing-impaired children have been reported in several other studies as well Monsen, 1978, Smith, 1975). They tend to parallel data depicting auditory speech feature recognition by similar groups of hearing-impaired children. The implication is that the ability to produce intelligible speech is related in a general way to the ability to perceive its spectral and prosodic qualities, although many hearing-impaired children learn to produce numerous speech qualities that they cannot hear (Gold, 1975; Smith, 1971).

It is acknowledged that most severely and profoundly hearing-impaired children depend to a considerable extent on their vision for language learning and for speech communication. Lipreading plays a major role in speech perception and also a part in certain aspects of speech learning (as in perception of an instructor's articulatory pattern;

Jenson, 1971). Accordingly, this discussion will include the possibilities and limitations of lipreading as a speech perception and feedback mode. Then we will examine ways in which attention to acoustic cues from a hearing aid can benefit a hearing-impaired child during combined auditory-visual perception of speech.

DISTURBANCES IN THE COMMUNICATION CHAIN

The communication chain, in both its acoustic and optical channels, can be disturbed in many ways (Erber, 1979b). The accuracy of message transmission and reception depends upon the nature and extent of the disturbance.

The Lack of Acoustic Feedback

Normally hearing children can monitor themselves through acoustic feedback, and the initial stages of language development normally depend on hearing for this purpose. Although a hearing-impaired infant often begins to babble at an age comparable to that of normally hearing infants, babbling soon may cease because the infant cannot monitor himself easily through an acoustic or an optical feedback system. That is, the hearing-impaired child normally cannot lipread himself as he produces speech and therefore cannot easily substitute a visual feedback system for acoustic feedback.

Thus, the period of development during which the infant is optimally suited to learn spoken language can be disturbed seriously by hearing loss. Unless educational programs stress the early training of audition and lipreading, the hearing-impaired child will begin to rely on a formal or informal set of gestural language symbols, and this shift of attention may hinder later acquisition and/or organization of spoken language.

The Inefficiency of Visemes for Conveying Information

Typically, hearing-impaired children are unable to perceive all of the sounds of speech accurately through hearing and so substitute visual perception of articulation for the auditory perception of certain speech sounds. The linguistic symbols thought to be used in lipreading are the visually observable positions[1] of the lips, teeth, tongue, and the surrounding facial surfaces. Visual perception of an articulatory position

---

[1] Although transitional movements, as well as articulatory positions, are important for visual perception of speech, these, typically, are not incorporated into theoretical analyses of visible speech features.

alone, however, usually is insufficient for the accurate recognition of a speech element. For example, a closure of the lips, considered by itself, has no linguistic value; it even may signal an absence of communication. If lip closure is perceived in combination with a subsequent lip opening, however, this lip position then becomes a visible marker of an articulatory gesture which corresponds to a particular set of phonemes in English (/p, b, m/).

It has been suggested that the visually observable units of speech articulation be called "visemes" (i.e., homophenes, clusters; Fisher, 1968). These visemes can convey linguistic information in a similar way as do the phonemes of a language. Most speakers, however, do not consciously create visemes as they talk, but instead speak to generate acoustically correct sounds. Thus, visemes are unconscious byproducts of speech production. Although visemes usually are unnoticed by hearing people, they can function as useful linguistic symbols for those with hearing impairments (see Alich, 1967).

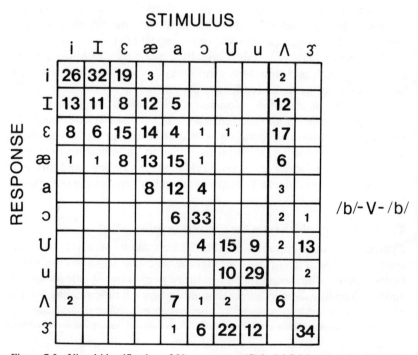

STIMULUS

	i	I	ɛ	æ	a	ɔ	U	u	ʌ	ɝ
i	26	32	19	3					2	
I	13	11	8	12	5				12	
ɛ	8	6	15	14	4	1	1		17	
æ	1	1	8	13	15	1			6	
a				8	12	4			3	
ɔ					6	33			2	1
U						4	15	9	2	13
u							10	29		2
ʌ	2				7	1	2		6	
ɝ					1	6	22	12		34

(RESPONSE — vertical label on left)

/b/-V-/b/ (right side label)

Figure 7.2   Visual identification of 20 consonants (C) in /a/-C-/a/ context by 6 hearing-impaired children. Results are given in the form of a confusion matrix. Stimuli were presented under conditions of frontal illumination by a talker who articulated carefully (Reproduced with permission from Erber, 1974c).

Unfortunately, visemes are less efficient language symbols than are phonemes (speech sounds) or graphemes (printed letters) for several reasons: 1) numerous speech sounds are produced by similar, visible speech movements (e.g., /f, v/); 2) some speech gestures occur deep within the oral cavity and are not easily visible to the observer (e.g., phonation, velar closure); and 3) coarticulation influences the visibility of many speech articulations; some visemes that can be identified in isolation become indistinguishable in combination. For example, in the word *needles*, the phonetic elements /d/, /l/ and, /z/ blend to form one viseme.[2]

In this way, approximately 40 English phonemes are reduced to about 9 to 14 visemes in conversational speech (see Jeffers and Barley, 1971). These visemes correspond to consonants that typically are confused with one another because certain speech features, such as voicing and nasality, are not visually apparent (e.g., /t, d, n/) and to vowels that commonly are confused because of similarities in degree of lip spread or rounding (e.g. /ɪ, ɛ / and /ʊ, u/). The resulting ambiguities in the optical code may require the young deaf child, in effect, to learn about a 40-phoneme spoken language system through a sensory channel that transmits considerably fewer than that number.

INFORMATION AVAILABLE THROUGH LIPREADING

In spite of this apparent obstacle to communication, numerous hearing-impaired children do learn speech and language mainly through lipreading—assisted by acoustic cues from a hearing aid, by natural gestures, by written material, and by help from a teacher.

What sort of information regarding speech production is available through lipreading? It is well known that consonants can be distinguished categorically on the basis of their points of articulation (e.g., labial, alveloar, velar; Figure 7.2), although consonant recognition is affected by vowel context (Erber, 1971; Pesonen, 1968). The consonants that are confused visually with one another generally are those that differ on the basis of voicing or manner of articulation (Erber, 1972a). Apparently, under good illumination conditions, even inexperienced lipreaders can learn to distinguish reliably among the places of consonant articulation (Erber, 1972a), and little specific practice seems required to reach this level of competence (Walden et al., 1977).

---

[2] One might argue that all of the articulatory configurations in this difficult word are perceived by the lipreader as a single viseme.

Accurate classification of consonant visemes, however, requires good optical conditions (Erber, 1971, 1974a). Lipreaders seem to vary considerably in ability to accurately identify vowels, although they have little difficulty distinguishing between spread (front) and rounded (back) categories; the two types of lip pattern form very distinct visemes. But they may misidentify vowels produced in neighboring articulatory (lip shape) positions (Figure 7.3). Vowel identification is relatively unaffected by distance, light level, or optical clarity (Erber, 1971, 1974a). Although vowel articulation may appear ambiguous, a gross mouth shape usually can be categorized correctly even under extremely poor optical conditions.

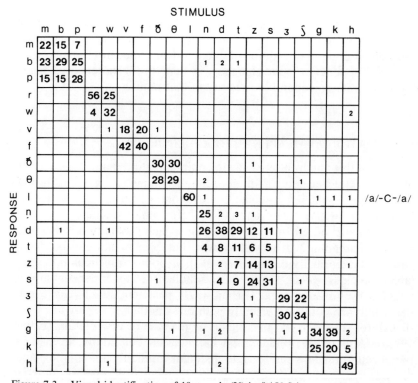

Figure 7.3.   Visual identification of 10 vowels (V) in /b/-V-/b/ context by 5 profoundly hearing-impaired children. Results are given in the form of a confusion matrix. Stimuli were presented under conditions of frontal illumination by a talker who articulated carefully.

Words

Longer words, such as spondees, tend to be more intelligible visually than are shorter words, such as monosyllables (Erber, 1971, 1974a). Two-syllable words with either iambic or trochaic stress are intermediate in intelligibility. It seems that if more (stressed) syllables are in a word, then more visible cues are available for its identification. Our experience suggests that a very important factor contributing to a word's intelligibility is the degree to which its articulatory pattern is optically unique, that is, the extent to which the word looks different from other words in the language (see Argila, 1978).

Sentences

Short, syntactically simple sentences tend to be visually more intelligible than are long, complex sentences (Clouser, 1977). Complicated syntactic transformations that can occur in sentences, such as embedded clauses, passive verb constructions, negatives, multiple subjects or objects, question forms, or various combinations of these are more difficult to lipread (Schwartz and Black, 1967). Many deaf children seem to have the least difficulty with sentences of the form subject-verb-object (-prepositional phrase), probably because this construction is one of the most basic and is introduced early during their education.

A major problem in lipreading sentences is that the coarticulation of speech elements often makes it difficult for the lipreader to specify word boundaries, especially where reduced stress in syllables affects the clarity of articulatory gestures. To isolate words, the lipreader must rely on vision for perception of speech rhythm and word emphasis, as well as refer to memory for probable word sequences.

AUDITORY AND AUDITORY-VISUAL PERCEPTION

Numerous studies have indicated that the acoustic speech perception skills of severely hearing-impaired children differ considerably from those with profound hearing impairments, especially regarding the ability to recognize the spectral qualities of speech components (see Risberg, 1976). For instance, many severely hearing-impaired children can distinguish certain low-frequency vowels and consonant qualities nearly as well as can those with normal hearing (Boothroyd, 1967; Erber, 1972a; Pickett and Martin, 1968; Pickett and Mártony, 1970), and so can understand simple words (e.g., numbers, spondees) with high accuracy (Erber, 1974b). In contrast, because profoundly hearing-impaired children have difficulty discriminating sounds of neighboring frequency (Risberg, Agelfors, and Boberg, 1975), they generally are poor at distinguishing the spectral qualities of vowels and consonants (Boothroyd, 1976; Erber, 1972a; Risberg, 1976), and so cannot recognize even common words (Erber, 1974b, 1979b). Profoundly hearing-impaired children, in fact, seem to perceive little more than the overall intensity patterns of amplified acoustic speech signals through appropriately selected hearing aids (Erber, 1972b, 1979a; Zeiser and Erber, 1977). Several studies have suggested that they do not hear at all, but instead detect amplified acoustic stimuli through vibrotactile receptors in their ears (Boothroyd and Cawkwell, 1970; Nober, 1967). These two capacities for perception of amplified speech, 1) auditory spectral discrimination, mainly on the basis of low-frequency cues, by the severely hearing-impaired; and 2) (vibrotactile) envelope perception by the profoundly hearing impaired, differ greatly, especially when combined with lipreading for speech perception. Undoubtedly, an important reason for observed differences in the communicative progress of hearing-impaired children is the discrepancy in their auditory abilities.

It appears that moderately and severely hearing-impaired children are able to achieve high levels of oral communication skill. Under good optical and acoustic conditions they can perceive place of articulation for consonants and lip shape cues for vowels through lipreading, and also complementary voicing, manner of articulation, and formant information through low-frequency hearing. As a result of obtaining through one sensory modality that which is not available through the other, their speech comprehension by combined auditory-visual reception usually is quite high (Numbers and Hudgins, 1948; Prall, 1957; Thornton and Erber, 1979) and they quickly acquire oral language skills.

Profoundly hearing-impaired children, on the other hand, experience more difficulty in speech communication. Although they also receive place of articulation and lip shape information through lipreading, amplification provides mainly supplementary cues to them in the form of speech intensity patterns. Voicing, nasality, and numerous postdental articulatory cues often are not apparent. The important factor seems to be whether the child receives amplified acoustic information through his ears that complements or only supplements the cues that are available to him through lipreading.[3]

---

[3] Recent work suggests that much of this supplementary acoustic information contained in the speech waveform envelope is redundant with the visible articulatory feature of mouth opening (area of aperture; see Erber, 1979a). Nevertheless, the acoustic supplement is useful to the lipreader (Erber, 1972b).

PERCEPTION AND SPEECH FEEDBACK

Audition is the normal feedback mode for speech acquisition. The way in which a severely or profoundly hearing-impaired child learns to produce speech is complicated by the fact that he hears many speech elements only after considerable spectral transformation by his hearing aids and ears; some sounds of speech may not be audible at all. If the child is to succeed as an oral communicator, he or she must develop an effective, personal method for monitoring and controlling speech as he or she produces it. For speech elements that are audible and distinguishable (e.g., /u, a/), the child may use remnants of hearing for feedback. To monitor the production of other, less audible speech units (e.g., /f/), the child may attend to articulator position, vibration, and/ or pressure. At other times, he or she may rely on memory (without conscious attention to feedback) to generate automatic articulatory sequences that previously were learned mainly by reference to a teacher's instructions (e.g., /st/). Each feedback mode may play a role in monitoring and controlling a different set of speech elements. In fact, it is likely that a hearing-impaired child's self-monitoring strategies will vary with successive speech segments in an utterance (see Figure 7.4).

Many profoundly deaf children learn to produce acoustically intelligible speech in spite of serious limitations in their auditory self-monitoring systems. How do they accomplish this? Educators have developed a variety of special instructional techniques and instruments to help deaf children identify speech patterns that approximate normal articulation. Optical techniques include nodding, smiling, or gesturing when the child produces correct speech (Calvert and Silverman, 1975); providing cues for invisible articulatory features through a phonetic sign system (Schulte, 1978); allowing the child to watch a mirror for changes in oral or facial images (see Pflaster, 1979); or providing the child with electromechanical devices that detect and display a visible pattern analogous to particular aspects of speech, especially voicing and nasality cues (Boothroyd et al., 1975). Acoustic techniques include amplifying and presenting the speech signal through a hearing aid to the child's ears (Pollack, 1970) or processing the speech waveform before amplification in order to match the acoustic signal more appropriately to the child's limited auditory system (e.g., peak-clipping, compression, vocoding, frequency-shifting: see Villchur, 1978). Tactile techniques include allowing the child to place his hand(s) on his own face or throat while speaking (Calvert and Silverman, 1975) or feeling amplified speech patterns delivered by a single vibrator (Schulte, 1978)

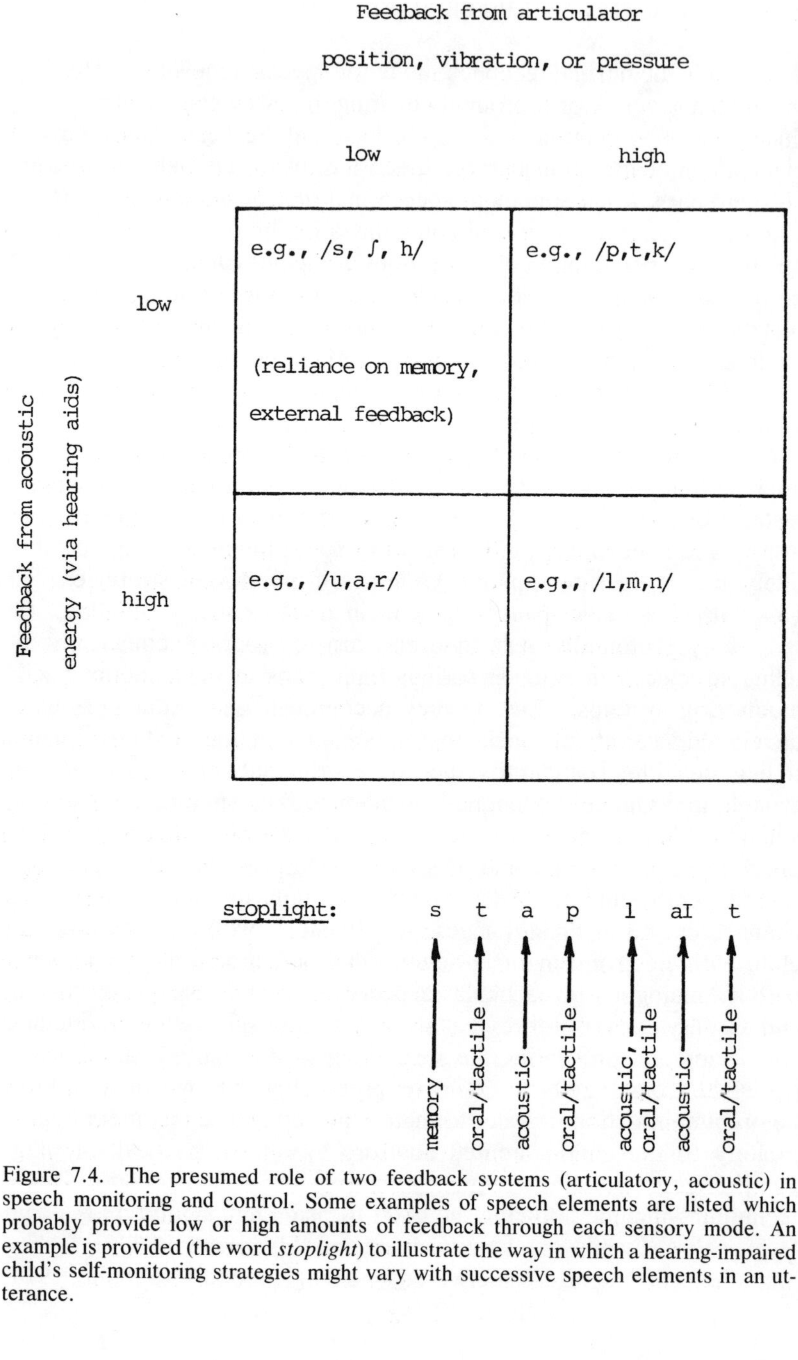

Feedback from articulator

position, vibration, or pressure

low   high

| | low | e.g., /s, ʃ, h/

(reliance on memory,
external feedback) | e.g., /p,t,k/ |
| | high | e.g., /u,a,r/ | e.g., /l,m,n/ |

(left vertical label) Feedback from acoustic energy (via hearing aids)

stoplight: s   t   a   p   l   aI   t

memory   oral/tactile   acoustic   oral/tactile   acoustic, oral/tactile   acoustic   oral/tactile

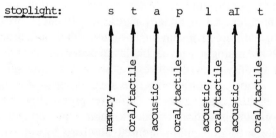

Figure 7.4.   The presumed role of two feedback systems (articulatory, acoustic) in speech monitoring and control. Some examples of speech elements are listed which probably provide low or high amounts of feedback through each sensory mode. An example is provided (the word *stoplight*) to illustrate the way in which a hearing-impaired child's self-monitoring strategies might vary with successive speech elements in an utterance.

or a set of tactile stimulators, each activated by a particular sound quality (Sparks et al., 1979).

Our spoken language, although perhaps encoded and stored in articulatory terms, is transmitted acoustically, and if normally hearing listeners receive these acoustic signals as distorted or intermittent, then they will not be able to reconstruct the child's intended messages. All of the compensatory methods listed above are intended to help the child judge the correctness of his sound patterns, and so identify and continue to produce speech that is acoustically intelligible to people with normal hearing. To transfer this ability to everyday conversation, however, the child must eventually learn to substitute personal (or portable) feedback systems and internal production criteria for those special techniques on which he previously relied.

DEMONSTRATION, PERCEPTION, AND IMITATION IN SPEECH LEARNING

Perception and development of spoken language during daily communication depends on the effective use of sensory information. Several authors have described speech teaching methods that attempt to exploit available sensory inputs (see Calvert and Silverman, 1975; Ling, 1976). Because speech production in both normally hearing and hearing-impaired children typically is learned through perception and imitation of a parent or teacher's speech models, instruction strategies have evolved which formalize and/or systematize the demonstration-perception-imitation approach, considering the child's sensory limitations in the normally primary mode (hearing) and ways in which secondary modes (vision, touch) can provide alternate avenues for speech learning.

In one approach (Ling and Ling, 1978), the capabilities of the various sensory systems are examined, and speech models are provided to the children in a specified sequence: auditory, auditory-visual, visual (alone), and visual-tactile (see Figure 7.5). When the child's auditory capacity is adequate for perception, an acoustic model will be sufficient, and the child will learn to match the utterances of an instructor whose mouth is covered during speech practice (see Beebe, 1953; Pollack, 1970). Some speech features, however, are very difficult to teach successfully to particular hearing-impaired children through the auditory sense alone, and optical or tactile cues such as those described previously can be provided as substitutes.

The following sequence frequently is employed in speech instruction: 1) the teacher demonstrates correct speech production; 2) the

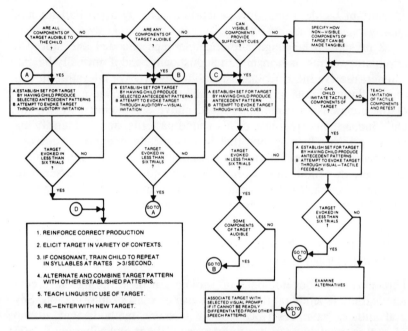

Figure 7.5.   Suggested sequence through which a clinician may employ a child's various sense modalities to teach speech (Reproduced with permission from Ling and Ling, 1978).

child perceives and attempts to remember this; 3) the child imitates the teacher's model; 4) while producing this speech pattern, the child perceives his own vocal output; 5) the child compares the imitation with a recalled image of the model utterance and judges similarity and thus correctness of his or her speech.

To summarize, development of speech through imitation depends on perception of a model as well as perception of one's own utterance. The child's speech perception, however, is not itself perceivable by the teacher, and so cannot be taught simply by modelling the required behavior. Rather, one usually teaches perception by the following sequence: 1) the instructor shows the child a repertoire of responses (or discovers those already known by the child); 2) the instructor associates a stimulus with each response; 3) he or she presents one of these stimuli with a request to respond; 4) the child chooses from among the alternatives; 5) the instructor rewards correct responses and points out (or ignores) the incorrect responses. If the child frequently responds correctly, the instructor can assume that the desired perceptual learning has taken place. If incorrect responses are common, one concludes that the child is having difficulty learning, or that the instructor has incorrectly presented the perceptual task. During instruction, stimulus and response complexity may be varied according to the child's success or difficulty with the perceptual activity (see Erber, 1976, 1977, 1979b).

Because the basic perceptual process is not overt, but is hidden from the instructor's (and child's) view, most learning must be inferred. Even the child's degree of attention to the task often must be inferred from his external behavior. In some instances, a child's head and body may be oriented properly, although in fact he or she is not watching or listening to the teacher. Considerable teaching experience is required to make correct inferences regarding a child's capacity for learning perception and thus production of speech through each sensory mode.

It is obvious that speech perception and production are closely interrelated, although the direction of the dependency is far from clear. They are but two of the many components of learning spoken language. And so, subdividing and labeling teaching or learning activities into "auditory training," "lipreading practice," "articulation drill," and so on, seem quite artificial and perhaps restrictive to the child in his acquisition and retention of speech-oriented skills. We need to develop methods that smoothly blend all of these to achieve the most effective instruction.

REFERENCES

Alich, G. W. 1967. Language communication by lipreading. In Proceedings of the International Conference on Oral Education of the Deaf (Vol. 1). A. G. Bell Association for the Deaf, Washington, D.C.
Argila, C. A. 1978. A computer simulation of lipreading. Doctoral dissertation, Santo Tomas University, Philippines.
Beebe, H. 1953. A Guide to Help the Severely Hard of Hearing Child. Karger, New York.
Boothroyd, A. 1967. The discrimination by partially hearing children of frequency distorted speech. Int. Audiol. 6:136–145.
Boothroyd, A. 1976. Influence of Residual Hearing on Speech Perception and Speech Production by Hearing-Impaired Children. S.A.R.P. Report #26. Clarke School for the Deaf, Northampton, Mass.
Boothroyd, A., P. Archambault, R. E. Adams, and R. D. Storm. 1975. Use of a computer-based system of speech training aids for deaf persons. Volta Rev. 77:178–193.
Boothroyd, A., and S. Cawkwell. 1970. Vibrotactile thresholds in pure tone audiometry. Acta Otolaryngol. 69:381–387.
Calvert, D. R., and S. R. Silverman. 1975. Speech and Deafness. A. G. Bell Association for the Deaf, Washington, D.C.
Clouser, R. A. 1977. Relative phoneme visibility and lipreading performance. Volta Rev. 79:27–34.

144   Erber

Erber, N. P. 1971. Effects of distance on the visual reception of speech. J. Speech Hear. Res. 14:848–857.

Erber, N. P. 1972a. Auditory, visual, and auditory-visual recognition of consonants by children with normal and impaired hearing. J. Speech Hear. Res. 15:413–422.

Erber, N. P. 1972b. Speech envelope cues as an acoustic aid to lipreading for profoundly deaf children. J. Acoust. Soc. Am. 51:1224–1227.

Erber, N. P. 1974a. Effects of angle, distance, and illumination on visual reception of speech by profoundly deaf children. J. Speech Hear. Res. 17:99–112.

Erber, N. P. 1974b. Pure-tone thresholds and word-recognition abilities of hearing-impaired children. J. Speech Hear. Res. 17:194–202.

Erber, N. P. 1974c. Discussion of sensory capabilities. In R. E. Stark (ed.), Sensory Capabilities of Hearing-Impaired Children. University Park Press, Baltimore.

Erber, N. P. 1976. The use of audio tape-cards in auditory training for hearing impaired children. Volta Rev. 78:209–218.

Erber, N. P. 1977. Developing materials for lipreading evaluation and instruction. Volta Rev. 79:35–42.

Erber, N. P. 1979a. Speech perception by profoundly hearing-impaired children. J. Speech Hear. Disord. 44:255–270.

Erber, N. P. 1979b. Optimizing speech communication in the classroom. In A. Simmons-Martin, and D. R. Calvert (eds.), Parent-Infant Intervention. Grune & Stratton, New York.

Fisher, C. G. 1968. Confusions among visually perceived consonants. J. Speech Hear. Res. 11:796–804.

Gold, T. 1975. Perception and production of prosodic features by hearing-impaired children. Paper presented at the meeting of the American Speech and Hearing Association, November, Washington, D.C.

Jeffers, J., and M. Barley. 1971. Speechreading. Charles C Thomas, Springfield, Ill.

Jenson, P. M. 1971. The relationship of speechreading and speech. In L. Connor (ed.), Speech for the Deaf Child: Knowledge and Use. A. G. Bell Association for the Deaf, Washington, D.C.

Ling, D. 1976. Speech and the Hearing-Impaired Child: Theory and Practice. A. G. Bell Association for the Deaf, Washington, D.C.

Ling, D., and A. Ling. 1978. Aural Habilitation. A. G. Bell Association for the Deaf, Washington, D.C.

Monsen, R. B. 1978. Toward measuring how well hearing-impaired children speak. J. Speech Hear. Res. 21:197–219.

Nober, E. H. 1967. Vibrotactile sensitivity of deaf children to high intensity sound. Laryngoscope 77:2128–2146.

Numbers, M. E., and C. V. Hudgins. 1948. Speech perception in present day education for deaf children. Volta Rev. 50:449–456.

Pesonen, J. 1968. Phoneme communication of the deaf. Finn. Acad. Sci. 151(Series B):2.

Pflaster, G. 1979. Mirror, mirror on the wall. . . ? J. Speech Hear. Disord. 44:379–387.

Pickett, J. M., and E. S. Martin. 1968. Some comparative measurements of impaired discrimination for sound spectral differences. Am. Ann. Deaf 113:259–267.

Pickett, J. M., and J. Mártony. 1970. Low-frequency vowel formant discrimination in hearing-impaired listeners. J. Speech Hear. Res. 13:347–359.

Pollack, D. 1970. Educational Audiology for the Limited Hearing Infant. Charles C Thomas, Springfield, Ill.

Prall, J. 1957. Lipreading and hearing aids combine for better comprehension. Volta Rev. 59:64–65.

Risberg, A. 1976. Diagnostic rhyme test for speech audiometry with severely hard of hearing and profoundly deaf children. KTH Q. Prog. Rep. 2–3:40–58.

Risberg, A., E. Agelfors, and G. Boberg. 1975. Measurements of frequency discrimination ability of severely and profoundly hearing-impaired children. KTH Q. Prog. Rep. 2–3:40–48.

Schulte, K. 1978. The use of supplementary speech information in verbal communication. Volta Rev. 80:12–20.

Schwartz, J. R., and J. W. Black. 1967. Some effects of sentence structures on speech reading. Centr. States Speech J. 18:86–90.

Smith, C. 1971. Hearing measures and speech intelligibility in deaf children. Paper presented at the meeting of the American Speech and Hearing Association, November, Washington, D.C.

Smith, C. R. 1975. Residual hearing and speech production in deaf children. J. Speech Hear. Res. 18:795–811.

Sparks, D. W., L. A. Ardell, M. Bourgeois, B. Wiedmer, and P. K. Kuhl. 1979. Investigating the MESA (Multipoint Electrotactile Speech Aid): The transmission of connected discourse. J. Acoust. Soc. Am. 65:810–815.

Thornton, N. E., and Erber, N. P. 1979. Auditory-visual speech perception by hearing-impaired children. Hearing Aid J. 32(6):32–33.

Villchur, E. 1978. Signal processing. In M. Ross, and T. G. Giolas (eds.), Auditory Management of Hearing-Impaired Children. University Park Press, Baltimore.

Walden, B. E., R. A. Prosek, A. A. Montgomery, C. K. Scherr, and C. J. Jones. 1977. Effects of training on the visual recognition of consonants. J. Speech Hear. Res. 20:130–145.

Zeiser, M. L., and N. P. Erber. 1977. Auditory/vibratory perception of syllabic structure in words by profoundly hearing-impaired children. J. Speech Hear. Res. 20:430–436.

CHAPTER 8

TACTILE STIMULATION IN SPEECH RECEPTION: EXPERIENCE WITH A NONAUDITORY CHILD

Moise H. Goldstein, Jr., Adele Proctor, Laura Bulle, and Hiroshi Shimizu

CONTENTS

The disability of hearing loss is especially costly when it precedes the acquisition of language. Modern practice is to give the prelingually deaf child intensive preschool training starting at the time of detection, often at age one year or younger. The child's progress in language acquisition is quite dependent on the nature and degree of hearing loss. Those with enough residual hearing to be helped by a conventional hearing aid usually do well. Their perception and production of speech are reasonably good. On the other hand, profoundly deaf children may receive only limited benefit from a conventional hearing aid, if any, and usually fail to achieve satisfactory speech perception and production (Boothroyd, 1970; Erber, 1974).

    The long-range goal is to develop a wearable, skin-stimulating communication aid for the prelingually, profoundly deaf individual (Goldstein and Stark, 1976). Usefulness of such an aid may depend considerably on when and how the cutaneous signal is provided. From a number of points of view it seems important to start speech communication training early. Not only is it valuable to gain training time, but the child's ability to learn language and speech production changes with age. It is desirable to give the profoundly deaf child training during the years in which language acquisition occurs in the hearing child. Moreover, the sensory input from the aid should be available during all waking hours. Ideally, the aid would be worn throughout each day as a conventional hearing aid is worn by someone with good residual hearing. (This ideal was not achieved in the pilot work presented here.)

The transformation of the acoustic signal from the aid's microphone into a signal for stimulation of the skin requires consideration of patterned stimulation, multipoint stimulation, or a combination of the two (Scott et al., 1977); and location of the stimulator—hairy skin versus glabrous skin, and so on. Additionally, the transformation of the acoustic signal, which is a unidimensional function of time, to a suitable signal in time and two-dimensional place for stimulating the skin must be considered.

It occurred to us that we would obtain information important in terms of our long-range goals if we built a simple, wearable vibrotactile aid for one or more profoundly deaf children. Practical considerations dictated that we work with one subject.

One question this study could answer was whether vibrotactile stimulation is well tolerated by a young deaf child. Would the stimulation be aversive? pleasant? neutral? Secondly, if the child would tolerate a wearable aid, would daily use be helpful in the development of speech communication? The results of our experience with one child are presented in terms of observations, standardized test scores, and anecdotes. Thirteen training sessions were videotaped and 35 were audiotape recorded. A detailed analysis of the recordings and details of the standardized tests, and so on, will be presented in another report (Proctor and Goldstein, in press).

SUBJECT SELECTION

Some factors important in subject selection were: 1) age at the time a hearing loss was identified; 2) type of educational management; 3) communication philosophy of the subject's teachers; 4) educational philosophy and child rearing practices of parents; 5) parental attitude toward subject's deafness, their prior training and counseling; 6) parent-child interaction; 7) birth order of subject in family, number of siblings, subject's interaction with siblings, acceptance of deaf child by siblings, and vice versa; and 8) willingness of family to maintain a schedule of home visits. It is assumed that the deaf subject would have parents and siblings with normal hearing.

Based on audiological records of children seen at the Johns Hopkins Hospital (including results of scalp-recorded auditory-evoked responses (AER)), age-appropriate experimental subjects were located. An initial home visit was scheduled with both parents present during which the project was explained, the device was demonstrated, and the clinician had an opportunity to assess parental cooperation and the general home environment. Information was given to the school about the project and the school was asked to provide information about the child. After parents agreed to have their child participate in the project, the project therapist arranged for routine home visits and coordinated management with all other professionals involved with the child.

Although the long-range goal was to develop a wearable aid that could be provided to an infant less than 1 year old, the age criterion was shifted upwards because the younger child is less capable of providing a voluntary response and is less easily conditioned to perform particular tasks. Furthermore, with an older infant it is possible to communicate requirements of a task more readily, allowing use of tests such as the Peabody Picture Vocabulary Test. Finally, the parents of an older deaf child generally will have adjusted to and become more accepting of the child's handicap. The parents have received more counseling and have more knowledge about available therapeutic techniques.

The Subject: History and Audiological Information

T.K., a female, was born on January 13, 1975 and weighed 8 lbs., 12 oz. The mother had a normal pregnancy, but labor was complicated by a maternal urinary tract infection and 101° fever. Because of the mother's infection, the child was treated with ampicillin and gentamycin for 5 days after birth, which is the assumed etiology of the hearing loss. During T.K.'s early infancy, her mother questioned the baby's hearing because of lack of reaction to sounds. When her mother brought T.K. to the Johns Hopkins Hospital Hearing and Speech Center on October 20, 1975 (age 9 mo.), she reported that T.K. had never responded to any kind of sound. T.K. has no older siblings. A younger male sibling was born in 1976 and has normal hearing.

Behavioral observation audiometry using sound field stimuli revealed no detectable response. No startle reflex was elicited. In order to validate the results of behavioral observation audiometry, AER audiometry was performed with T.K. under sedation. No brain stem response to clicks was obtained at 85 dB hearing level (HL) bilaterally. Recording of the slow vertex response at 500 Hz, 1000 Hz, and 2000 Hz showed response only to the 500 Hz tone at 110 dB HL. A clear response was obtained to vibrotactile stimulation.

T.K. was placed in a parent-infant program; her parents received counseling about her management; and snap-ring earmolds were made for use with a powerful, body-type hearing aid.

Subsequently, she was given a body-type hearing aid with a Y-cord. Her mother encountered no difficulty getting T.K. to wear the hearing aid, and thought that the child could hear with amplification. When T.K. was nearly 13 months old, conditioned orienting response (COR) audiometry was attempted but no conditioning was established, either because the conditioned stimulus was not audible or because the child did not attend to the test sounds. None of the amplified sounds startled the child.

At age 16 months, she was conditioned in COR audiometry only for frequencies of 125 Hz and 250 Hz at sound field intensities of 95 dB sound pressure level (SPL) and 100 dB (SPL), respectively. These low-frequency acoustic stimuli are known to evoke vibratory responses. In fact, COR thresholds at 125 dB and 250 Hz showed little or no change with her hearing aid on.

The audiometric results remained unchanged during the follow-up evaluations. At 39 months, an audiogram was obtained by play audiometry which validated previous test results. T.K. responded to vibratory stimuli resulting from a high-intensity, low-frequency pure tone presented through a loudspeaker, but never responded when pure tones were presented through TDH-39 earphones.

Pure tone thresholds with the vibrotactile device were 70 dB hearing level (HL) from 250 Hz to 2000 Hz.[1] With the wearable vibrotactile device T.K. responded to voice at 65 dB sound pressure level (SPL). Figure 8.1 shows her wearing the vibrotactile aid vest with binaural body-type hearing aids.

THE AID

The aid is worn as a vest (Figure 8.2). The vibrotactile stimulator from a bone conduction hearing aid which has good low frequency response is spring loaded to press gently on the user's sternum (breast bone).

---

[1] The thresholds for acoustic stimuli obtained with T.K. wearing the vibrotactile device were dependent on the sensitivity (adjust threshold) setting. This adjustment sets the minimum signal that will activate the device. In practice, it is set so that background noise will seldom activate the device.

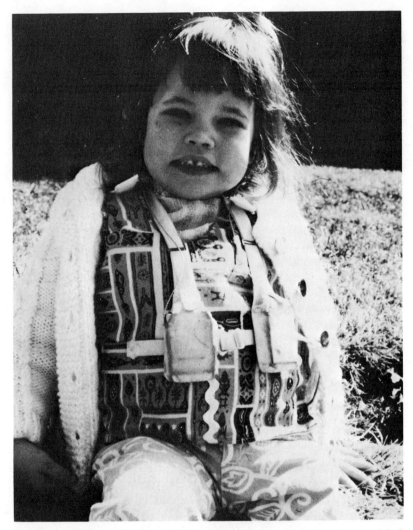

Figure 8.1.   T.K. wearing the vest. The vest is covered with a bright print material. On top of the vest her binaural hearing aids may be seen.

The miniature electret type microphone is clipped to a shoulder strap of the user's clothing. It is a nondirectional microphone (Knowles BT-1750) which picks up sounds in the user's vicinity as well as the user's vocalizations. The power pack consists of four 1.2 volts rechargeable Ni Cad cells, which run the aid for at least 10 hours without recharging.

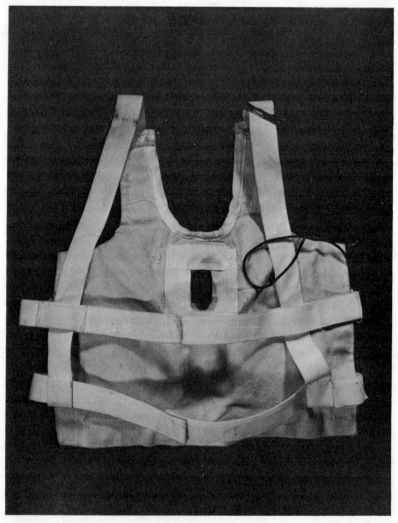

Figure 8.2.   Back view of the vest with vibrotactile device. The vibration stimulator of the Radioear B-72 bone conduction hearing aid is evident in the center of the vest. It is spring-loaded to push gently against the sternum.

The heart of the electronics is an envelope detector (Figure 8.3), which is a modification of an electronic system employed by Beguesse (1976). The envelope signal was multiplied by a 250-Hz sinusoid to produce a signal appropriate for skin stimulation.

Unless the device has a sensitivity floor (or threshold), ambient noise (e.g., room noise) will cause the vibrator to be continually active.

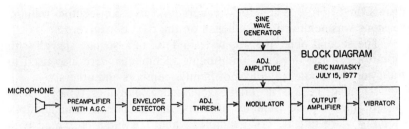

Figure 8.3.   Block diagram of electronics of the vibrotactile device.

For this purpose, an adjust threshold control determines the lowest level of sounds which will be sensed. It was usually set from 60 dB to 70 dB SPL. The dynamic range of the device need not be high because the dynamic range of the vibrotactile sense is low relative to that of the auditory system. The device has a linear range of about 20 dB SPL.

The device needs automatic gain control (AGC) so that loud, close voices will not overdrive it and so that it can pick up soft or distant voices. The AGC used yielded an input dynamic range from approximately 35 dB SPL to 90 dB SPL. The onset time constant of the AGC was 5 msec, and the offset time constant was 12 sec. Thus, gain is reduced quickly for high level stimulation, but does not recover in the pauses in speech.

TRAINING PROCEDURE

The overall objective of the training sessions was to develop communication behavior in this profoundly deaf child through the use of the vibrotactile aid. Initial objectives with the shelf model vibrotactile device were: 1) to develop consistent responses to acoustic stimuli; 2) to associate the vibration of the device with a variety of sound sources, particularly speech of others; 3) to associate the vibration of the device with the child's own vocalization; and 4) to increase the rate and quality of the child's vocal productions.

T.K. had training sessions at school and at home. Her mother participated in all sessions. At school her teacher was always present. At home her father and younger brother were often present. The project therapist was present at many sessions at home and at school. She made audiotape or videotape recordings of most of the sessions she attended.

First, conditioning techniques were used to train T.K. to respond to auditory (vibratory) stimuli produced by sound toys such as bells, drums, and horns. When 100% accuracy in two consecutive training sessions was achieved, work began on the next objective.

The second objective was to train T.K. to associate speech with vibrations of the device. Conditioning techniques were also used to train her to respond to voices of family members and others.

Because there is no tactile vocabulary, activities typically suggested for auditory training, auditory discrimination, and auditory memory were taught. For example, when T.K. was presented with loud-soft sounds for tactile discrimination, she was asked, "Do you hear it? Is it loud? Is it soft?" That is, when T.K. sensed an acoustic stimulus vibrotactically, she was told she "heard" it. As a result she came to associate the vibrotactile sensations with hearing. The audiological work-up at 39 months mentioned above included a test when she was wearing the vest. At first, with vest and no conventional hearing aid, she failed to respond. With the ear molds in place and the conventional hearing aid turned off, however, T.K. began to respond to the vibrotactile stimulation.

For the third objective (to have T.K. associate the vibration of the device with her own vocalizations), imitation tasks were employed emphasizing number of syllables, duration and pause time, and intensity. She was required to imitate her mother, father, teacher, and other adults who participated in training sessions. In structured and unstructured sessions, adults imitated T.K.'s productions as well. During all training sessions, T.K. was required to look at the speaker, but no particular emphasis was placed on lips. Once she associated vibratory sensation with her own vocalizations, both conditioning and imitation tasks were used to increase the rate and quality of T.K.'s vocal utterances, which met the fourth objective.

These initial training routines used the shelf model for which the vibrator was placed in her hand. She did not demonstrate hand preference and during sessions she was allowed to change hands.

Throughout the early training the authors stressed what the device was for, how it was to be used for communication, and that communication, that is, vocal with appropriate gestures, would be rewarding. This first phase was also used to establish the basis for learning routines of turn-taking and other situational and socially appropriate communicative behaviors believed to establish the basis for language acquisition (Bruner, 1975; Hardy and Hardy, 1971; Miller, 1978; Rees, 1978; Yoder and Reichle, 1977).

With the same overall objectives, new language-oriented training objectives were established when the wearable vest model became available: 1) to develop a basic receptive language vocabulary; 2) to comprehend a variety of syntactical constructions; 3) to produce sounds and words in the basic lexicon and in progressively longer utterances; and 4) to continue to develop positive social behavior through parent counseling.

Speech and language activities suggested for the hearing-impaired child (e.g., Ling, 1976; Northcott, 1977; van Uden, 1977) were introduced in this phase. At home, emphasis was placed on a conversational and experiential approach, whereas a more structured, grammatical approach was used at school.

RESULTS

No formalized speech and language tests could be administered directly to the child at the start of the project, because of her inability to speechread or generally to comprehend verbal directions. Only those preschool language tests requiring parent interview and clinical observation of her behavior were completed at that time.

At the start of the project (October 3, 1977) observations at home and school revealed that T.K.'s vocal repertoire was limited to requests using vowel-like and nasal sounds. Other consonants noted to occur sporadically were /h/, /d/, /w/, and /b/-like sounds. T.K. was judged to be a "quiet child" who relied heavily on gesture for communication. Her mother reported she could not recall T.K. going through a babbling stage.

Receptively, T.K. could associate five words (ball, baby, shoe, car, and apple) with picture cards and real objects when presented one at a time. These responses were not consistent, however, and she could perform this task only when the words were presented by her mother.

In retrospect, the first 5 weeks of training with the vibrotactile device were crucial to our work. In this period the shelf model was used, with T.K. holding the vibrator in her hand. After 1 week of training, she exhibited consistent responses to auditory stimuli. After 2 weeks of training, a significant increase in the amount of vocalization occurred. After 5 weeks of training, she clearly exhibited an association of vibration of the device with her own vocalizations when she initiated vocalization while holding the vibrator. When her vocal behavior stopped she stared at the vibrator with a surprised look, initiated vocalization again, paused, looked at the vibrator with surprise again, and so on. This self-initiated routine continued for at least five vocalized rounds. Then she looked at her mother and the therapist with delight and indicated that she wanted each of us to imitate her.

For the first 7 months we did not attempt to use formal tests to measure her progress in order to: 1) maintain as natural an atmosphere as possible in the training sessions; 2) eliminate the possibility of teaching the test items due to constant repetition; and 3) reduce the level of frustration encountered when she could not understand what was required of her in a testing situation. Our testing was designed to coincide with the formal testing usually done at the end of a school year. We believed it important to measure this child's behavior with those instruments that are accessible to therapists and teachers and frequently used to evaluate language behavior in normal and language-impaired populations.

After up to 9 months of training with the device (3 months use of the shelf model followed by up to 6 months use of the wearable vest model) the subject's language skills were measured independently by the teacher at school without the device, and by the therapist at home, using the device. Hearing aids were worn with gain turned on during all testing. Use of the vest stopped at age 42 months.

Vocabulary Growth

A record of T.K.'s understanding of single words presented by adults and other children at home and at school was kept by teacher, therapist, and mother. A word was listed only if T.K. consistently responded appropriately more than three times and demonstrated through action, gesture, or vocalization that she understood. For a word to be recorded, two of the three observers had to list it independently. Words accompanied by additional cues, for example, hand gestures, were included if the cue was considered appropriate to the communicative situation for hearing people. Words were frequently embedded in a variety of syntactical constructions.

Figure 8.4 shows vocabulary growth, in which a semilogarithmic plot indicates a nearly logarithmic growth from age 36 months to 42 months, when use of the vest stopped.

During that period, T.K.'s receptive vocabulary approximately doubled each month. This rate of vocabulary development presents a pattern similar to that observed in hearing children (Benedict, 1976; Ling and Ling, 1978; McCarthy, 1954).

Two important observations may be made about T.K. in the 10 months following introduction of the vibrotactile device. First, her speechreading ability changed significantly. For example, at the end of this period she was able to understand and follow verbal directions for test taking. Secondly, whatever benefits T.K. derived from training with the vibrotactile device were carried over to her unaided speech

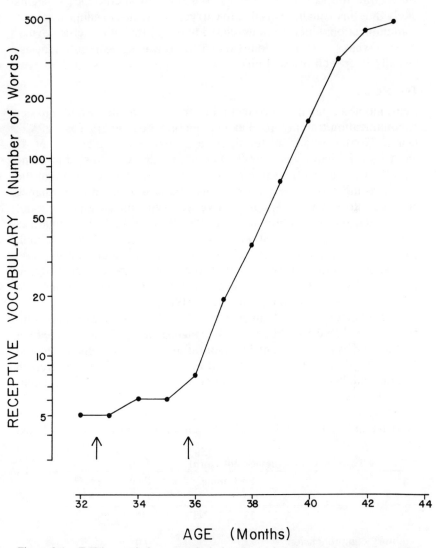

Figure 8.4.   T.K.'s vocabulary growth during the period covered in this report. The arrow on the left indicates initial use of the shelf model vibrotactile device. The arrow on the right indicates changeover to the wearable vest. For a word to be counted as being in her vocabulary, two of three observers (teacher, therapist, mother) had to list it independently.

communication. That is, her receptive and productive competence were quite the same with and without the vibrotactile aid. It seems likely that this equality was due to carryover and not to gains in speech communication which were unrelated to use of the vibrotactile device. After 6 weeks (1978) without the aid there was some regression, especially in speech production.

Test Results

Eight months after the introduction of the vibrotactile device into her communication training, the Peabody Picture Vocabulary Test (PPVT; Dunn, 1965) was administered. At a chronological age (CA) of 41 months, T.K. had a test age (TA) of 30 months when tested at home with the device and the same score when tested at school without the device, using two different forms. This contrasts with her performance at 33 months CA when she had a five-word vocabulary and could not understand the instructions to take the PPVT. Table 8.1 summarizes the results of the PPVT and other clinical tests administered at school, and Table 8.2 the results of the same tests administered at home.

Another clinical instrument that could not be directly administered to the child at the start of the project was the Preschool Language Scale (PLS; Zimmerman, Steiner, and Evatt, 1969).

Three scores are obtained from the PLS test, "auditory comprehension," "verbal ability," and "language age." Tests at school at 40 months CA rated T.K. at 37.5 months auditory comprehension, and 27 months verbal ability. At home at age 42 months CA she scored 38 months and 28 months on the auditory comprehension and verbal ability scales, respectively.

The Receptive-Expressive Emergent Language (REEL) scale (Bzoch and Leaque, 1971) and the Preschool Attainment Record (PAR;

Table 8.1. Tests at school (device not worn)

Test	Pretraining CA	Pretraining TA	Post-training CA	Post-training TA	Gain
PPVT	33	CNT	41	30	
PLS					
Auditory comprehension	33	CNT	40	37.5	
Verbal ability	33	CNT	40	27	
Language age	33	CNT	40	32.3	
REEL					
Receptive language	33	10	40	28	18
Expressive language	33	14	40	31.5	17.5
Combined language	33	12	40	29.7	17.7
PAR	32	37.9	40	50.6	12.7

Table 8.2.   Tests at home (device worn)

Test	Pretraining CA	Pretraining TA	Post-training CA	Post-training TA	Gain
PPVT	33	CNT	41	30	
PLS					
Auditory comprehension	33	CNT	42	38	
Verbal ability	33	CNT	42	28	
Language age	33	CNT	42	33	
REEL					
Receptive language	33	10	42	30	20
Expressive language	33	14	42	33	19
Combined language	33	12	42	31.5	19.5
PAR	33	37.9	42	51	13.1

Doll, 1966) were completed both pre- and post-training with the device. Results of both of these scales, which are based on direct observation of the child's performance and/or information gained through parent and teacher interview, revealed significant improvement in T.K.'s communicative and social behavior.

The REEL test is based on a rationale that there is a universal and, therefore, predictable pattern of receptive and expressive language during the first 36 months of human life. The presence, absence, or transition of both receptive and expressive language functions is scored. The REEL test was administered at school when T.K. was age 33 months CA (before training with the vibrotactile device) and when she was 40 months CA. Receptive language ages were 10 months and 28 months, respectively, and expressive language ages were 14 months and 31.5 months, respectively. Thus, the gain over the 7-month period was 18 months for receptive language and 17.5 months for expressive language. The same test given at home, with a pretraining and post-training time of 9 months resulted in a 20-month gain for receptive language and a 19-month gain for expressive language.

Hearing-impaired children generally score higher in expressive language and lower in receptive language on the REEL scale than on the PLS. This is because they are given expressive credit for self-talk during play, asking for help with personal needs, attempting to tell about experiences using jargon and words, and so on, on the REEL. At the same time the PLS penalizes them in verbal ability for failure in sentence repetition, digit repetition, correct sound pronunciation, and so on, in which they generally lag behind their hearing counterparts.

It is worth noting that analysis of the REEL results revealed that no regression occurred when pre- and postvibrotactile training scores were compared.

The PAR measures aspects of physical, social, and intellectual achievement through the use of the parent interview and behavioral observation. At 33 months CA, before vibrotactile training, T.K. received an attainment age of 37.9 months; after 7 and 9 months of training she received attainment ages of 50.6 months and 51 months, respectively.

Clearly, T.K.'s age measure on this test was significantly higher than for other language-based tests. The physical area contains aspects of ambulation and manipulation, and the social area includes rapport and communication and responsibility. High ratings in these areas appear to contribute to the high score. As a direct result of the attainment of language skills and communicative ability, T.K. at 40 months and 42 months CA was an extremely independent child who interacted freely with people. These and other aspects of her outgoing personality may be particularly reflected in the social area. In the PAR, however, the most progress was observed to occur in the intellectual area which includes information, ideation, and creativity. The growth in the intellectual area of this test was consistent with the growth trend as measured by other language-based tests.

Speech Production

It is difficult to report receptive language abilities without reference to relevant features of expressive skills. With respect to production, the device made T.K. aware of communication through speech and increased her ability to vocalize. T.K. learned that she could produce speech, and thus control her environment.

Although T.K.'s vocalizations increased in frequency within the first week of therapy, it was not until later that intelligible productions occurred. An early intelligible production was "orange," produced 6 weeks after training. Oranges were then used as tangible reinforcers during subsequent training.

The device helped reduce the lip smacking noted in bilabials /p/, /b/, and /m/, and aided in her differentiation of one-, two-, and three-syllable productions, her attainment of the concept of long versus short sounds, and of loud versus soft sounds, and the production of inaudible phonemes, for example, /p/, /b/, /t/, and /d/. The vibrotactile device aided in the production of a variety of consonant-vowel (CV) and CVC combinations, affected her rate of production, improved breath control, and affected change in voice quality, primarily loudness.

The gains in speech production did not keep pace with her speech reception and comprehension. At the end of the project, T.K. spent 6 weeks without the device, and her teacher noted a significant difference in intelligibility and voice quality. When the feedback provided by the device was removed, T.K. could not continue to monitor her productions consistently and began to regress in speech production. She had not learned to habituate patterns, particularly for consonants.

Over the observation period, mother, therapist, and teacher had consistently noted the immediate effects of the device on the loudness level of her vocalization. Without the vibrotactile feedback, her voice could become abnormally loud, but would be moderated as soon as she had the device. Furthermore, T.K. could maintain this moderation for 2 to 3 days without the device.

Social Effects

At the beginning of the 1977–78 school year T.K. was a challenging child with whom to work, despite 2 years prior training in a parent-infant program. She was manipulative, frequently rejecting materials and activities designed to interest her. The previous teacher's report described her as "very willful with frequent temper outbursts." Much of this behavior can be attributed to a breakdown in communication. T.K. neither understood much of what was being said to her, nor could she make her wishes known to others. The frustration was great and resulted in temper tantrums.

Not long after she started using the vibrotactile device, T.K.'s receptive and expressive communication skills improved and gradual but constant change was noted in her behavior. As she began to understand certain things expected of her and could, in turn, exert influence over others through speech and language, she became more reasonable. There were fewer temper displays, she was happier and calmer than before, and she began to interact with other adults and children, taking the initiative in communication and play. Through counseling and as T.K. progressed, her parents became less anxious and more optimistic. A more relaxed attitude, as well as improved ability to handle their child's behavior and communication, significantly altered the home situation. The parents became adept at home carryover and reinforcement of language skills. With improved communication skills, positive aspects of T.K.'s personality began to emerge. She became a very personable and outgoing little girl, exhibiting a sense of humor, a cooperative nature, and a desire to please others. Her tolerance of limitations and rules improved as her ability to understand the explanations improved. This change in behavior and personality significantly contributed to her learning at home and school, and with each new skill added, her behavior improved.

DISCUSSION

The long-range goal is to develop a tactile aid for the profoundly deaf that would provide a substitute sensory input for the lost auditory input (Bach-y-rita, 1972). The visual system is this kind of sensory substitute when a nonauditory person speechreads.

The simple wearable device provided T.K. did *not* act as a sensory substitute. Her speech communication performance by every measure employed was as good without the device as with it. It seems likely, however, that her impressive gains in speech and language competence are in part attributable to experience with the vibrotactile device.

There are two main reasons the sensory substitution approach was not really tested here: 1) the device was worn 1 or 2 hours a day, not all the child's waking hours; and 2) single-channel skin stimulation probably cannot provide a rich enough input for sensory substitution during the critical periods of language learning. It is worth mentioning that Saunders is using a vocoder-type belt stimulator with deaf school children (see Saunders, Hill, and Simpson, 1976). He uses electrotactile stimulation and appears to have solved the main problems others have had with that approach. Another group (Sparks et al., 1978, 1979) has been experimenting with a raster-type electrocutaneous input.

One question to be answered was how a child would accept a vibrotactile aid. T.K.'s acceptance of vibrotactile stimulation was indicated at the start of the school year following the one described in the present report. Her teacher requested the shelf model device for use in voice production training. When it was brought to the school in September, T.K. greeted it with delight, like a fond friend. She vocalized, feeling the vibration, and passed the vibrator around the table so that others could do the same.

Although not a substitute for hearing, the vibrotactile input was effective in the development of this subject's comprehension of spoken language. Clinical results may have implications for those who suggest that comprehension precedes production (Benedict, 1978; Gleitman, Shipley, and Smith, 1978; Newport, Gleitman, and Gleitman, 1975; Shatz, 1975; Shipley, Smith, and Gleitman, 1979). For a profoundly deaf child such as T.K., the device provided awareness of speech; that is, she learned when speech sounds were present, and then visually searched the immediate environment to identify the speaker. Once she had learned to identify who the speaker was, she began to focus on what the speaker said.

With the device, T.K. could respond to speech at 65 dB SPL (normal conversational level), and the need for people to scream at her or constantly touch and pull her to get her attention was eliminated. After using the device for an average of 15 hours per week for 5 weeks, T.K. could search her immediate environment and tune in to the appropriate speaker. This in itself greatly relaxed the communicative situation at home for parents, relatives, and T.K. herself. This was contrasted with her behavior at the start of the project when speech and/or sound had very little, if any, meaning for her.

For children with profound hearing loss, understanding the rhythmical patterns of speech is most difficult. We believe the device was particularly useful in providing suprasegmental aspects of speech such as duration, rhythm, and loudness. The vibratory patterns which she felt and used in conjunction with watching the speaker(s) probably enhanced her learning of speechreading skills. Also, T.K. learned to speechread well from watching profiles, particularly of mother, father, and teacher.

Erber (1977) has suggested that vision is the main compensatory sense used for speech perception in the profoundly deaf child and that the vibratory sense is most beneficial as an aid to lipreading. We believe our clinical test results support this concept. The device provided suprasegmental information (tactile) concurrent with the visual display of the human face (speechreading), which provided segmental information. The variety of natural communicative situations in which she was placed served as positive reinforcers when T.K. demonstrated that she understood a particular word or task. The device seemed to speed up the process of learning speechreading and she was able to carry over the benefits to times when she was not wearing the vest. That is, after she learned certain relationships through using the device, she consistently used the information in appropriate contexts: she was able to speechread easily when not using the device (see Table 8.1).

Tables 8.1 and 8.2 show consistency of results obtained in the home setting and at school. Test performance was not dependent on wearing the vibrotactile device, and results were robust enough not to be greatly affected by setting or by the person administering the tests. The comparison of test results obtained at 33 months CA and at 40 to 42 months CA shows a dramatic gain. It is this gain and the great increase in receptive vocabulary and expressive language skills that reinforce our qualitative belief that the vibrotactile device has been useful in T.K.'s development of speech communication skills.

CONCLUSIONS

As a result of our preliminary work with one nonauditory child, we can say:

1. A wearable tactile device can make the child aware of sound and speech and her ability to produce speech. This awareness can ease the communicative situation by helping her understand what is being said and making her speech more intelligible to others.
2. A single channel vibrotactile device, used in conjunction with traditional oral teaching techniques, can aid in developing receptive language skills, particularly vocabulary acquisition, and speechreading.
3. The gains in receptive and expressive speech communication made using the vibrotactile aid are carried over to speech communication without the aid.
4. Clinical tests are useful as measures of language change, reinforcing our qualitative judgment that the device was helpful.
5. Using home therapy as well as school therapy allows opportunities to develop better methods of quantifying observations. Most important, it encourages parents to be good observers and reporters.

ACKNOWLEDGMENT

Initial work on this project was supported by the National Foundation, March of Dimes. We gratefully acknowledge contribution of funds and facilities by the Electrical Engineering Department, Johns Hopkins University; the White Oak School, Baltimore County; the Hearing and Speech Clinic of the Johns Hopkins Hospital; and the Department of Speech Pathology and Audiology, Northeastern University. Eric Naviaski was responsible for the final electronic design and fabrication of the vibrotactile device. Dr. Goldstein's long-range research project with the aim of developing a wearable cutaneous speech communication aid for the deaf is supported by the National Science Foundation and the Rehabilitation Engineering Center, Gallaudet College.

REFERENCES

Bach-y-rita, P. 1972. Brain Mechanisms in Sensory Substitution. Academic Press, New York.
Beguesse, I. M. 1976. A single channel tactile aid for the deaf. Master's thesis, Massachusetts Institute of Technology, Cambridge, Mass.
Benedict, H. E. 1976. Language comprehension in 10 to 16 month old infants. Doctoral dissertation, Yale University, New Haven, Conn.
Benedict, H. 1978. Language comprehension in 9–15 month old infants. In R. Campbell and P. Smith (eds.), Recent Advances in the Psychology of Language. Plenum Press, New York.

Boothroyd, A. 1970. Distribution of Hearing Levels in the Student Population of the Clarke School for the Deaf. S.A.R.P. Report #3. Clarke School for the Deaf, Northampton, Mass.

Bruner, J. 1975. The ontogenesis of speech acts. J Child Lang. 2:1–20.

Bzoch, K. R., and R. Leaque. 1971. Receptive-Expressive Emergent Language Scale. Tree of Life Press, Gainesville, Fla.

Doll, E. 1966. Preschool Attainment Record. American Guidance Service, Inc., Circle Pines, Minn.

Dunn, L. M. 1965. Peabody Picture Vocabulary Test. American Guidance Service, Inc., Circle Pines, Minn.

Erber, N. P. 1974. Discussion of sensory capabilities. In R. E. Stark (ed.), Sensory Capabilities of Hearing Impaired Children. University Park Press, Baltimore.

Erber, N. P. 1977. Speech perception by profoundly deaf children. Paper presented at the Research Conference on Speech Processing Aids for the Deaf. May, Washington, D.C.

Gleitman, L., E. Shipley, and C. Smith. 1978. Old and new ways not to study comprehension. J. Child Lang. 5:501–519.

Goldstein, M. H., and R. E. Stark. 1976. Modification of vocalizations of preschool deaf children by vibrotactile and visual displays. J. Acoust. Soc. Am. 59:1477–1481.

Hardy, W. G., and M. P. Hardy. 1971. Lecture notes. Courses in philosophy of language and aural rehabilitation. The Johns Hopkins University, Baltimore.

Ling, D. 1976. Speech and the Hearing-Impaired Child: Theory and Practice. A. G. Bell Association for the Deaf, Washington, D.C.

Ling, D., and A. Ling. 1978. Aural Habilitation. A. G. Bell Association for the Deaf, Washington, D.C.

McCarthy, D. 1954. Language development in children. In L. Carmichael (ed.), Manual of Child Psychology. Wiley, New York.

Miller, J. 1978. Assessing children's language behavior. A developmental process approach. In R. L. Schiefelbusch (ed.), Bases of Language Intervention. University Park Press, Baltimore.

Newport, E., L. Gleitman, and H. Gleitman. 1975. A study of mother's speech and child language. Papers Rep. Child Lang. Dev. (Stanford Univ.) 10:111–117.

Northcott, W. H., 1977. Curriculum Guide: Hearing-Impaired Children—Birth to Three Years—And Their Parents. A. G. Bell Association for the Deaf, Washington, D.C.

Proctor, A., and M. H. Goldstein. Development of lexical comprehension in a profoundly deaf child using a wearable, vibrotactile communication aid. Language, Speech and Hearing Services in Schools. In press.

Rees, N. 1978. Pragmatics of language: Application to normal and disordered language development. In R. L. Schiefelbusch (ed.), Bases of Language Intervention. University Park Press, Baltimore.

Saunders, F. A., W. A. Hill, and C. A. Simpson. 1976. Speech perception via the tactile mode: Progress report. Conference Record of IEEE International Conference on Acoustics, Speech, and Signal Processing, New York.

Scott, B. L., C. L. DeFilippo, R. M. Sachs, and J. D. Miller. 1977. Evaluating with spoken text a hybrid vibrotactile-electrotactile aid to lipreading. Paper presented at the Research Conference on Speech Processing Aids for the Deaf. May, Washington, D.C.

Shatz, M. 1975. How children respond to language. Papers Rep. Child Lang. Dev. (Stanford Univ.) 10:97–110.

Shipley, H., C. Smith, and L. Gleitman. 1979. A study in the acquisition of syntax: Free responses to verbal commands. Language 45:322–342.

Sparks, D. W., L. A. Ardell, M. Bourgeois, B. Wiedmer, and P. K. Kuhl. 1979. Investigating the MESA (Multipoint Electrotactile Speech Aid): The transmission of connected discourse. J. Acoust. Soc. Am. 65:810–815.

Sparks, D. W., P. K. Kuhl, A. E. Edmonds, and G. Gray. 1978. Investigating the MESA (Multipoint Electrotactile Speech Aid): Segmental features of speech. J. Acoust. Soc. Am. 63:246–257.

van Uden, A. 1977. A World of Language for Deaf Children. 3rd Ed. Swetsand Zeitlinger, Amsterdam and Lisse.

Yoder, D. E., and J. E. Reichle. 1977. Some current perspectives on teaching communication functions to mentally retarded children. In P. Miffler (ed.), Research to Practice in Mental Retardation: Education and Training, Vol. 2. University Park Press, Baltimore.

Zimmerman, I. L., V. G. Steiner, and R. L. Evatt. 1969. Preschool Language Scale. C. E. Merrill, Columbus, Ohio.

ASSESSMENT OF SPEECH PRODUCTION AND PERCEPTION

CHAPTER 9

SOME COMMENTS ON SPEECH ASSESSMENT WITH DEAF CHILDREN

János Mártony and Tekla Tunblad

CONTENTS

The primary aim of this chapter is to summarize the major points of speech assessment with hearing-impaired and deaf children and to outline the requirements for an expanded speech assessment procedure, wherein speech is evaluated with both language proficiency and the general ability to communicate with verbal language. (The term *verbal language* is used for spoken and written languages, differentiated from manual languages, which are produced by hand and face movements.)

As teachers in a Swedish school for the deaf, the authors address the application of speech assessment procedures to the Swedish school system. Therefore, it is necessary to describe briefly the differences between the Swedish school system and those in Great Britain and the United States. In Sweden there are three possible school programs for hearing-impaired children: 1) classes for normally hearing students with individually integrated hearing-impaired children (mainstreaming); 2) partially hearing units (classes) in schools for normally hearing children; and 3) schools for severely hard-of-hearing and deaf children.

The criteria for choosing the type of school program are not only audiological (generally, children with average thresholds at 500 to 2000 Hz better than 90 to 95 dB attend partially hearing units, and those with poorer hearing levels attend schools for the deaf), but also depend on the child's verbal language competence and potential for coping

169

with an entirely oral education. Parents also have great influence in choosing the school programs for their children.

The aim of the Swedish educational system is to make hearing-impaired pupils bilingual, that is, they must have competence in a manual language (genuine Swedish sign language) as well as in a verbal language (Swedish). Both languages are used for teaching in school. This bilingual model is rather new and it is not yet consistently practiced by every teacher. The consequence of this inconsistency is that contrasts and differences between such genuine sign language and Swedish (or signed Swedish) are not made clear and, therefore, a mixture of these two languages is accepted in the classroom.

School attendance in Sweden is compulsory beginning at age 7. The home guidance and preschool program has no general curriculum, so that by age 7 hearing-impaired children have rather different levels of language proficiency. Early reading is generally included in the preschool work but there is no systematic speech training. The children's home situations also vary greatly, in that parents are using genuine sign language, signed Swedish with or without speech, or speech only. In approximately 24% of the families at our school the mother tongue, if a spoken language, is not Swedish.

WHAT DO WE WANT TO MEASURE AND WHY?

How realistic are we when judging the speech quality of a hearing-impaired or deaf child? Either we see only deviations and errors of speech which would have to be corrected on all possible occasions— or we consider the speech good, even though the child will not be understood when speaking to someone other than the classroom teacher or parents. Speech assessment provides a more objective measure of the speech quality of the speaker and some data important to improve the pedagogic work. Speech assessment should 1) measure speech quality and describe errors; 2) make a diagnosis of underlying reasons for the occurrence of errors; and 3) develop a speech training program based on the results.

When measuring speech quality and errors, the entire speech production process should be studied, including breathing, phonation, segmental features, and suprasegmental features. Breathing during speech refers to breathing technique, phonation, and planning of articulatory activity (see Whitehead, this volume). Characteristics of phonation, such as voice quality and pitch level, should be observed. Segmental features are the speaker's phonological system and its phonetic realization (see Fisher et al., this volume). Suprasegmental features include speech tempo, pausing, coarticulation, duration, stress, intonation, nasality, and pharyngealization (see Stevens, Nickerson, and Rollins, this volume).

When making a diagnosis of the underlying reasons for speech errors one should deal with three different considerations. There is a lack of linguistic knowledge; for example, the student does not know the important difference between "a" and "å" (/a/ and /o/), between short and long speech sounds, or that different intonation contours and stress patterns have different meanings. Additionally, there is a lack of knowledge about production; for example, the student does not know how to produce the difference between /ş/ and /ç/. Difficulties also exist in control, that is, there is no internal feedback of the speaker's own production. The speaker may know theoretically how to produce /u/ or /o/ but not know whether the tongue position or jaw opening is precisely correct when producing the vowel because he or she is not using internal feedback signals.

Levitt and Stromberg (this volume) categorized speech errors of hearing-impaired speakers into three groups: 1) errors typical for all hearing-impaired speakers; 2) errors typical for students of one school, and 3) individual errors. The following observations can be made upon comparing our groups of errors with those of Levitt and Stromberg. Errors of the first type are those for which internal control is difficult to learn (e.g., onset time in stops), or for which there are no simple explicit language rules (e.g., speech rhythm). Errors also occur when the teaching methods used at one specific school are not sufficiently adequate. In our experience this usually results from a lack of linguistic knowledge or knowledge of production. The following case study exemplifies different reasons for speech errors.

A student (age, 12;9, hearing loss, 105 dB, no hearing aid used) read a list of long Swedish vowels (/b/-V syllables, 4 repetitions in random order). The material was videotaped and presented to two groups of sophisticated listeners (teachers of the hearing impaired). The first group lipread the speaker (no audio signal) and made a phonemic transcription of the vowels. They correctly identified 55% of the material (Figure 9.1A) which is within the normal range (Mártony, 1974). The results indicated that /i/ and /e/ are produced with a somewhat larger jaw opening. For other vowels the visual articulation was normal.

The second group of subjects listened to and transcribed the vowels (with no videotaped signal). The subjects did not know which vowel was intended. The results of the listening test, shown in Figure 9.1B, indicated that /i/ and /e/ were perceived as a more open vowel such as [ɛ]. All five of the rounded vowels were perceived as rounded back

/b/-V

SUBJECT: M   AGE 12.9 YEARS ♀

A. LIPREADING:

55%

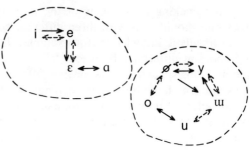

B. AUDITORY
PERCEPTION

42%

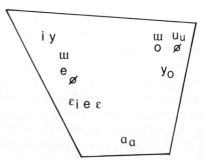

C. ARTULATION
IDENTIFICATION   CORRECT LIPROUNDING

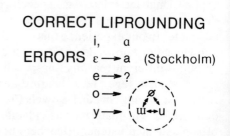

1.) KNOWS HOW TO PRODUCE "i" BUT DOESN'T DO IT.

2.) NO KNOWLEDGE ABOUT BACK VOWEL TONGUE POSITION.

Figure 9.1.   Results of vowel test for a hearing-impaired speaker. A, Result of lipreading of the speaker's vowels. Lines and arrows show typical confusions, the dotted lines show typical confusions for normal hearing native speakers. B, Result of auditory perception and phonetic transcription of vowels. Smaller letters show place of the correct Swedish vowels; larger letters show the intended vowel. The place of the letter gives the phonetic quality. C, Result of identification of articulatory pictures of different vowels.

vowels, and the tongue height was incorrect. The articulatory parameters of jaw opening and tongue height can be separated by comparing the results of the visual-only and auditory-only perception tasks.

The student identified articulatory pictures (midsagittal section and "en face") for different vowels to check her knowledge of articulation. She correctly discriminated between unrounded and rounded vowels (Figure 9.1C). All /i/ and /a/ articulations were correctly identified. When /ɛ/ was identified as /a/ this was accepted as no error because /ɛ/ is realized as /e/ in Stockholm Swedish. No rounded vowels were correctly identified. In summary, the data show that the speaker had correct articulatory knowledge of /i/ but not enough articulatory control to correctly produce it. The speaker also had insufficient knowledge of tongue position and height for the rounded vowels. (A similar but simplified procedure can be used in the speech clinic for making diagnosis: the student reads one unknown random word list while the teacher lipreads or listens; no audio or video recording is necessary.)

When planning speech training and correction we can utilize a hierarchy of statements, such as good aerodynamic control is necessary for phonation; good phonation is necessary for speech production, and so on. However, there are other possible ways to begin: 1) work with speech features which most improve intelligibility or naturalness; 2) work on those speech errors that make speaking difficult for the child; or 3) work with speech errors that are easy to correct. This gives the child positive reinforcement and motivation for continuing speech work.

There are not enough research data which show the importance of different speech features for intelligibility and naturalness of speech. However, Florén (1980) showed some correlations of general speech intelligibility to vowel and consonant quality. Florén recorded the speech of 24 students (ages 15 to 17; hearing loss greater than 95 dB$_m$) at the Manilla School for the Deaf in Stockholm. The recorded material included: 1) lists of long vowels in /b/-V syllables for measuring vowel quality (e.g., bi, be, ba); 2) a list of rhyming words for measuring voiced/voiceless ("pil-bil, får-vår"), nasal/nonnasal ("läsa-näsa"), and continuant/noncontinuant ("sår-tår-står") consonant features; and 3) a list of simple questions for the reversed Helen test. The Helen test (see Ewertsen, 1973) is used to measure audiovisual perception of hearing-impaired subjects. The subjects answer simple questions. A correct answer gives a quick measure of the person's speech perception ability. In the reversed Helen test the hearing-impaired speaker reads a question aloud, for example, "How much is 2 plus 2?" "What color is a lemon?" If normally hearing subjects give the correct answers to most of the questions, this indicates that the speech has been understood and that the communicative quality is sufficient. In Florén's (1980) study, a group of trained listeners were asked to identify the vowels and consonants (forced-choice situation) and answer the questions.

Figure 9.2 shows the correlation between vowel quality (percentage of vowels correctly perceived) and general speech quality (percentage of sentences correctly perceived). The data are corrected for guessing (11% for vowels). There is a correlation between vowel quality and speech quality. Correct vowel quality, however, is not important for speech quality. As is shown in Figure 9.2 the sentence perception is rather high, with about 50% vowel perception.

Figure 9.3 shows the correlation between consonant feature quality and general speech quality. The data are corrected for guessing (44.4% for consonants). The correlation between correctly perceived

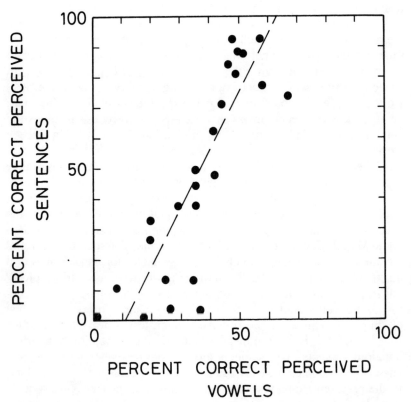

Figure 9.2.   Perception of vowels and questions in speech of 24 hearing-impaired speakers (corrected for guessing).

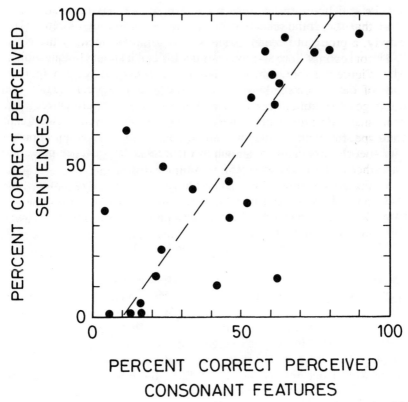

PERCENT CORRECT PERCEIVED
CONSONANT FEATURES

Figure 9.3.   Perception of some consonant features and questions in speech of 24 hearing-impaired speakers (corrected for guessing).

consonant features and general speech quality is not as good as between vowels and speech, but Figure 9.3 shows that good consonant quality is important for speech quality. This investigation is not complete because it lacks data on the influence of prosody on speech quality, but it can give some help in the planning of speech training.

SOME COMMENTS ON SPEECH ASSESSMENT

The question is often raised whether to use spontaneous speech or lists of words, phrases, and sentences in speech tests. When we measure the segmental features, prepared material can be used, which makes the assessment easier. In addition to assessment of the overall quality of speech, the contrast between speech sounds or speech features is important. Therefore, minimal pairs in prepared speech material can be very useful. If the speaker does not produce a contrast, for example, between voiced and voiceless stops (/b/-/p/), different voiceless fricatives (/ş, ʃ, ç/), or long-short vowels (/si:l, sil:/), it should be determined whether the speaker is able to perceive the contrast in minimal pairs and whether he or she knows the linguistic importance of these contrasts. Written stimuli can be used for this purpose and the child can be questioned as to whether he or she can explain the meaning of some contrasts, for example, the meaning of "sil" /si:l/ (strainer) and "sill" /sil:/ (herring), or make a sentence with "banan" (banana; the path). The use of minimal pairs might be an indicator of the speaker's phonological system. For diagnosing underlying causes of speech errors, evaluation of the variation in phonetic context is important. For example, we are using lists of words and phrases with different vowel and consonant contexts for measuring voice quality.

In the assessment of segmental features, both phonemic (broad) and phonetic (narrow) transcription have to be made to allow us to describe the speaker's phonological system and its realization. It is also necessary to observe articulation (lip, jaw, and tongue movements). It is therefore important to record not only the acoustic signal but also the visual part of the articulation. We prefer that the listeners do not know the words in advance when they perform the phonemic transcription (the material is totally or partially unknown). For example, in our vowel test the listener knows that there will be words of the type /m/-V-/r/ ("myr-mor-mår") but is not informed of the order of the vowels.

We prefer to use spontaneous speech samples (instead of word lists) when we measure the nonsegmental features. In this case, special emphasis must be placed on the evaluation of breathing, phonation, coarticulation, speech tempo, and prosody. With reference to prosody, two different types of speech modes can be observed: 1) articulatory mode, in which the speech is based on the articulation of a sequence of sounds; and 2) prosodic mode, in which the speech is grouped by the prosody in "pitch contours." If the speaker uses the prosodic mode, then this might be an indication that he or she is conscious of the importance of the prosody and is probably able to perceive it by hearing.

When it is not possible to elicit an adequate spontaneous speech sample, the child can be given a written sentence to read and sign using a genuine sign language (to ensure comprehension). The child should then be asked to say it again without the text. If this procedure does not produce an appropriate sample, it can be an indication of verbal language retardation, central language disorders, memory disorders, or it also could be due to a lack of training.

The measurement of the general intelligibility of speech is rather complex. A practical method is the reversed Helen test, as described earlier. What we have described here covers a good method of speech assessment as it exists today. We have to ask, however, whether this kind of assessment is sufficient and, if not, what additions are necessary.

WHY SPEECH ASSESSMENT?

In general terms, the speech assessment should provide us with a measure of the oral communication abilities of a hearing-impaired person and how to improve these abilities with pedagogical work. This implies that we also have to measure factors important for communication and not only speech. These are 1) communication ability and motivation for communication in sign language; 2) verbal language on the lexical, syntactical, and phonological level; 3) communication ability, that is, speech production and perception; 4) motivation for oral communication; 5) audiological data on hearing capacity, including etiology of hearing loss; and 6) other data on secondary handicaps (language dysfunction, motor disorder) and psychological test results (memory span, pattern recognition, etc.). When all these factors are taken into consideration, speech and speech training will then be integrated into the bilingual situation of a hearing-impaired child.

SOME COMMENTS ON THE
PEDAGOGICAL ASPECTS OF SPEECH ASSESSMENT

One of the main questions in speech correction is where to begin. This problem has already been discussed. A second question is how the speech samples should be evaluated. We need a type of normalized speech quality pattern for hearing-impaired children of different ages. This speech quality pattern could then be used to determine which production level we can expect from children of different ages. Apart from the chronological age, speech quality is also dependent on other very important factors: 1) previous language and speech work in verbal and manual language; 2) speech perception capability; 3) ability profile (e.g., general learning ability, motoric ability, spatial ability, etc.); 4) language used at home; and 5) hearing capacity. If the speech quality is below the expected level there is one possible explanation, namely, that the optimal learning period has been missed. Sensory deprivation makes learning of speech production and perception even more difficult for older children. Therefore, it is important when planning future speech work that, in addition to a recommendation regarding what to work on, advice should be given on how intensely speech training should be performed. The pedagogical recommendations should include language learning, perceptual training (auditory, visual, and tactile speech reception), and technical aids for speech production and perception.

To summarize, after assessments are completed, recommendations should be given concerning 1) language training; 2) speech training; 3) coordination of perception training and speech production; 4) amount of training; and 5) technical aids.

CONCLUSIONS

Our assessment program is somewhat unrealistic in that a great proportion of the school time would be spent on testing rather than teaching. More detailed assessment of language and speech could be conducted by the clinic teacher. Hearing capacity, secondary handicaps, ability profile, and so on, can be tested by audiologists or psychologists, respectively. Many of these tests would not require frequent repetition.

The classroom teacher, responsible for all of the pedagogical work in the class, must have a broad knowledge of the students. He or she has to be familiar with the results collected by other members of the evaluation team (clinic teacher, audiologist, psychologist). A good deal of personal observation is also necessary. All of these factors are important for choosing training programs, and so on. The teacher will have to observe the pupils in the following aspects: 1) cognitive aspects and language comprehension; 2) preferred communication mode (sign language, signed Swedish, spoken language, and language spoken at home); 3) frequency of spontaneous verbal communication; 4) speech perception ability (auditory, visual, tactile) in spontaneous communication; 5) use of hearing aid(s); 6) speech production ability and speech mode (articulatory or prosodic mode); 7) use of voice and speech to call for attention, in conversation with other school mates, and in communication with hearing-impaired children and hearing adults; and 8) memory and perception of sequences.

Knowledge about all of these factors and others is necessary in order to organize the school work and the teaching time. Teachers with this kind of implicit and/or explicit knowledge of all pupils can plan for excellent school work, but it is not an easy job. With these comments on speech assessments, the authors hope to draw attention to the necessity for further observation and test development to improve verbal language teaching in schools for hearing-impaired and deaf children.

REFERENCES

Ewertsen, H. W. 1973. Auditive, visual, and audio-visual perception of speech: Operation Helen. First preliminary report. The State Hearing Center, Bispebjerg Hospital, Copenhagen.
Florén, Å. 1980. Some measurements on speech quality of deaf speakers. Unpublished manuscript, University of Stockholm.
Mártony, J. 1974. On speech reading of Swedish consonants and vowels. STL-OPSR 2–3:11–33.

CHAPTER 10

EVALUATION OF SPEECH

Arthur Boothroyd

CONTENTS

When the speech of a hearing-impaired individual is evaluated, several questions may be asked. For example:

1. How effective is the speech in terms of communicating the intended message?
2. How accurate are the sound patterns when compared with those of normally hearing talkers?
3. If there are acoustic inaccuracies, to what extent do they contribute to any lack of effectiveness?
4. What are the underlying motor behaviors which cause the acoustic inaccuracies?
5. Why did the individual develop these motor behaviors?

The purpose of this chapter is to review our ability to answer these questions in the light of current knowledge about normal and pathological speech.

THE NATURE OF SPEECH

Before discussing evaluation, it is appropriate to define speech itself. In fact the word *speech* is used in different ways by different people (and even in different ways by the same person at different times). The following definition is proposed:

> Speech is a system of movements that generate patterns of sound. These movements, and the resulting sounds, represent linguistic structures that in turn represent conceptually organized thoughts. Speech is used for communication among human beings. The linguistic structures fulfill their purpose when they permit a listener to generate the same thoughts as exist in the mind of the talker. The speech patterns fulfill their purpose when they permit a listener to generate the same linguistic structures as exist in the mind of the talker.

This may seem like an unnecessarily complicated definition, but verbal communication is complicated. To evaluate speech one must consider its acoustic aspects, its motor aspects, and its linguistic aspects, as well as the active role of the listener in the communicative process.

This last point — the role of the listener — cannot be overstressed. In the communication of linguistic structures, both talker and listener generate language. Each is selecting specific linguistic structures from an internal linguistic repertoire. The difference between talker and listener lies in the source of control for the selection process. In the case of the talker, control comes from within. In the case of the listener,

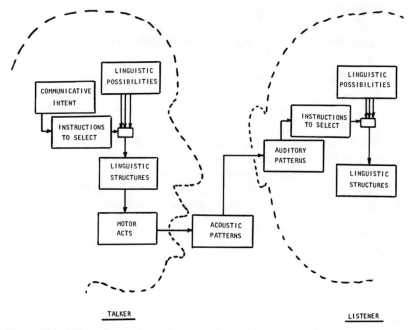

Figure 10.1. The process of speech communication. Note that both talker and listener are generating language.

the process of selection is temporarily guided by the speech patterns of the talker. This concept of speech as "instructions to select" from an internal repertoire is central to an understanding of human communication (see Cherry, 1961). The process is illustrated in Figure 10.1.

EVALUATION OF EFFECTIVENESS

When measuring the effectiveness of speech one is asking, essentially, how well a listener can generate the intended linguistic structures on the basis of acoustic signals generated by the talker. At first sight it should be easy to answer this question. One would simply give the talker some sentences, words, or speech sounds to produce and ask a listener to write down what was said. Because the listener is an active participant in this process, however, our results may be influenced as much by his or her skills and experience as by the speech abilities of the talker.

To complicate things further, the results will be affected by linguistic, semantic, and situational redundancy, because these determine the informational load placed on the acoustic signals.

Yet another problem arises in considering the origin of the linguistic structures. Translating written language into spoken language is very different from translating one's own thoughts into spoken language, and the two processes may result in different kinds of speech behavior.

In devising tests of effectiveness, researchers have adopted a variety of approaches to the problems just discussed.

Hudgins Word Intelligibility Tests

Hudgins (1949) used groups of listeners who were previously unfamiliar with the speech of the deaf and gave them sufficient practice to reach a learning plateau. For linguistic structures he chose words in isolation. The subject under investigation read a phonetically balanced list of words, and the listeners, without the support of context, tried to write down what they heard. Hudgins demonstrated a high correlation between scores obtained with isolated words and those obtained with sentences.

Magner Intelligibility Test

Magner (1972) chose to measure the intelligibility of words in sentence context. She wrote 600 sentences of roughly equal length, containing vocabulary and structures of the type used with deaf children in written language exercises. Each child reads six sentences which are then audited by six students attending a training program for teachers of the deaf. Intelligibility is measured as the percentage of words correctly identified.

Spontaneous Speech Samples

Ling and Milne (1981) reported a procedure in which samples of conversation are dubbed onto a listening tape and audited by persons previously unfamiliar with the speech of the deaf. Intelligibility score is the percentage of words correctly identified.

Intelligibility Ratings

Subtelny and Johnson of NTID modified intelligibility rating scales previously developed at Gallaudet College. Sophisticated listeners audit a recording of the subject's reading of a standard paragraph and estimate the intelligibility on a 5-point scale (Subtelny, 1977).

Articulation Tests

The standard articulation test in which it is determined whether the subject "has" various speech sounds in his or her repertoire, is a test of effectiveness. The linguistic structure is the phoneme. The sounds can be isolated, in words, in read sentences, or in spontaneous speech. The listeners are usually sophisticated and may base scores on their own perceptions or may try to make inferences about the perceptions of unsophisticated listeners. This kind of testing is obviously more analytic than the four described above.

Feature Tests

Boothroyd and Gorzycki (1977) developed a "micro" test of effectiveness in which listeners had only to decide which of two alternative phonemes was intended. They used this procedure to assess adequacy of /s/ - /ʃ/ contrasts and voiced/voiceless distinctions. Suitable test design rendered the results independent of linguistic context and they were also shown to be independent of listener experience.

Another feature test, developed by Nickerson, Stevens, and Rollins (1979), focuses on intonation contours. Low-pass filtering is used to eliminate segmental information and auditors must choose which of several phrases, of equal length but different stress patterns, was intended.

The above procedures vary considerably in terms of validity, reliability, and efficiency. In some cases, information on these three important parameters is just not available. To make matters worse, very little is known about the relationships among scores obtained from these various tests.

ACOUSTIC EVALUATION

When we perform acoustic evaluation of an individual's speech we are essentially asking: How do the acoustic patterns compare with those of normally hearing talkers?

We may perform the evaluation in two ways — by instrument or by ear. Instrumental analysis has the advantage of objectivity. Unfortunately, it tends to provide more information than we can use and offers no clues as to which acoustic parameters are important and which are trivial. Evaluation by ear permits one to focus on the critical features of acoustic patterns but is inherently unreliable. It is in the nature of speech perception to seek the appropriate interpretation of acoustic patterns in spite of their inaccuracies. It takes years of "ear training" before listeners can reliably attend to and identify these inaccuracies.

The results of acoustic evaluation may be expressed in both physical and psychological terms. One describes the stimulus; the other describes the sensation it evokes.

Long Term Vowel Spectrum   This depends on larynx waveform and resonances in the chest, pharynx, nose, and mouth. It is perceived in terms of voice quality (see Figure 10.2).

Aperiodic Noise in Voiced Sounds   This is caused by turbulence of air escaping through the glottis and is perceived in terms of "breathiness" (also illustrated in Figure 10.2).

Time Patterns   One can measure such things as the average speech rate (in syllables per second), the ratio of voiced to voiceless segments, the ratio of speech to silence, and the relative durations of sounds, syllables, and pauses. These parameters are perceived in terms of rate, fluency, rhythm, stress, and syntactic boundaries.

Fundamental Frequency   One can measure average fundamental frequency, which is primarily responsible for perceived pitch. The changes of fundamental frequency over time can also be measured. These changes are perceived in terms of intonation and convey such information as emotional content, syntactic boundaries, stress, and emphasis (see Figure 10.3).

Vowel Spectra   The formant patterns of individual vowels can be measured and compared. These parameters are perceived in terms of vowel quality (see Figures 10.4 and 10.5).

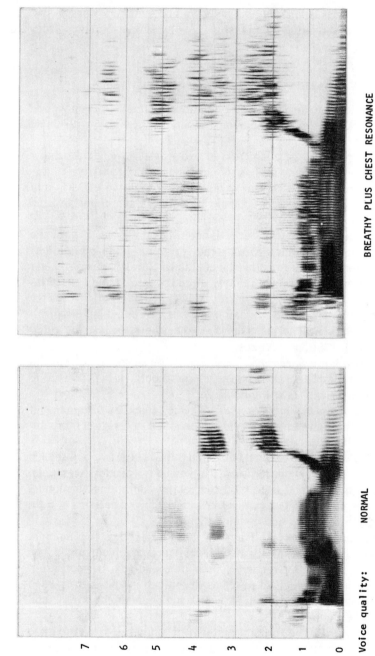

Voice quality: NORMAL   BREATHY PLUS CHEST RESONANCE

Utterance: "Who are we?"

Figure 10.2.   Broad band spectrograms of "Who are we?" spoken by an adult male with normal laryngeal function, and with an excessively breathy voice. Note that, in addition to the aperiodic noise produced by breathiness, there is a loss of definition of the first formant. This is caused by a reduction of sound reflections from the glottis and the partial replacement of oral resonance by chest resonance.

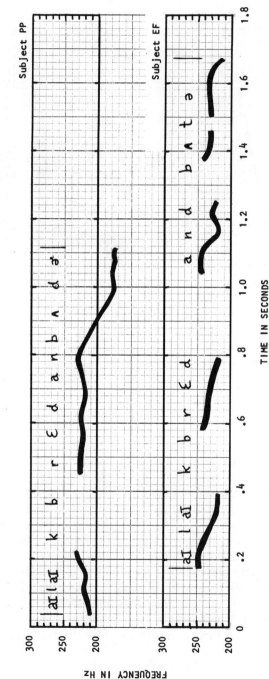

Figure 10.3.   Fundamental frequency contours of two 14-year-old girls. Both subjects have normal values of average fundamental frequency, but the timing and intonation contours in the lower tracing are abnormal. Subject PP has a 75-dB hearing loss and has acquired speech auditorily. EF has a 113-dB hearing loss and has acquired speech nonauditorily. These contours were prepared by tracing the fifth harmonic in narrow band spectrograms.

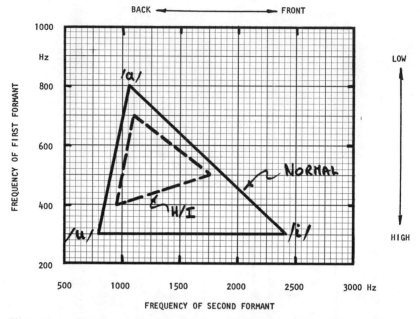

Figure 10.4.   Comparison of first and second formant frequencies for the vowels /u/, /a/, and /i/ in two subjects. AB is an adult male with normal hearing. RG is an adult male with a hearing loss of 105 dB, acquired at age 22 months. These data were obtained from broad band spectrograms (see Figure 10.5).

Consonant Spectra and Time Patterns   These are perceived in terms of a consonant system with underlying features such as voicing, continuance, and place of articulation.

Formant Transitions   The mutual acoustic influence of contiguous segments is perceived in terms of fluency and concatenation.

Although sound spectrographs and other instrumental aids to speech analysis have been available for many years, they have not been used very much by the professions serving deaf children.[1] There are several practical reasons. For example, the equipment is expensive, the tests are time consuming, and interpretation of results requires considerable expertise in acoustic and physiological phonetics. One of the most serious deterrents, however, is lack of knowledge. It is not yet known exactly which acoustic features are essential to the integrity of speech, how much variation there is among normal speakers, and how much deviation from the norm is permissible in hearing-impaired speakers. This topic is further complicated by the fact that acoustic

[1] A notable exception is to be found in the work of Monsen (1977).

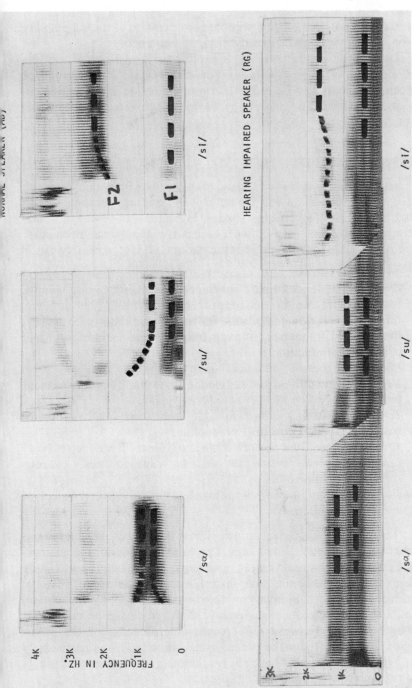

Figure 10.5. Broad band spectrograms used to derive formant frequencies for Figure 10.4. Note that, in addition to a restricted range of variation in formants, there are several other ways in which the spectrograms of RG differ from those of AB. For example, formant transitions are less apparent, formants are less well defined, and the vowels are much longer.

criteria cannot be established without consideration of the adaptability of the listener — a point already discussed at length.

Despite these shortcomings, it is clear that instrumental analysis has much to offer in the description and diagnostic evaluation of speech. It should also be noted that a combination of critical listening and spectrographic analysis is a very effective technique for ear training.

MOTOR EVALUATION

Having determined that the acoustic patterns of an individual's speech differ in some important way from the norm, one may reasonably ask: What are the motor behaviors that account for the deviant acoustic patterns? It would be very simple if each part of the speech mechanism were responsible for a single acoustic parameter. Unfortunately this is not so.

1. *Breathing* influences timing, fundamental frequency, voice quality, vowel spectra, and consonant production.
2. *Laryngeal function and posture* influence breathing, voice quality, fundamental frequency, formant frequency, formant clarity, and consonant production.
3. *Pharyngeal posture* influences voice quality.
4. *Velar function and posture* influence voice quality and consonant production.
5. *Tongue movements and posture* influence voice quality, formant frequencies, and consonant production.
6. *Jaw movements and posture* influence formant frequencies.
7. *Lip movements and posture* influence formant frequencies and consonant production.
8. *Coordination of the above* influences virtually every aspect of speech production.

This complex web of relationships between speech physiology and speech acoustics can, if understood properly, be an aid to diagnosis. For example, hypernasal vowels, plosive/nasal substitutions, and weak fricatives can all have the same underlying cause: failure to close the velopharyngeal port. Similarly, a combination of choppy speech and imploded stops suggests excessive use of glottal closure to control air flow. Sometimes, however, inferential determination of the motor origins of an acoustic error can be very difficult. This is particularly true when two or more motor errors combine to influence a single acoustic parameter, such as voice quality.

Possibilities for direct observation of speech movements and postures are limited. The lips and the jaw, and to a certain extent the tongue, can be seen, but to explore beyond this one must use such techniques as: x-ray, fluorography, electromyography, laryngoscopy, fiber optics, palatography, volume measurement by use of a body plethismograph, measurement of air flow, or measurement of oral or esophageal air pressure. Although these techniques will continue to play an important role in speech research, their potential application in the clinic is limited.

More appropriate to the clinic are compromise techniques such as measurement of glottal waveform from changes of electrical impedance across the larynx (Fourcin and Abberton, 1971), detection of surface vibrations (Stevens, Kalikow, and Willemain, 1975), and measurement of air flow from mouth and nose (Hudgins, 1934). At the present time most clinical evaluations of motor function are performed by inference on the basis of listening. When this is done by persons with inadequate ear training or insufficient knowledge of speech, the results can be grossly misleading.

CAUSATIVE EVALUATION

If 1) the effectiveness of a child's speech has been measured and found to be low; 2) acoustic analysis has been performed and the results have been interpreted in physiological terms; and 3) the deviations have been identified—particularly those most responsible for poor intelligibility; it would be wise to ask one more question before defining developmental or remedial targets and pursuing a course of training. Why does this individual talk the way he or she does? The basic cause is obviously impaired hearing, but superimposed on this must be other causes, because the same hearing loss in another individual by no means results in the same speech characteristics.

Answers to this question must largely be inferential and their formulation requires years of practical experience. Some possibilities are: inadequate use of residual hearing, specific characteristics of the residual hearing, specific teaching techniques (pedagogogenesis), and/or hypertonicity resulting from negative emotional reactions to the speech act. Sensitivity to the issue of genesis may help teachers to avoid remedial approaches that will simply perpetuate the cause of the problem.

PROBLEMS AND NEEDS

Speech evaluation has been discussed in terms of four major questions: How effective is the speech? How accurate are the acoustic patterns?

How accurate are the speech movements? What is the cause of deviant speech patterns?

The ability to answer these questions across a broad spectrum of hearing-impaired children is, at the time of writing, poor. Only a handful of people have the knowledge, the experience, the expertise, and the instrumentation to carry out in-depth evaluation and even then there will be many questions left unanswered.

One of the problems is limited knowledge. A complete understanding of the complex relationship between speech movements and speech acoustics has not yet been achieved. Even more seriously, the relationship between speech acoustics and speech intelligibility is not yet understood fully. (See Nickerson and Stevens, 1980, for a detailed treatment of this topic.) This last problem is complicated by the fact that intelligibility is influenced as much by the listener as by the talker.

It is clear, therefore, that there is more to learn about normal and deviant speech, and that reliable and efficient evaluation procedures are also needed. But this would only help the handful of experts to do a better job. New research — indeed, existing research — will not have practical impact until it is transferred to the teachers and therapists who work with children. The amount of knowledge that is needed by persons who teach hearing-impaired children, and the pitifully inadequate mechanisms by which they must try to acquire it is overwhelming.

The greatest need, in the opinion of the author, is for inservice training. This should not be of the watered-down, sporadic, guest-lecturer type, but must provide opportunities for the people who need the information and the people who have the information to interact, over a protracted period of time, in the "hands on" solution of practical problems with real children. Only then will the accumulated knowledge of decades soak into the fabric of educational practice and find meaningful application.

REFERENCES

Boothroyd, A., and P. Gorzycki. 1977. Sibilant Articulation in Hearing Impaired Children. S. A. R. P. Report 29. Clarke School for the Deaf, Northampton, Mass.
Cherry, C. 1961. On Human Communication. Wiley, New York.
Fourcin, A. J., and E. Abberton. 1971. First applications of a new laryngograph. Med. Biol. Illus. 21:172–182.
Hudgins, C. V. 1934. A comparative study of the speech coordinations of deaf and normal subjects. J. Genet. Psychol. 44:3–48.
Hudgins, C. V. 1949. A method of appraising the speech of the deaf. Volta Rev. 51:597–601, 638.

Ling, D., and M. Milne. 1981. The development of speech in hearing impaired children. In F. Bess, B. A. Freeman, and J. S. Sinclair (eds.), Amplification in Education. A. G. Bell Association for the Deaf, Washington, D. C.

Magner, M. E. 1972. A speech intelligibility test for deaf children. Clarke School for the Deaf, Northampton, Mass.

Monsen, R. B. 1977. Toward measuring how well hearing-impaired children speak. J. Speech Hear. Res. 21:197–219.

Nickerson, R. S., and K. N. Stevens. 1980. Approaches to the study of the relationship between intelligibility and the physical properties of speech. In J. Subtelny (ed.), Speech Assessment and Speech Improvement for the Hearing Impaired. A. G. Bell Association for the Deaf, Washington, D. C.

Nickerson, R. S., K. N. Stevens, and A. M. Rollins. 1979. Research on Computer Based Speech Diagnosis and Speech Training Aids for the Deaf (Report 4029). Bolt, Beranek & Newman, Cambridge, Mass.

Stevens, K. N., D. N. Kalikow, and T. R. Willemain. 1975. The use of a miniature accelerometer for detecting glottal waveforms and nasality. J. Speech Hear. Res. 18:594–599.

Subtelny, J. D. 1977. Assessment of speech with implications for training. In F. H. Bess (ed.), Childhood Deafness: Causation, Assessment and Management. Grune & Stratton, New York.

CHAPTER 11

ASSESSMENT OF SPEECH PRODUCTION AND SPEECH PERCEPTION AS A BASIS FOR THERAPY

John Fisher, Angela King, Ann Parker,
and Richard Wright

CONTENTS

The controversial subject of developing and improving the speech of hearing-impaired children has received much previous attention in the form of textbooks on methodology (see Calvert and Silverman, 1975; Ewing and Ewing, 1954; Haycock, 1933; Ling, 1976). There is also a substantial body of literature which describes patterns found in the speech of hearing-impaired children and adults (Connor, 1971; Hudgins, 1934; Hudgins and Numbers, 1942; Levitt and Smith, 1972; Levitt, Smith, and Stromberg, 1976; Markides, 1970; Monsen, 1976; Smith, 1975). Teachers have been presented with strong claims for disparate approaches to speech development. Yet there is much evidence that, regardless of method, the speech of many profoundly deaf children is unintelligible (Conrad, 1979; Markides, 1970). Furthermore, certain unnatural speech patterns are considered to be the result of teaching methods (Clark, 1975).

It is more difficult, however, to find detailed accounts of the rationale and planning of speech work suitable for individual children. The application of the more theoretical research literature to the practical problems of how to improve a particular child's speech is not always obvious. The basis for such planning should be a detailed assessment of each child's needs; but, for reasons discussed below, the methods that have been used by many investigators to describe the speech patterns found in groups of hearing-impaired children are not necessarily appropriate for assessment of individuals.

Clearly, there is a need for normative data within a population of hearing-impaired children against which to judge the progress of individuals. However, the assessment of speech production and perception serves three distinct purposes. It provides: (1) a basis for planning remedial speech work for individual children; (2) a means of evaluating the results of particular therapeutic programs by assessing the relevant aspects of speech before and after remedial work, with individual children or groups; and (3) information for a general description of the speech perception and production of a defined population based on details from a large number of assessments. Much of the published literature has concentrated on the last purpose and it is difficult to abstract information relevant to other aims because categories are oversimplified and too general. This chapter begins with the first aim of assessment and discusses the description of individuals' speech. It is the most relevant area for the teacher and speech-language pathologist and, it is argued, only by developing satisfactory procedures for individuals can the researcher gather valid information about linguistically relevant patterns found in groups of people.

ANALYSIS OF SPEECH

Limitations of Error Analysis

A popular type of analysis of the speech of hearing-impaired people is the "error" analysis which compares tokens produced by hearing-impaired speakers with an inventory of adult normal speech targets (often particular phonemes as realized in particular words). A speech sound in a word is classified as "correct" or not; errors are often subdivided into substitutions (the incorrect sound produced is recognized as an allophone of an English phoneme other than the target sound, e.g., an adult normal /k/ is realized as /tʰ/, distortions (the produced sound not being a possible realization of an English phoneme, e.g., the voiced bilabial implosive /ɓ/ for adult normal /b/), and omissions. Data analyzed in this way form the basis of a description of the number of errors of a particular type in the speech of individuals and groups, and have provided interesting information about typical error patterns in the speech of the hearing impaired. Classically, the profoundly deaf speaker produces fewer place-of-articulation errors than either manner-of-articulation or voiced/voiceless errors (see Hudgins and Numbers, 1942; Levitt, 1971; Levitt and Smith, 1972; Levitt et al., 1976). To some extent, the technique can be applied to prosodic features, such as voice quality and pitch.

The technique of analysis of errors, however, has some serious limitations of both a theoretical and a practical nature (see list below and Grunwell, 1975; Ingram, 1976; King and Parker, 1980; and Monsen, 1976), meaning that the validity and usefulness of some results are questionable. These limitations include:

1. Assumption of normal system with only phonetic level errors
2. Articulatorily (speech production) based
3. Predominantly segmental analysis; little on prosodics
4. Prosodic analysis is usually at the phonetic level, for example, there are few references in the literature to the contrastive use of the falling nuclear tone (see Ashby, 1978) but many to poor voice quality
5. Structural (syntagmatic) analysis is rarely made in detail since comparison is of child's single phonetic level tokens with the adult normal phonemic inventory
6. Assumes consistency in child's productions; often only one token for a word is elicited
7. Ignores interaction with other levels of speech production and perception

The basis of error analysis is linguistically unsound because it ignores the possibility that hearing-impaired speakers may not simply have "errors" in speech but may be employing a system which differs from the adult normal model both at the phonetic (or realization) level and at the phonological level (Grunwell, 1975; King and Parker, 1980; Monsen, 1976). If this is the case, then a simple mapping of the production of a hearing-impaired speaker onto the phonemic inventory of the normal speaker of English will be as inappropriate as attempting

Table 11.1.   Examples of patterns in the speech of hearing-impaired children

Adult normal system			
Sounds contrasted	Example	Child's speech	Description	Notes
p b m	pen Ben men	b b b	System reduction; here the adult-normal 3-term contrast is reduced to one term in the child's production.	Work concentrates on system expansion at the phonologic level, and is based on checking and then training the child's ability to perceive the contrasts which provide meaning differences in language, before working on production.
b	Ben	b ɓ (implosive p' (ejective) mb	Each production is different; whereas the adult normal system produces a voiced bilabial plosive consistently for this word, certain features in the child's system are in free variation.	Error analysis of only one of these examples could have produced any one of three different results (correct, distortion, or substitution), all of which would have been misleading. Speech work concentrates on stabilizing consistent use of phonetic contrasts in the child's productions.

p	pike, pen, pan	b	Phonologic-level contrast is maintained by the child, although phonetic-level realization is abnormal.	Broad transcription might have failed to acknowledge child's consistent use of a contrast. In this case, to familiar listeners, the contrasts will be intelligible (though abnormally produced) and speech therapy may concentrate first on other areas of the child's production in which the phonologic system is reduced.
b	bike, Ben, ban	ɓ (implosive)		
m	Mike, men, man	~b (prevoiced)		
p	pan	p	Contrast is maintained but not all features are normal; in this case, bilabial place is appropriately contrasted with labiodental.	Error analysis from tape or broad transcription may fail to note good use of place contrast and record [p] in both cases ('substitution'). The important fact that the lipreader sees an appropriate contrast is lost.
f	fan	p̪ (labiodental)		

to transcribe French, Turkish, or Arabic using only English phonemic symbols. Furthermore, in some cases such an approach could lead to inappropriate attempts to "correct" speech.

For example, the speaker who produces voiced bilabial implosive /ɓ/ in the word *bin* may be described as producing a distortion error; production of voiced bilabial plosive /b/ in *pin* is described as a substitution error. But if these two errors are produced consistently by one speaker, the important fact to capture in the descriptive analysis is that the voiced/voiceless contrast for this speaker is maintained. In other words, at the phonological level, the linguistic contrast is intact even though the phonetic realization is not normal. Work to correct the more serious of the errors (the voiced bilabial implosive) to a /b/ will clearly, in this case, reduce the speaker's contrastive system and, therefore, reduce speech intelligibility rather than improve it. An analysis of the speech of hearing-impaired speakers which accounts for this type of pattern is not as simple as error analysis and requires trained listeners, but it reveals many more interesting and relevant patterns at the phonological level, some of which are illustrated in Table 11.1. Furthermore, it allows a more comprehensive analysis of prosodic features at both levels (phonetic and phonological) and, where other linguistic levels are included, provides a more realistic framework within which to plan remediation.

Levels of Linguistic Analysis

Assessment requires a framework of categories within which speech is described. Many workers have relied for this purpose on a traditional separation of "language" from "speech" or "articulation" (Ewing and Ewing, 1954; Ling, 1976). This dichotomy is theoretically unsound and causes unnecessary practical difficulties. For example, if intonation contours are described without reference to systematic contrasts of syntax and meaning (see Ashby, 1978; O'Connor and Arnold, 1961), their linguistic role for the hearing-impaired speaker is ignored. A more appropriate framework is provided by the well-established convention in linguistics of a hierarchy of levels for analyzing spoken language (speech): semantic, syntactic, phonological, and phonetic (Lyons, 1968; Malmberg, 1968; Robins, 1964; de Saussure, 1966).

The limitations of the error analysis approach and the need for systematic and detailed assessment at all linguistic levels lead to a rather different approach to the assessment of speech production and speech perception. The procedure described below is intended to provide a detailed account of the child's abilities at phonetic and phonological levels as a basis for comparison with tests at other levels

(Crystal, Fletcher, and Garman, 1976; Reynell, 1977) in order to select priorities for speech therapy.

ASSESSMENT OF SPEECH PRODUCTION

Requirements of an Assessment Procedure

It is essential that the material collected for assessment of speech production is tape recorded to a high standard so that thorough transcription and analysis can be carried out. To be capable of fulfilling the three goals listed above, assessment must follow a consistent, repeatable procedure that is comprehensively applicable to children at various stages in development of overall language ability. The language sample should include various levels of complexity, and both systematically elicited and spontaneous speech. Material collected must be capable of being analyzed at all linguistic levels. Similarly, assessment of receptive abilities should include different linguistic levels.

The part of the assessment concerned with the segmental aspects of speech involves particular requirements which bear examination in more detail. The main reason for assessing speech production and perception is to provide a basis for planning remedial work. Our assessment therefore describes the contrastive system used in the child's own speech and compares these contrasts with the contrasts of the adult normal system. This procedure is quite different from a nonlinguistic item-by-item comparison of the elements of the two systems, which would exclude the child's own phonology. Structural (syntagmatic) relations are also analyzed and compared. Programs of therapy can then be planned specifically to expand the child's system and make it more consistent. We place heavy emphasis on auditory training as an initial stage in each therapy program on the grounds that maximum use of residual hearing to discriminate speech sound contrasts will give the child the most efficient means of monitoring his or her own production. Therefore, the assessment of speech perception, like that of speech production, is designed to be a basis for planning therapy. Before beginning auditory training, one should assess the child's present ability to discriminate and to label syllables which differ along the acoustic dimensions cueing adult normal phonemic contrasts.

The assessment of speech production and perception is designed to encompass suprasegmental aspects as well as speech sound system and structure. Within the suprasegmental category is included not only phonetic level features such as voice quality and overall pitch or timing, but also an examination of the use of prosodic features to make linguistic contrasts. This is compared with the adult normal system of contrastive intonation.

In order that assessments may be compared, both for an individual child at different times (e.g., before and after a program of therapy) and between children or between defined groups (e.g., children in different educational environments), it is essential that from the detailed analysis an unambiguous set of descriptive categories may be derived. This is achieved in part by using assessors who are not only phonetically trained, but also have considerable experience in listening to the speech of hearing-impaired people, and who are employing prescribed levels of transcription and an agreed, consistent terminology. It is also assisted by having a preset format for recording the results of analysis. Format is dictated by what is already known, from practical experience and from existing research, about the common differences between the speech of hearing-impaired people and that of people with normal hearing. But it also allows for discrepancies from predicted patterns. A standard set of descriptive categories enables comparison of assessments, checking by other assessors, and checking against physical speech measurements.

Material for Assessment of Speech Production

The tape-recorded material collected for assessment includes single words, sentences, utterances with contrastive patterns of sentence stress, stories, and spontaneous speech.

One hundred single words are elicited using a set of color pictures. In addition, 10 of them are elicited a second time as a check on productive consistency. If the child fails to produce a word spontaneously, imitation is used and this is noted on the transcription sheet. For children who have little spontaneous production even at the single word level, a shortened list is employed. The selection of words was made according to two main criteria: (1) the words were within the vocabulary of the majority of 5- to 12-year-old hearing-impaired children in the schools in which we work, and (2) the set of words included minimal or nearly minimal pairs for each syllable-initial consonant contrast in the adult normal system and for the range of vowel contrasts. A range of word structures was also included.

Twenty sentences are elicited by recall from the written form (look, remember, speak). The sentences are short, familiar classroom expressions, varying in grammatical structure.

Utterances with contrastive patterns of sentence stress are elicited by asking questions about a set of pictures, attempting to evoke similar replies but with the stress in different positions in the sentence. For example, "Is Pat wearing blue *trousers?*" to elicit something like "No! She's wearing a blue *dress,*" paired with "Is Pat wearing a *red* dress?" to get back something like "No, a *blue* dress."

A short, written text of a story is used at a language level appropriate for a normally hearing 6- to 7-year-old child. It includes many items from the single word list to allow comparison between production of a word in isolation and in connected speech. The text is accompanied by a picture sequence, allowing various options of telling, reading, and retelling, depending on the abilities of the particular child.

For the spontaneous speech sample all children are asked to count to 10 and recite the days of the week. A sample conversation is recorded also, with prompting questions or use of objects or pictures if necessary. For children whose spoken language is extremely restricted, an imitation procedure is adopted incorporating nonsense words with different patterns of syllable rhythm, pitch change, names of familiar objects and classmates, and familiar classroom phrases. A sample assessment form, with description of the format in which the analysis is recorded, is given in the Appendix.

Transcription

To perform the phonological analysis described above, it is necessary to transcribe narrowly the set of single words, sometimes using new symbols for sounds not used as segments in known languages. This level is needed for a full description of the child's system and to reveal those instances in which a contrast is preserved, but with abnormal phonetic realizations. Similarly, it is necessary to transcribe prosodic features in a way that does not assume use of a normal pitch-based system of contrastive intonation.

For hearing-impaired children, it is important that a transcription be made at the time of recording, and a second one from tape, or at least that the initial transcription be checked against the auditory information from the recording. The point is that the phonological system of a hearing-impaired person is often more complete visually than auditorily. For example, articulatory movements may be made in the absence of either phonation or air stream, particularly at the ends of words, resulting in no auditory effect. Vowels may also be more distinguishable visually, and so on.

ASSESSMENT OF SPEECH PERCEPTION

Speech production assessment alone, however detailed, provides a limited view of speech communication ability; an important part of any assessment is an evaluation of receptive ability. Various tests exist for language comprehension at higher linguistic levels (in Britain, for example, the Reynell Developmental Language Scales; Reynell, 1977) but work at phonetic and phonological levels, which is particularly important where the primary impairment is in auditory perception of speech patterns, has been confined to the use of word and sentence lists for error analysis. The lists are primarily designed for comparison of scores under different listening conditions (see Levitt et al., 1978, for a review). Where the aim is to assess pattern perception as a basis for remedial auditory and speech production training, there is a need for tests of the contrasts important in speech communication, that is, the contrasts relevant at the phonological level of language.

Requirements of Perception Tests

To be capable of performing a detailed assessment of phonological level the tests must meet several criteria. The tests must evaluate specific features, that is, a single contrast is to be the stimulus variable. Specific linguistic levels involved in task success should be clearly identified. Small increments in degree of contrast must be available to allow measurement of small changes in performance. The input must be speech-like to allow speech-mode processing.

Testing children aged 3 years and older requires consideration of the cognitive demand and attention requirements of tasks. The cognitive demand should be as simple as possible, with appropriate training procedures and a method to test subject task competence. It must be possible to divide the task into short sections (5 minutes or less), with free control of stimulus interval within the sections.

The task must also allow for attention control to know the child is attending, and to restore attention as well as confidence control if needed. The task must be comfortable and rewarding, and allow for appropriate—occasionally massive—doses of positive reinforcement.

Testing hearing-impaired children introduces extra considerations. A consistent method should be used to ensure optimum stimulus amplitude for each child. If necessary, the entire job of task training and running the test should be possible without requiring verbal or sign language skills on the part of the child. Finally, to be used practically, the test should require minimum equipment. Our goal was a test to be run by one person using one cassette deck and a speech trainer for amplification.

Existing Tests

Attempts to perform a detailed investigation of auditory performance generally fall into two categories: psychophysical measures and natural speech. Psychophysical testing includes measures of thresholds, discrimination limens, and so on, on purely physical dimensions, usually using nonspeech sounds. The natural speech category refers to discrimination or labeling on real speech items. The problem is that with psychophysical tests the stimulus is specified but little can be said about the relation to speech perception; but with natural speech little can be said about what there is physically in the stimulus which is significant for task success or failure. Our solution is to use synthetic speech items, so that physical differences can be related to speech sound contrasts.

Contrasts Tested

We have devised and used tests covering both prosodic and segmental contrasts. Prosodic tests include a one- versus two-syllable test differing in amplitude contour, and a rising versus falling pitch test varying in extent of pitch change. Segmental tests include an open versus closed vowel test varying separation between the first and second formants; b-w: plosive versus approximant, varying transition rate; b-m: plosive versus nasal, varying bandwidth and prevoicing; and b-d: place contrast, varying direction of the second formant transition.

Procedure

Consideration of related procedures (Danhauer and Singh, 1975; Godfrey and Millay, 1976; Graham and House, 1971; Pickett et al., 1972; Tallal, Stark, and Curtiss, 1976) and experience with preceding tests at University College London (Fourcin, 1976; Fourcin et al., 1978) led to a paradigm including same-different tasks and labeling tasks. The same-different task was used because of low perceptual and cognitive demand, well-defined response expectation (right versus wrong responses), and the possibility of dividing the test into subtests of fixed difficulty level, with efficient strategies for ending the test at each level and for moving between levels. For the labeling task a very abbreviated test, made up only of the items from the extremes of the test continuum, was constructed as a practical supplement to the discrimination test.

Children were tested using a Connevans Speech Trainer. Pure tone detection and discomfort thresholds were established using standard procedures (Martin et al., 1976). Within the child's usable region, presentation level was varied according to performance, gradually increasing the presentation level in 5-dB steps until performance no longer improved.

Training was developed to establish that the child had the concepts of same and different, that the concepts could be applied to sequentially presented visual stimuli, and that the child could then transfer to auditory stimuli. A pointing response was elicited, preventing extra auditory distraction. A flexible policy regarding feedback was used, both to control attention and response bias and to provide positive reinforcement. Feedback was given after each response except for a few children, at the discretion of the tester, when it was considered that feedback was causing the child to be anxious. Attention was also focused and rewarded by use of simple reward games. At the difficulty level causing performance to drop below 75% correct, an easier level was reintroduced to check attention and fatigue.

Test Population

Normally hearing children in three age groups (3 to 4, 7 to 8, 10 to 11) were tested in a pilot study with 12 subjects; a second pilot study tested both normally hearing (12 subjects) and partially hearing (20 subjects) at the same school. Finally, for 3 successive years the tests have been incorporated into the annual assessment procedure at a school for profoundly deaf children, where the authors attempted tests on about 25 children aged 4 to 12. All subjects in the normally hearing groups had passed the standard school screening tests for hearing.

Results

Previous tests (Fourcin, 1976), especially those that measured labeling of fully randomized stimuli along a test continuum, were unsuitable because of the length of the test and lack of method to detect and control attention. As a result only two-thirds of the tests yielded enough data to compare performance on the extremes of the test variable. In addition, performance was random in about 70% of cases. The same-different discrimination tests lead to a statistically reliable result in about 95% of the trials, and performance is nonrandom in 80% of the results on the two easiest tests (one versus two syllables and open versus close vowels), dropping to 15% nonrandom performance on the b-d test, which was the most difficult.

Comparisons of test scores for normally hearing, partially hearing, and profoundly deaf subjects showed considerable similarity for the results on the normally hearing and partially hearing groups, which tended to cluster their scores at the more difficult end of the range. The profoundly deaf children tended to span the range, always with at least some children's scores being right at the very easy (very poor discrimination) end of the range.

A comparison between discrimination and labeling for the same subjects showed that in two-thirds of the cases, failure to label coincided with failure to discriminate. The remaining one-third were those interesting subjects who could discriminate but not label. Had we been

Table 11.2.   Relation of production assessment to perception test scores

Average scores		Test				
		Open/close vowels	b/w	b/m	One/two syllables	Pitch rise/fall
Children	Normally hearing	9	6	4	7	9
	Profoundly deaf	8	1	2	6	1
Child A	Test	8	1	Cannot do	Cannot do	Cannot do
	Production	Good contrast	Adult normal three-term contrast reduced to one term—plosive	Cannot do	Deletes unstressed syllables, adds extra final syllables	No consistent use of pitch contrastively
Child B	Test	9	3	5	7	1
	Production	Good contrast	Maintains contrast by closure plus liprounding for /w/	Nasal/non-nasal used in free variation	Has good speech rhythm	Some use of a fall on nucleus; often uses length
Child C	Test	9	6	6	8	5
	Production	Good contrast	Complete and consistent contrast	Complete and consistent contrast	Has good speech rhythm	Can consistently use falls, especially when reminded

testing labeling only, we would have judged this one-third of cases as incapable of making the contrast, when in fact they could make the contrast at the level of auditory discrimination, with their failure to label attributable to a higher level linguistic problem.

The relation of perception to production is most relevant on an individual basis. In Table 11.2 scores on five tests are presented for three children, all profoundly deaf, aged 11 or 12. The table includes a brief synopsis of the relevant portion of the assessment of speech production for those same children. In most cases, high scores for the perception tests are paired with the presence of the corresponding phonological contrast in production.

CONCLUSIONS

The phonetic assessment of speech production and perception which we have described gives a comprehensive analysis of a child's speech as a basis for planning remedial work, but leaves open certain questions about the relation between reduced and abnormal speech sound systems and abnormal prosodics on the one hand, and intelligibility on the other. More information is required about factors affecting improvement in intelligibility, so that decisions about remedial priorities can be better founded. Elsewhere the authors have reported the results of a project which attempted to relate assessment results to a specific program of intervention (King and Parker, 1980).

It is important to reiterate that any test procedures and results are only an abstraction from the total picture of the communicating child. The authors have suggested that the notion of interacting levels of linguistic analysis is a more appropriate framework than the speech/ language dichotomy. The test procedures we have described concentrate on the phonological and phonetic levels, and we think these procedures provide a basis for speech work within the overall context of language.

ACKNOWLEDGMENTS

The work described here has been funded by several bodies at various times. For several years, support was granted at University College London by the Medical Research Council. We would like to thank the National Deaf Children's Society, the National Research Trust for Speech Therapy, the Camden and Islington Area Health Authority, and the Inner London Education Authority. The continuing work is based at and supported by the Royal National Institute for the Deaf, U.K.

REFERENCES

Ashby, M. G. 1978. A study of two English nuclear tones. Lang. Speech 21:326–336.
Calvert, D. R., and S. R. Silverman. 1975. Speech and Deafness. A. G. Bell Association for the Deaf, Washington, D. C.
Clark, M. H., 1975. Teaching speech to profoundly deaf children. Paper presented at the National Deaf Children's Society Conference, London.
Connor, L. E. (ed.). 1971. Speech for the Deaf Child: Knowledge and Use. A. G. Bell Association for the Deaf, Washington, D. C.
Conrad, R. 1979. The Deaf School Child: Language and Cognitive Function. Harper & Row, London.
Crystal, D., P. Fletcher, and M. Garman. 1976. Grammatical Analysis of Language Disability: A Procedure for Assessment and Remediation. Edward Arnold, London.
Danhauer, J. L., and S. Singh. 1975. Multidimensional Speech Perception by the Hearing Impaired: A Treatise on Distinctive Features. University Park Press, Baltimore.
DeSaussure, F. 1966. Cours de Linguistic Generale. Payot, Paris.
Ewing, I. R., and A. W. G. Ewing. 1954. Speech and the Deaf Child. Manchester University Press, Manchester, England.
Fourcin, A. J. 1976. Speech patterns for deaf children. Speech and Hearing: Work in Progress. University College London, London.
Fourcin, A. J., S. Evershed, J. Fisher, A. B. King, A. Parker, and R. D. Wright. 1978. Perception and production of speech patterns by hearing-impaired children. Speech and Hearing: Work in Progress. University College London, London.
Godfrey, J. J., and K. Millay. 1976. Perception of formant transitions by hearing-impaired subjects. Paper presented at the meeting of the American Speech and Hearing Association, November, Houston.
Graham, L., and A. House. 1971. Phonological oppositions in children: A perceptual study. J. Acoust. Soc. Am. 49:559–566.
Grunwell, P. 1975. The phonological analysis of articulation disorders. Br. J. Disord. Commun. 10:31–42.
Haycock, G. S. 1933. The Teaching of Speech. A. G. Bell Association for the Deaf, Washington, D. C.
Hudgins, C. V. 1934. A comparative study of the speech coordination of deaf and normal subjects. J. Genet. Psychol. 44:3–48.
Hudgins, C. V., and F. C. Numbers. 1942. An investigation of the intelligibility of the speech of the deaf. Genet. Psychol. Monogr. 25:289–392.
Ingram, D. 1976. Phonological Disability in Children. Edward Arnold, London.
King, A., and A. Parker. 1980. The relevance of prosodic features to speech work with hearing-impaired children. In F. M. Jones (ed.), Language Disability in Children: Assessment and Remediation. MTP Press, Lancaster, England.
Levitt, H. 1971. Speech production and the deaf child. In L. E. Connor (ed.), Speech for the Deaf Child: Knowledge and Use. A. G. Bell Association for the Deaf, Washington, D. C.
Levitt, H., M. J. Collins, J. R. Dubno, S. B. Resnick, and R. E. C. White. 1978. Development of a Protocol for the Prescriptive Fitting of a Wearable

Master Hearing Aid. Communication Sciences Laboratory Research Report 11. City University of New York, New York.

Levitt, H., and C. R. Smith. 1972. Errors of articulation in the speech of profoundly hearing-impaired children. J. Acoust. Soc. Am. 51:102–103 (Abstract).

Levitt, H., C. R. Smith, and H. Stromberg. 1976. Acoustic, articulatory and perceptual characteristics of the speech of deaf children. In G. Fant (ed.), Speech Communication Seminars, Vol. 4. Wiley, New York.

Ling, D. 1976. Speech and the Hearing Impaired Child: Theory and Practice. A. G. Bell Association for the Deaf, Washington, D. C.

Lyons, J. 1968. Introduction to Theoretical Linguistics. Cambridge University Press, London.

Malmberg, B. 1968. The linguistic basis of phonetics. In B. Malmberg (ed.), Manual of Phonetics. North Holland Publishing Co., Amsterdam.

Markides, A. 1970. The speech of deaf and partially-hearing children with special reference to factors affecting intelligibility. Br. J. Disord. Commun. 5:126–140.

Martin, M. C., B. C. Grover, J. J. Worrall, and V. Williams. 1976. The effectiveness of hearing aids in a school population. Br. J. Audio. 10:33–40.

Mártony, J., and P. E. Nordstrom. 1975. On vowel production in deaf children. Paper presented at the VIIIth International Congress of Phonetic Sciences, Leeds.

Monsen, R. B. 1976. The production of English stop consonants in the speech of deaf children. J. Phonetics 4:29–41.

O'Connor, J. D., and G. F. Arnold. 1961. Intonation of Colloquial English. Longmans, London.

Pickett, J. M., E. S. Martin, D. Johnson, S. Brandsmith, Z. Daniel, D. Willis, and W. Otis. 1972. On patterns of speech feature reception by deaf listeners. In G. Fant (ed.), Proceedings of the International Symposium on Speech Communication Ability and Profound Deafness. A. G. Bell Association for the Deaf, Washington, D. C.

Reynell, J. 1977. The revised Reynell Developmental Language Scales. National Federation for Educational Research, Northampton, England.

Robins, P. 1964. General Linguistics: An Introductory Survey. Longmans, London.

Smith, C. R. 1975. Residual hearing and speech production in deaf children. J. Speech Hear. Res. 18:795–811.

Tallal, P., R. E. Stark, and B. Curtiss. 1976. Relation between speech perception and speech production impairment in children with developmental dysphasia. Brain Lang. 3:305–317.

Appendix
Sample Assessment Form

Revised Phonetic Assessment 1979	School/Hospital	Name
Copyright Angela King and Ann Parker	Date of Recording	Assessed by

Summary and Comparison with Previous Assessment

When pages 2 and 3 have been completed, the main points should be summarised.

If there has been a previous assessment, a comparison should be made at this stage, and the results should be described in relation to the speech work which has been done.

Suggestions for Speech Therapy

A detailed plan should be given when appropriate.

Other assessments (for example, speech perception and comprehension tests, syntactic analysis) may be revelant to phonetic and phonologic work, and should be referred to at this point.

PROSODIC FEATURES

Airstream Mechanism for Speech

Is an egressive pulmonic air stream always used for speech, or do other mechanisms occur? If implosives, ejectives, or clicks occur, are they phonologically contrastive? (see segmental description).

Is breath abnormally retained or wasted?

Voice

Describe the voice quality: normal, creaky, breathy, whisper, tense.

Does the voice quality vary?

Is overall pitch appropriate, or not?

Are there marked pitch fluctuations which are not related to meaning?

Is pitch-range restricted compared to that of a normal speaker of the same age?

Is the voice inappropriately loud, or quiet, or are there marked fluctuations in loudness?

Does involuntary voicing occur? Does devoicing of words or syllables occur?

PROSODIC FEATURES (*Continued*)

Overall Timing and Rhythm

Is overall rate of utterance normal? If not, are there any particular features associated with this, such as prolonged vowels, word-by-word utterance with breaths in between, extra syllables, or speaking like the written form?

Is speech rhythm normal (i.e., stress-timed) or does other timing operate (e.g., syllable-timing or "speech-sound" timing)?

Intonation Patterns

Describe the characteristic patterns found for single words, read and spontaneous sentences.

Is pitch change used normally in a contrastive system of intonation, or is there any other systematic way of marking sentence-stress (for example, additional length on nuclear syllable)?

Other Comments

Note any other features, such as overall hypernasality.

SEGMENTAL FEATURES

Vowel System

The phonologic system and structure, and phonetic realisations, are described in comparison with the adult normal model.

Does the speech have the contrastive system as the adult normal model? What are the phonetic-level realisations of these contrasts, and are they consistent?

Note differences between single words, read sentences, and spontaneous speech.

Consonant System
Place Contrasts

Do the structural relationships correspond to those in normal speech; for example, is normal assimilation found? Or do other relationships, such as "consonant harmony," occur?

Include comments on the effect of nonsegmental features where they are relevant; for example, masking of vowel contrasts by nasality.

Manner Contrasts

(NOTE: *a different format may be appropriate for certain children with very idiosyncratic or greatly reduced systems*)

Voice/Voiceless
Contrast

Other Comments

CHAPTER 12

PATTERNS OF PERFORMANCE IN SPEECH PERCEPTION AND PRODUCTION

Joanne D. Subtelny

CONTENTS

From preceding chapters in this volume it is apparent that those interested in habilitation of the hearing impaired have recognized the basic need to assess varied parameters of communication in order to plan an intelligent course of training. This chapter restricts the focus of assessment to consider patterns of performance in perception and production, and to discuss their relevance in aural rehabilitation.

For the past 2 or 3 decades, investigators have studied relationships between pure tone thresholds and word recognition ability (Beasley and Rosenwasser, 1950; Elliott, 1963; Kryter, Williams, and Green, 1962; Mullins and Bangs, 1957; Ross et al., 1965; Young and Gibbons, 1962) in efforts to discover predictive relationships between pure tone thresholds and speech perception. The results consistently showed that subjects with similar pure tone thresholds varied in their word recognition ability. As a result, it was generally concluded that speech perception, as indicated by performance in word recognition, could not be predicted reliably from pure tone audiometric data.

This rather disappointing status and the persistent need to understand relationships between pure tone sensitivity and auditory perception of speech, or potential to develop it, encouraged continued research utilizing phoneme and feature recognition rather than word recognition to specify perception. Results reported by Cox (1969), Lawrence and Byers (1969), and Pickett et al. (1972) have been summarized as follows: "While the probability of making recognition errors

is certainly greater the more severe the hearing impairment, the phonemes and features actually confused seem to be remarkably similar
regardless of nature and extent of the hearing impairment" (Walden
and Montgomery, 1975, p. 445). The analysis of consonant confusions
consistently showed that information about voicing and manner of articulation is transmitted rather well to most hearing-impaired listeners,
but perception of place of articulation usually is severely affected by
hearing impairment.

More recently, test materials and analysis procedures were improved. As a result, patterns of performance in auditory perception of
phonemes and features have been identified with differences in the
degree and configuration of loss as defined by pure tone testing (Bilger
and Wang, 1976; Wang, Reed, and Bilger, 1978). Thus, clinical predictions of potential to improve perception now seems to be on a much
firmer basis. Guidelines and procedures also have been provided, making it possible to plot changes in perception by features and phonemes
incident to auditory training and/or hearing aid fitting.

Investigators have studied speech production in hearing-impaired
subjects utilizing articulation testing procedures (Hudgins and Numbers, 1942; Markides, 1970; Smith, 1975) to describe patterns of error.
Although similar error patterns have been reported in the speech of
different groups of hearing-impaired children (Levitt et al., 1978), Markides (1970) reported both the frequency and type of error varied with
the degree of hearing loss.

Thus, patterns of performance in phoneme perception and in phoneme production have been found to be significantly related to hearing
loss. Despite these data, relationships between phoneme perception
and production are not clearly understood. Nor do we currently understand how the perception-production relationship is affected by variable degrees of hearing loss. Recognizing that phonemes and features
are in some respects rather well differentiated acoustically and phys-
iologically, it might be hypothesized (1) that some features would be
perceived with a higher degree of accuracy than others; (2) that features
perceived with greater accuracy would be produced more intelligibly,
and (3) that performance in both perception and production would be
related to the extent of hearing loss.

If any or all of these hypotheses were found to be supported, analysis of phoneme perception and production would appear to offer rather
rich diagnostic implications to assist in determining the objectives, procedures, and strategies to apply in efficient training of spoken communication. Considering this possibility, a group of 160 young adults

attending the National Technical Institute for the Deaf were randomly selected. Auditory and speech tests were administered to define phoneme perception and production, respectively. Students were then categorized by degree of hearing impairment to study relationships between perception and production as they relate to degree of hearing loss. Data secured from this study will be summarized to formulate diagnostic implications.

METHOD

Subjects were subdivided into four groups based upon tests of auditory discrimination. The group descriptions appear in Table 12.1.

The Phoneme Identification Test Series (Jones et al., 1976) was used to evaluate both consonant perception and production. This test (Sims and Montgomery, 1977), consisting of 64 consonant-vowel items, includes four repetitions of 16 consonants paired with the vowel /ɑ/.[1] The test was administered under headphones at the student's most comfortable listening level. The student's task was to identify the stimulus consonant from a set of 16 possible responses presented on an opscan sheet. Responses were scored by computer to yield percentage correct for all consonants combined and for consonants categorized by manner, voicing, and place of production. Because place of articulation is the phonetic feature reported to be most susceptible to the effects of sensorineural hearing loss (Boothroyd, 1976; Pickett et al., 1972; Risberg, 1976), and is "virtually imperceptible" to persons with hearing losses in excess of 90 dB (Boothroyd, 1978), manner of production was selected as the singular basis for categorizing consonants in this study.

The validity and reliability of the Phoneme Identification Test material used to assess consonant intelligibility was evaluated at NTID and found to be satisfactory for research purposes (Whitehead, 1978). Subjects read the syllables on the Phoneme Identification Tests while the therapist recorded responses on the opscan sheet. No visual or auditory modeling was provided during testing. If an utterance could not be phonetically categorized after two repetitions, no response was recorded for that item. Tests were scored by computer to yield the total percentage of consonants intelligibly produced and percentages for consonants categorized by manner.

---

[1] Although the Phoneme Identification Test (PIT) Series is limited to consonant-vowel syllables, it appears to be a valid test because PIT scores correlate ($r = 0.78$) with scores achieved on the Modified Rhyme Test.

Table 12.1   Sample descriptors and hearing characteristics

Group	Number	Descriptor		Discrimination (%)	PTA[a] (dB)	Cut-off[b] (Hz)
A	38	≥50% identification of key words within sentences	Mean	69.47	74.27	6750
			SD	11.67	14.31	1950
B	61	<50% identification of key words within sentences	Mean	24.93	85.03	5200
			SD	12.88	13.46	2900
C	17	≥50% identification of spondees	Mean	0	94.88	3110
			SD		9.38	2140
D	44	<50% identification of spondees	Mean	0	97.31	3480
			SD		22.33	2830

[a] PTA, Three-frequency pure tone average (500 Hz, 1000 Hz, 2000 Hz); SD, standard deviation.
[b] Cut-off, Upper limit of responses to pure tone testing.

RESULTS

The results of testing were first studied to obtain an overview of consonant perception and production without consideration of differences in manner. These data are shown in Figure 12.1. Several patterns of performance emerged when the means were compared for measures of consonant perception and measures of production with subjects grouped by degree of hearing loss.

First, mean scores for both perception and production became progressively lower as hearing loss increased from group A to group D. Second, it was also evident that scores for auditory perception were consistently lower than the corresponding scores for intelligible production in all four groups of subjects. Third, by comparing the degree of difference between means for perception and production for the groups, a progressive increase in degree of difference is shown to be associated with progressive increments in degree of hearing loss. The t values indicated the difference between perception and production were statistically significant in all four groups.

Coefficients of correlation between measures of consonant perception and production were low, but significant for subjects in group A ($r = 0.37$; $P < 0.05$) and for subjects in group B ($r = 0.40$; $P < 0.01$). No significant correlations between perception and production were revealed in groups C and D. Because subjects in these groups had profound hearing losses with very poor (if any) auditory perception, significant correlations between perception and production would not be anticipated. Little difference in consonant perception was revealed when measures for group C and group D were compared; however, much larger differences in perceptual skill (approximating 20%) were noted between groups A, B, and C.

In Figure 12.1, mean scores for groups A, B, C, and D are graphed for all consonants combined and for consonants grouped by the manner feature. By comparing the relative heights of the solid black areas, a pattern in perception is indicated for speakers in group A. Perception of nasals (Mean, 73%) and glides (Mean, 67%) is better than perception of plosives (Mean 58%) and fricatives (Mean 53%). On the basis of these data, it appears that there is about a 20% differential between nasal and fricative consonant perception.

In group A, the means for production are 15% to 20% higher than the corresponding means for perception for all manner features except for plosives where production (Mean, 92%) is much better (34%) than perception (Mean, 58%). For subjects in group B (pure tone average (PTA), 85 dB) the means for perception reflect much the same pattern

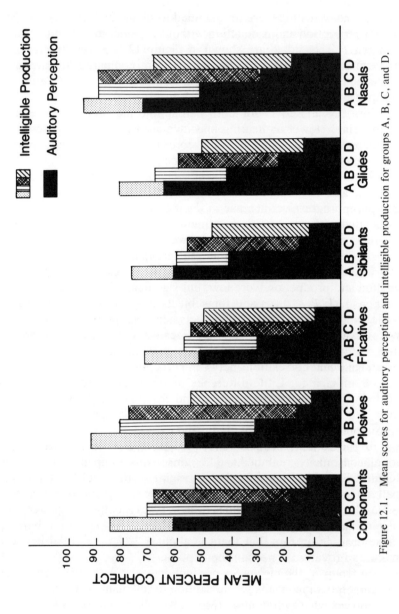

Figure 12.1.   Mean scores for auditory perception and intelligible production for groups A, B, C, and D.

shown for subjects in group A (PTA, 75 dB). By comparing the relative heights of the black bars for groups A and B, however, it becomes evident that the 10-dB greater hearing loss in group B resulted in 20% to 25% reduction in consonant perception for all manner features. Nasal (Mean, 52%), glide (Mean, 42%), and sibilant (Mean, 41%) perception, however, remained superior to perception for plosives and fricatives (Mean, 32%).

Mean scores for production in group B were lower (6% to 17%) than respective means for production in group A. The pattern of production in group B was also similar to that noted for group A, in the sense that nasal (Mean, 89%) and plosive (Mean, 81%) consonants were produced more intelligibly than other groups.

In group B the means for production are 20% to 35% higher than the associated means for perception of all manner features with the exception of the plosive group. Again, plosive production was much better (almost 50%) than plosive perception as was indicated in group A.

Perception of manner for subjects in group C with average losses of 95 dB also revealed a pattern with better perception for glide and nasal features. In group D perception for manner was just above the chance level for all manner groupings. Despite poor if any perception, the average student in groups C and D could still produce all manner features with about 50% intelligibility within a simplified syllable context. However, nasal and plosive production in group D was noticeably lower than for the other three groups.

CLINICAL IMPLICATION

In overview, these findings show that patterns of performance in auditory perception and production are revealed when consonants are grouped by the manner features and when subjects are grouped by hearing level. Production skill was always observed to exceed skill in perception. This finding clinically suggests that students can learn to produce some consonants intelligibly even though they may never be able to identify them auditorily.

Because some manner features are perceived and produced with greater accuracy than others and because the relationship between perception and production varies with degree of loss, it is strongly recommended that diagnosis involve separate analyses of consonant perception and production so that these relationships can be studied within the reference of subject's degree of hearing loss. Through this type of analysis, the clinician can determine whether training should focus on perception or production or involve training in both. The recommended analysis also helps to identify target features for improvement, and provides base line data which permit the clinician and client to determine changes in performance incident to training.

These diagnostic implications may be clarified by discussing several individual subjects. In this discussion, information accumulated before and after training is included to indicate the relative impact of training on consonant perception and production. Measures of consonant perception and production secured before and after training are graphed for Speaker 42 in Figure 12.2. This speaker had a discrimination score of 28%, and a pure tone average (PTA) of 88 dB, with cutoff of 8 kHz. This speaker was from group B and his hearing characteristics are typical of subjects in that group.

In comparison with the group B means, it is apparent that Speaker 42 had comparatively poor perception of plosives, fricatives, and sib-

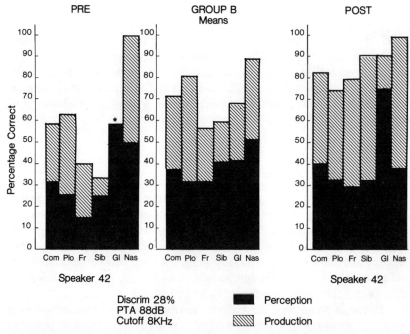

Figure 12.2. At far left and far right, measures are graphed for consonant perception and production before and after Speaker 42 received training. Respective scores are graphed for all consonants combined (Com) and for consonants grouped by manner; plosive (Plo), fricative (Fr), sibilant (Sib), glide (Gl), and nasal (Nas). Means for measures of consonant perception and production for subjects in group B with similar degrees of hearing loss are graphed in the center to facilitate comparisons between individual measures and group means. * Perception and production for glides in the pretraining status were equal.

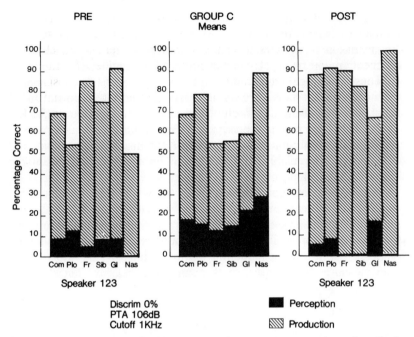

Figure 12.3.   At far left and far right, measures for consonant perception and production are graphed for Speaker 123 before and after receiving training. Respective scores are shown for all consonants combined and for consonants grouped by manner. Means for measures of consonant perception and production for subjects in Group C with similar degrees of hearing loss are graphed in the center to facilitate comparisons between individual measures and group means.

ilants before training. The slashed areas show that less-than-average production skill was associated for these three groups of consonants. By comparing pretherapy data with the averaged data, it also becomes apparent that this speaker had good perception of glides, but production did not exceed perception. Compositely, observations suggested that therapy should combine auditory training and production training focused on plosives and fricatives.

The measures secured for Speaker 42, after receiving 28 hours of individualized training, appear at the right in Figure 12.2. The solid and slashed areas plotting measures of perception and production for fricatives and sibilants indicate substantial improvement was achieved in both areas. Note also that glide perception and production improved, but nasal consonant perception regressed slightly.

Another example may be used to illustrate less favorable gains in perception as illustrated by Figure 12.3. Speaker 123 had no discrimination for speech, a pure tone average of 106 dB with cutoff at 1 kHz.

These hearing characteristics fit the criteria established for group C. Average measures for subjects in group C are graphed at the center. A comparison of individual measures and group means suggest that perception might be slightly improved for glides and nasals; however, prognosis for this gain would not appear good. Prognosis would appear much better if therapy were focused to improve production of nasal and plosive consonants. In both of these areas of production, Speaker 123 was below average in performance. Post-training measures for perception and production show perception for nasals and plosives did not improve appreciably; but significant improvement in producing these two consonant groups was realized.

Analogous data for Speaker 12 is shown in Figure 12.4. This speaker had 64% discrimination and a pure tone average of 68 dB with cutoff at 8 kHz. These characteristics in hearing, which fit criteria established for group A, indicate a very good prognosis to improve consonant perception and production, both of which fall far short of the mean measures for speakers with comparable hearing. The data ob-

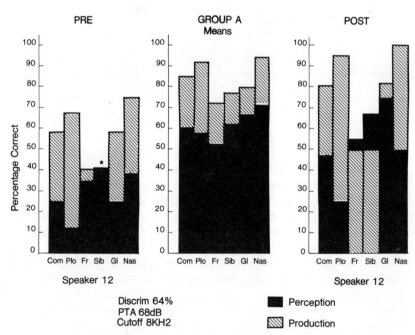

Figure 12.4. Pre and post scores for consonant perception and production graphed at left and right for Speaker 12. Means for measures of consonant perception and production for subjects in Group A with similar degrees of hearing loss are graphed at center to facilitate comparisons between individual measures and group means.

tained for this speaker also showed a high incidence of stop-fricative confusion, indicating a need for a strong auditory approach in training to improve both perception and production for stops and fricatives. Confusion for these two manner features was reduced after training; production was also improved for stops and fricatives.

In the post-therapy status graphed in Figure 12.4, it is interesting to note that fricative and sibilant perception exceeded production. This observation indicates that the 50% level of intelligibility in producing fricatives and sibilants could be improved with additional training. In this case, the post-training deficit in production of frication does not appear to be related to faulty perception, but rather to motoric deficiencies.

IMPACT OF TRAINING ON PERCEPTION AND PRODUCTION

One might justifiably criticize diagnostic implications and statements regarding the impact of training on perception and production which have been based upon the analysis of three students differing in degree of hearing loss. Mindful of this limitation, it seems appropriate to summarize briefly a study undertaken specifically to evaluate the impact of training on speech perception and production. In this study, 79 NTID students representing a rather broad range of speech and hearing skills participated. Pure tone averages in the better ear ranged from 65 to 120 dB with a mean of 94 dB. Discrimination scores ranged from 0% to 64% with a mean of 11.05% and a standard deviation (SD) of 16.22. Over half of the students (57%) had no discrimination for speech as assessed by key word recognition in the CID Everyday Sentences. Ninety percent of the students were using hearing aids all or most of the time during the interval of study.

In order to evaluate both consonant and vowel perception within word context, the Modified Rhyme Test (House et al., 1965) and a vowel test developed by Horii (1969) were administered. These tests were also used to secure measures of intelligibility for vowels and consonants in word context. The speech samples were recorded and played to five experienced listeners who wrote each word as understood. The responses of the five listeners were then averaged to yield single scores for intelligibility.

The data extracted from these auditory and production tests are presented in Table 12.2. The difference between mean scores for perception of vowels (Mean, 50%) and production of vowels (Mean, 53%) is very slight before training. Measures secured after training revealed slight but significant improvement was achieved in perception ($P <$

Table 12.2 Difference between perception and production before and after training (N = 79)

Measurement	Before training (%)			After training (%)		
	Perception	Production	Difference	Perception	Production	Difference
Vowels[a] (Vowel test)						
Mean	49.92	52.92	−3.00	52.49	57.33	−4.84
SD	22.80	19.41		23.24	19.52	
Consonants[a] (Modified Rhyme test)						
Mean	37.17	58.75	−21.58	41.98	68.66	−26.68
SD	17.39	13.73		18.65	12.06	
Consonants[b] (Phonetic Identification test)						
Mean	20.15	56.64	−36.49	21.58	71.05	−49.47
SD	14.20	23.49		17.53	23.96	

[a] Within word context.
[b] Within CV syllables.

0.05) and production ($P < 0.01$); however, the difference between perception and production for vowels remained minimal in comparison to the rather gross differences revealed for consonants within word and syllable contexts.

Data graphically displayed in Figure 12.5 show consonant production in word context before training (Mean, 59%) and after training (Mean, 69%) far exceeded consonant perception (Mean, 37% and 42%). Intelligible consonant production improved significantly ($P < 0.01$), approximating 10% to 12% on the average as a result of training. Improvement in perception of consonants improved also but to a much lesser degree ($P < 0.05$).

It should also be noted that consonant perception within word context was much better (Mean, 37% and 42%) than that within syllable context (Mean 20% and 22%). This difference in perception occurring as a function of context did not apply relative to consonant production, where rather slight differences in production were noted as a function of context. The variable vowel occurring within words and the symbolic value of the utterance aided consonant perception, but apparently did not facilitate intelligible production.

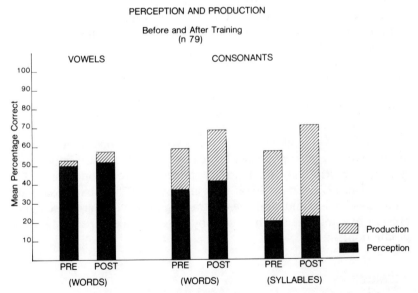

Figure 12.5. Mean scores, secured before and after speakers received training, are graphed for perception and production of vowels within word context. Mean scores are shown for consonant perception and production within word context and within syllable context.

Within word contexts, vowel perception was better than consonant perception: a finding reported by many investigators (Owens, Schubert, and Benedict, 1971; Oyer and Doudna, 1959). Contrary to what might be expected on the basis of perception, it is interesting to observe that vowel production was *not* better than consonant production. The comparatively better performance in vowel perception would seem to suggest good prognosis for improving vowel production. As reported, the results of our evaluation of therapy indicate that vowel production was improved minimally. Further study is needed to explain this consistent finding.

The overall results of this evaluation indicate that relatively large gains in consonant production can be achieved as a result of training. Smaller but significant gains in consonant perception were associated with improvements in production, but vowel perception and production improved minimally.

When the sample was subdivided on the basis of auditory discrimination, greater gains for most speech measures and for auditory discrimination were identified with students who had some discrimination ability. This finding is in agreement with the previous observations reported for individual subjects. Obviously, when some students with no discrimination are included within a large group of subjects, gross differences in response to auditory training would be anticipated. On a group mean basis, these very real differences in response to auditory training may be obscured.

In overview, the results of our evaluative efforts offer support for Ling's clinical statement that training in production will improve perception (Ling, 1976). In this respect, our results (Lieberth and Subtelny, 1978; Subtelny, Orlando, and Webster, 1980) are in agreement with those reported by Ling and Maretic (1971), and by Novelli-Olmstead (1979) and Osberger (this volume). Consistent gains in production and perception can be achieved if audiological information is used prescriptively to improve phoneme perception (Asp, 1975; Caccamise, 1973; Erber, 1974; Ling and Ling, 1978; Winitz, 1975) and if target selection and strategies in training production are based upon prescriptive information provided by assessing both perception and production.

REFERENCES

Asp, C. W. 1975. Measurement of aural speech perception and oral speech production in the hearing impaired. In S. Singh (ed.), Measurement Procedures in Speech-Hearing-Language. University Park Press, Baltimore.

Beasley, W. C., and H. Rosenwasser. 1950. Determining factors in composing and analyzing speech-hearing tests. Laryngoscope 60:658–679.
Bilger, R. C., and M. D. Wang. 1976. Consonant confusions in patients with sensorineural hearing loss. J. Speech Hear. Res. 19:718–748.
Boothroyd, A. 1976. Influence of residual hearing on speech perception and speech production by hearing-impaired children. S.A.R.P. Report 26. Clarke School for the Deaf, Northampton, Mass.
Boothroyd, A. 1978. Speech perception and sensorineural hearing loss. In M. Ross and T. Giolas (eds.), Auditory Management of Hearing-Impaired Children. University Park Press, Baltimore.
Caccamise, F. C. 1973. An analysis of hearing-impaired persons' responses to C/i syllables under three test modes. Doctoral dissertation, University of Washington, Seattle, Wash.
Cox, P. 1969. The identification of unfiltered and filtered consonant-vowel-consonant stimuli by sensori-neural hearing-impaired persons. Doctoral dissertation, University of Pittsburgh.
Elliott, L. L. 1963. Prediction of speech discrimination scores from other test information. J. Aud. Res. 3:35–45.
Erber, N. P. 1974. Pure-tone thresholds and word-recognition abilities of hearing-impaired children. J. Speech Hear. Res. 17:194–202.
Horii, Y. 1969. Specifying the speech-to-noise ratio: Development and evaluation of a noise with speech-envelope characteristics. Doctoral dissertation, Purdue University, Lafayette, Ind.
House, A. S., C. Williams, M. Hecker, and K. Kryter. 1965. Articulation testing methods: Consonantal differentiation with a closed response set. J. Acoust. Soc. Am. 37:158–166.
Hudgins, C. V., and F. C. Numbers. 1942. An investigation of the intelligibility of the speech of the deaf. Genet. Psychol. Monogr. 25:289–392.
Jones, K., R. Whitehead, J. Bancroft, and D. Sims. 1976. The performance of students at the National Technical Institute for the Deaf on an auditory speech perception test. Paper presented at the meeting of the American Speech and Hearing Association, Houston.
Kryter, K. D., C. Williams, and D. M. Green. 1962. Auditory acuity and the perception of speech. J. Acoust. Soc. Am. 34:1217–1223.
Lawrence, D. L. and V. W. Byers. 1969. Identification of voiceless fricatives by high frequency hearing-impaired listeners. J. Speech Hear. Res. 12:426–434.
Levitt, H., H. Stromberg, C. Smith, and T. Gold. 1978. The structure of segmental errors in the speech of deaf children. In D. L. McPherson (ed.), Advances in Prosthetic Devices for the Deaf: A Technical Workshop. National Technical Institute for the Deaf, Rochester, N.Y.
Lieberth, A., and J. D. Subtelny. 1978. The effect of speech training on auditory phoneme identification. Volta Rev. 80:410–417.
Ling, D. 1976. Speech and the Hearing-Impaired Child: Theory and Practice. A. G. Bell Association for the Deaf, Washington, D.C.
Ling, D., and A. Ling. 1978. Aural Habilitation: The Foundations of Verbal Learning in Hearing-Impaired Children. A. G. Bell Association for the Deaf, Washington, D.C.
Ling, D., and H. Maretic. 1971. Frequency transposition in the teaching of speech to deaf children. J. Speech Hear. Res. 14:37–46.

230   Subtelny

Markides, A. 1970. The speech of deaf and partially hearing children with special reference to factors affecting intelligibility. Br. J. Disord. Commun. 5:126–140.

Mullins, C. J., and J. L. Bangs. 1957. Relationships between speech discrimination and other audiometric data. Acta Otolaryngol. 47:149–157.

Novelli-Olmstead, T. 1979. Production and reception of speech by hearing impaired children. Master's thesis, McGill University, Montreal.

Owens, E., E. Schubert, and M. Benedict. 1971. Consonant phonemic errors associated with pure-tone configurations and certain kinds of hearing impairment. J. Speech Hear. Res. 15:308–322.

Oyer, H., and M. Doudna. 1959. Structural analysis of word responses made by hard-of-hearing subjects on a discrimination test. Arch. Otolaryngol. 70:357–364.

Pickett, J. M., E. Martin, D. Johnson, S. Smith, Z. Daniel, D. Willis, and W. Otis. 1972. On patterns of speech feature reception by deaf listeners. In G. Fant (ed.), International Symposium on Speech Communication Ability and Profound Deafness. A.G. Bell Association for the Deaf, Washington, D.C.

Risberg, A. 1976. Diagnostic rhyme test for speech audiometry with severely hard of hearing and profoundly deaf children. Speech Transact. Lab. Q. Prog. Status Rep. 2 3:40–58.

Ross, M., D. A. Huntington, H. A. Newby, and R. F. Dixon. 1965. Speech discrimination of hearing-impaired individuals in noise. J. Aud. Res. 5:47–72.

Sims, D. G., and A. A. Montgomery. 1977. Multidimensional analysis of auditory and visual perception among the profoundly hearing impaired. Paper presented at the meeting of the Acoustical Society of America, Miami.

Smith, C. R. 1975. Residual hearing and speech production in deaf children. J. Speech Hear. Res. 18:795–811.

Subtelny, J., N. Orlando, and P. Webster. 1980. Evaluation of speech training at the post-secondary level. In J. Subtelny (ed.), Speech Assessment and Speech Improvement for the Hearing Impaired. A.G. Bell Association for the Deaf, Washington, D.C.

Walden, B. E., and A. A. Montgomery. 1975. Dimensions of consonant perception in normal and hearing-impaired listeners. J. Speech Hear. Res. 18:444–455.

Wang, M. D., C. Reed, and R. Bilger. 1978. A comparison of the effects of filtering and sensorineural hearing loss on patterns of consonant confusions. J. Speech Hear. Res. 21:5–36.

Whitehead, R. 1978. Validity and reliability of phoneme identification test material to assess consonant production. Internal Report. National Technical Institute for the Deaf, Rochester, N.Y.

Winitz, H. 1975. From Syllable to Conversation. University Park Press, Baltimore.

Young, M. A., and E. V. Gibbons. 1962. Speech discrimination scores and threshold measurements in a non-normal hearing population. J. Aud. Res. 2:21–33.

DEVELOPMENTAL ASPECTS OF SPEECH PRODUCTION AND PERCEPTION

CHAPTER 13

RELATIONSHIP BETWEEN PRODUCTION AND PERCEPTION OF SPEECH: SOME DEVELOPMENTAL ISSUES

Claude Ruffin-Simon

CONTENTS

This chapter includes discussion of some aspects of the relationship between speech production and speech perception during the period of speech acquisition in a child's life. Experimental results referred to here may seem rather sketchy at first, but the consistent evidence emerging from these experiments suggests some challenging interpretations using the approach chosen here.

    Normal developmental aspects of speech production and perception are of crucial importance in their own right, in order to understand how speech is learned, and also for developing teaching programs for hearing-impaired children. It is necessary to know what a young normally hearing child is able to do in terms of pattern processing, cognitive development, and also motor development in order to know what can be expected from a hearing-impaired child of the same age. A therapeutic philosophy based on speech development in normally hearing children is likely to have a much firmer basis, and therefore, a better chance of success than one based on adult speech performances.

    The work described here was supported by grants from the Science Research Council and from the Medical Research Council of Great Britain to Professor Adrian J. Fourcin at University College London. The author was supported by the Medical Research Council of Great Britain during the writing of this chapter.

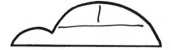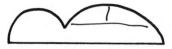

Figure 13.1.   Two visual patterns: part 1.

Pattern processing in speech is of great importance. Learning speech communication skills involves learning how to utilize (i.e., perceive and produce) auditory patterns in a systematic fashion. In order to discuss patterns and features it is first necessary to define what is meant by a pattern and to discuss some underlying issues.

A *pattern* is a set of features perceived and identified as a whole through a certain number of rules. Communication is based on the use of systems of patterns, which are in turn rule governed. In order to be used contrastively, patterns must not only be different, that is, discriminated perceptually, but they must be significantly different. In sum, they must be functionally different. We are dealing here not merely with a problem of discrimination, but with one of identification and labeling. Figure 13.1 provides an illustrative example of two visual patterns.

Both patterns could well be called "bug." Notice that the one on the left has a small head, compared to the one on the right, which has a large head. These two bugs are different and can be discriminated from each other. But they belong to the same category called "bug." Let us now add another feature to the small-headed bug—semi-circles, as shown in Figure 13.2.

The pattern on the right is now identifiable as a car. Of course, semi-circles, or wheels, are not the only distinguishing features between insects and cars, but the point is that one feature can change the labeling of a given pattern from one category to another. In this instance the semi-circles are the distinguishing feature. The same argument is true for auditory patterns, which can be represented visually for convenience by a time-frequency spectrum (i.e., a spectrogram) of the sound.

Figure 13.3 shows spectrograms of the naturally spoken sounds [bɑ], [dɑ], and [gɑ] produced by an adult male speaker. The areas of

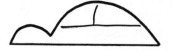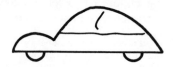

Figure 13.2.   Two visual patterns: part 2.

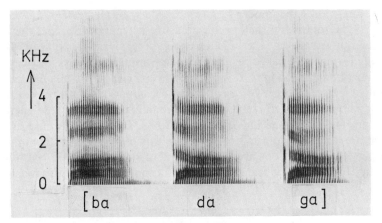

KHz

Figure 13.3.   Spectrograms of the syllables [ba], [da], and [ga] as spoken by a normally hearing adult male.

energy concentration, the black bars, are called formants. They represent the prominent features of the sound and thereby determine its auditory patterning. The main distinguishing feature between the spectral patterns of [ba] and [ga] is a rising onset, or transition, in the second formant of [ba] and a falling transition for [ga]. The analogy with visual patterns is not taken beyond this point, however, because we do not perceive the distinguishing auditory features independently of the whole as we do the visual features. In other words, the formant transitions distinguishing [ba] from [ga] are not audible per se.

It is important to remember that speech sounds are perceived auditorily as whole patterns and, although we do not perceive the features as such, they are the basis of our pattern discrimination and identification ability. The remainder of this chapter is concerned with the role of auditory pattern processing in speech acquisition. The intent is to compare aspects of the development of speech production to the development of speech perception, using an auditory perceptual approach.

THE DEVELOPMENT OF SPEECH PRODUCTION

The foundation of speech production is the production of a regular powerful voice, that is, laryngeal excitation. Although the vocal folds are in place and functioning in the infant at birth, they are not functioning well.

236   Ruffin-Simon

In Figure 13.4 the upper pair of traces show two aspects of the voice of a 27-day-old baby: the speech pressure waveform (Sp) and the laryngograph waveform (Lx). The laryngograph is a simple and safe electrical device that measures impedance variations across the larynx during phonation. The Lx waveform is a function of the degree of contact between the two vocal folds. At about 1 month of age, the baby can produce efficient regular phonation shown by the regular opening and closing action of the vocal folds. This is not the case, however, for the 2-day-old infant shown in this example. For this infant, the laryngeal vibrations are irregular and of small amplitude, as shown by the lower pair of traces. Substantial motor adjustments must be

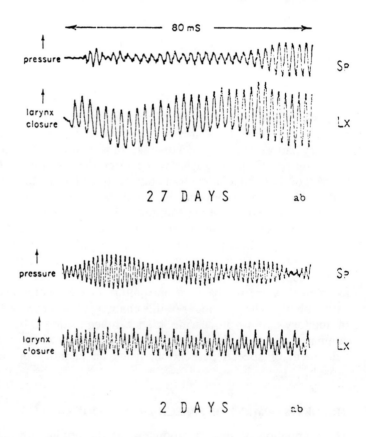

Fig. 1.

Figure 13.4.   Voice characteristics of a young baby at 27 days of age and at 2 days of age. In each pair of traces, the upper waveform represents the speech pressure waveform (Sp), and the lower trace represents the output of the Laryngograph (Lx), which is an indicator of the degree of larynx closure (from Fourcin, 1978; reproduced with permission).

made by the infant within the first 4 weeks of life in order to achieve efficient phonation. These adjustments could have been made simply on the basis of auditory feedback using the loudness component of the sound as a guide for more efficient phonation; that is, the infant may be using a simple auditory guide to achieve a complex sequence of motor skills. Having learned to produce a good voice excitation, infants must then learn to process and produce more complex patterns of speech sounds. The first few months of life seem to be spent simply learning how to extract patterns from the surrounding perceptual world. This process is clearly evident in the visual domain (e.g., Fanz, Fagan, and Miranda, 1975). It seems reasonable to assume that a similar perceptual development occurs in all sensory modalities including the auditory modality.

The infant probably spends the pre-babbling period, that is, the first 4 months of life, learning the task of extracting patterns from the surrounding speech sounds, starting with the patterns of intonation or fundamental frequency (F_o) patterns (Tonkava-Yampolskaya, 1969). There are several possible reasons for F_o patterns to be acquired before any other.

F_o patterns are more simplified and change more slowly than segmental speech patterns, that is, consonant-vowel transition patterns. Therefore, they may be easier to process than fast-changing and complex formant transition patterns such as those shown in Figure 13.3. Moreover, F_o represents the lowest frequency component of the speech signal, and it has been shown that young babies are much more sensitive auditorily to low frequencies than to high frequencies (Weir, 1976).

The next developmental stage is known as the babbling period. During the babbling period, infants will consolidate their pattern processing skills and build up a dictionary, so to speak, of corresponding auditory and motor patterns needed to produce primarily those sounds reinforced, vocally or otherwise, by the adult caretakers. Children eventually must organize a system of phonetic and phonological rules to generate sounds and combinations of sounds appropriate to their language environment, not to mention semantically acceptable messages. This stage represents the onset of systematic speech production, that is, the period of phonological development. In this period, which starts around 10 months of age, children use sounds in a systematic and contrastive fashion with a communicative purpose. They start using words to mean something.

The systematic nature of this period is reflected by the sequence of appearance of sound oppositions. There is now little doubt that there exists a tendency for the order of appearance to follow a similar pattern in many different language environments. This phenomenon is particularly noticeable for consonant sounds, mainly because research has been concentrated in this area for many years.

The general outline shown in Figure 13.5 gives an idea of this hierarchy of sound acquisition (Anthony et al., 1971; Fourcin, 1978). It must be pointed out, however, that there is a great deal of variability in the development of individual children. In general, the sequence is ordered in the place-of-articulation dimension as well as according to manners of articulation. The first consonants to appear are labials (i.e., /m/, /p/, /b/), then dental and alveolar consonants are acquired (i.e., /n/, /d/, /t/), and, finally, velar consonants appear (i.e., /g/, /k/, /ŋ/) (Jakobson, 1960). The first manner contrast to appear for each place of articulation is one between nasal and oral stops (e.g., /p,b/ and /m/). Note that certain alveolar sounds (e.g., fricative), appear later than some velar stops because of the interaction between place and manner of articulation in the developmental sequence. Only at the end of the second year do children produce systematic contrasts in the voicing dimension (e.g., between /p/ and /b/) and between stop and fricative consonants (e.g., between /t/ and /s/ or between /d/ and /z/). Two important questions can be raised at this point: why does phonological

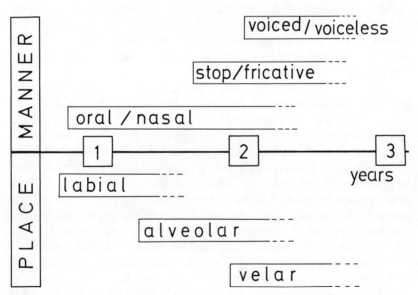

Figure 13.5. Overall sequence of sound acquisition in the period of phonological development.

development occur in this order—and how can we best account for
the developmental sequence?

THE PERCEPTUAL BASIS FOR THE
DEVELOPMENT OF SPEECH PRODUCTION

The hypothesis proposed here is that the primary basis for the first
stages of development is perceptual, especially auditory, and that the
hierarchy of appearance of sounds is largely due to auditory factors.
The obvious example is that of hearing-impaired children. Unfortunately, there are very few studies of the development of the phonological period in hearing-impaired children. Nevertheless, there is little
doubt that their speech does not develop normally because of the lack
of auditory feedback from their own productions and from those of
adults around them. In other words, in the case of hearing-impaired
children, the limitations of the perceptual system can prevent children
from developing adequate motor skills. The converse, however, is not
true: a defective motor control system does not prevent normal development of speech perceptual skills. Fourcin and Lenneberg (1973;
see also Fourcin, 1974) found that people with a congenital inability to
control their speech motor system and to produce any speech sounds
(cerebral palsied adults who did not go through the babbling period
during infancy), but with only slightly deficient hearing, are able to
process speech sounds auditorily in essentially the same fashion as
normally speaking and normally hearing adults. Their lack of motor
control over speech gestures in no way impairs their ability to learn
speech perception and labeling skills. In other words, the development
of the phonological system is heavily dependent on the normal development of the auditory perceptual system. As far as the order of sound
appearance is concerned, we need to look at the main auditory patterns
presented by the three categories of place of articulation: labial, alveolar, and velar.

Returning to Figure 13.3, which shows spectrograms of the three
syllables [bɑ], [dɑ], and [gɑ] produced by an adult male speaker, note
that in the case of [bɑ] (labial consonant), all the formants change in
the same direction, giving a simple uniform pattern. They also start at
low frequencies to which infants are sensitive at an early stage. The
formant pattern is slightly more complex in the case of [dɑ] (alveolar
sound). The upper formants F_2 and F_3 change in the opposite direction
from F_1 and start at high frequencies to which infants are less sensitive.
Finally, for the syllable [gɑ], the first formant rises, the second formant
falls, and the third formant rises, giving the most complex pattern of

all three. Moreover, velar consonants not only exhibit the most complex formant pattern, but they are also the most context sensitive. Their place of articulation, and therefore, their second and third formant patterning, is easily disturbed by their vocalic environment (e.g., see Halle, Hughes, and Bradley, 1957). Consequently, it is not surprising to find children processing simpler and more invariant patterns first—producing labials before alveolars, and alveolars before velars in their speech.

There is also direct perceptual evidence which supports this interpretation. In an earlier investigation (Simon, 1976) children were asked to identify synthetic speech-like stimuli that contrasted in the voicing dimension. We used three classes of stop consonants (labials, alveolars, and velars) in the initial position of monosyllabic words. In each experiment, children were given a forced choice between voiced and voiceless cognates. One very interesting result was that children's labeling was significantly more variable for velars than for alveolars or bilabials. A Kendall rank correlation test was performed on the standard deviations of the scores, and the coefficient of concordance W was significant at the 0.05 level (Simon, 1976). In other words, bilabials gave rise to more consistent responses than alveolars, which in turn were associated with more response consistency than velars. This result was interpreted to mean that the increasing pattern complexity of the three consonant classes influences significantly their perceptual difficulty, and consequently, the order in which children acquire those sounds. In sum, it appears that perceptual development starts with the simple patterns of bilabials in which the relevant acoustic features are concentrated in the low frequencies (low frequency burst and low frequency F_2 onset), and then moves to more and more complex patterns of alveolars and velars.

There are, of course, other perceptual factors which also come into play, especially in the visual domain. It is obviously easier to perform a gesture if one can see it performed first by someone else. Indeed, labial sounds, which are acquired first, offer enough visual cues for their place of articulation to be readily reproduced, even by profoundly hearing-impaired children. The place of articulation of alveolars, however, is hardly visible under normal circumstances, and that of velars is invisible under any circumstance. Consequently the visual factor is only of secondary importance as evidenced by the observation that blind children do not experience any remarkable difficulty in learning to speak.

Children may well be encouraged perceptually to learn consonants in a certain order, but we must keep in mind that they may also be constrained by their motor development, possibly in the place dimension and certainly in the manner dimension. As far as place of articulation is concerned, bilabials are produced by lip closure which results from the contraction of primarily one muscle, the orbicularis oris, whereas alveolars and velars involve the coordination of whole groups of muscles. We also know from misarticulation studies (Hall, 1938; Roe and Milsen, 1942; and especially Morley, 1965) that young children tend to "misarticulate" velars more often than they do alveolars or bilabials. Although it is difficult to assess the weight of the motor factor in the place dimension, it may well turn out to be very slight. Infants do produce perfectly clear velars during the babbling period, although they are not being used contrastively, nor, as far as we know, in a phonologically relevant context.

Motor factors probably play a greater role in the acquisition of manner contrasts. Stop consonants are of short duration and involve sudden articulator movements toward and/or away from complete closure of the vocal tract. Fricative consonants require the articulators to form a constriction of precise dimensions (Minifie, Hixon, and Williams, 1973) and to sustain it for several tens of milliseconds, sometimes over 100 msec. Consequently, the production of fricative consonants requires more control over the articulators than does the production of stop consonants. Indeed, for a given place of articulation, the acquisition of stops tends to precede the acquisition of fricatives (Anthony et al., 1971). This is also supported by results from misarticulation studies: fricatives and affricates are more likely to be misarticulated than plosives. Voicing oppositions are based on the very accurate timing of vocal fold adduction and vibration after the release of consonants (i.e., plosive burst or fricative noise). They depend on the exact control of laryngeal vibration onset. Only a few tens of milliseconds separate the onset of vibrations in voiced and voiceless cognates. It is not surprising, therefore, that voicing contrasts, although auditorily well defined, only appear relatively late in the speech development of a child. Studies of misarticulation also point out that voiced and voiceless consonants are more likely to be confused by young children than any other manner contrast.

Another interesting aspect of this development is that children will often find themselves unable, from a motor point of view, to reproduce an adult phonological contrast as they perceive it. They will nevertheless attempt to produce a contrast on the basis of other acoustic features that they can control at this stage but that do not appear in the adult contrast. For example, in a study of the speech production of British children between the ages of 3 and 14 (Simon, 1976) evidence was obtained suggesting that the younger children produced a distinguishing feature between /t/ and /d/, and to a lesser extent between other pairs of cognate stops which older children and adults do not utilize. This distinguishing feature was found to be a difference in the onset frequency of the second formant, which varies as a function of the place of articulation.

Figure 13.6 shows the difference in the onset frequency of F_2 as a function of age. This difference is quite large (500 Hz) for the 3-year-old children and disappears progressively as the children grow older. The trend was highly significant ($P < 0.001$ on a Pearson product moment correlation test). Young children "invent" their own acoustic distinguishing feature (F_2 transition) to make up for their motor inability to reproduce the perceived differences in the voice onset time that serve as a contrast between voiced and voiceless cognates. There is no doubt from previous work that very young children are able to discriminate and identify voiced and voiceless cognate pairs on the basis of voice onset time alone (Eimas et al., 1971; Simon and Fourcin, 1978). The authors hypothesize here that various individual strategies

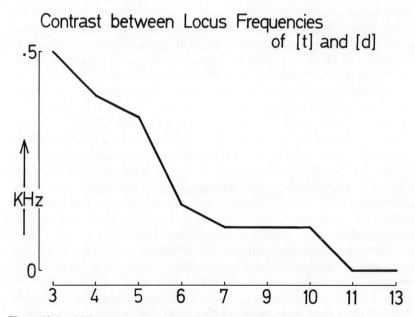

Figure 13.6.   Difference between the onset frequency of F_2 after the bursts of /t/ and after the bursts of /d/ plotted against the age of children who produced them.

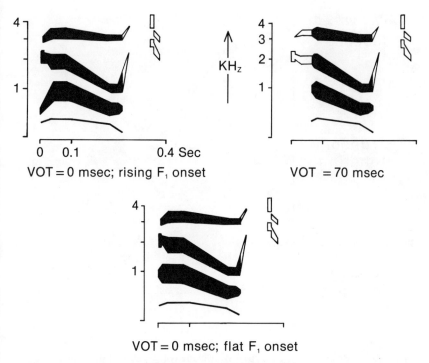

VOT = 0 msec; rising F₁ onset   VOT = 70 msec

VOT = 0 msec; flat F₁ onset

Figure 13.7.   Spectral characteristics of the synthetic voiced-voiceless stimuli "coat-goat." Formant width on the diagram corresponds to amplitude. The line below the first formant represents the fundamental frequency contour.

of this type will emerge from detailed longitudinal studies of children's speech development.

DEVELOPMENT OF SPEECH PATTERN LABELING

The development of speech patterning strategies is also reflected in the way young children learn to recognize speech patterns from their environment. Simon and Fourcin conducted a study (1978) to investigate how children learn to utilize basic acoustic cues in their labeling of a pair of cognate stimuli varying in only one dimension. These data make it clear how limited children are by the lack of refinement of their perceptual mechanisms and how progressive their perceptual learning turns out to be, contrary to widely accepted opinions.

Figure 13.7 shows the spectra of the stimuli used in the experiment. The variable of interest lies in the voicing dimension. The two variable

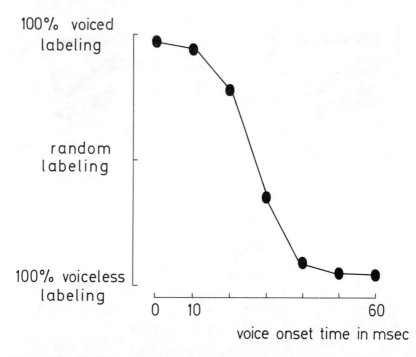

100% voiced
labeling

random
labeling

100% voiceless
labeling

0   10   60

voice onset time in msec

Figure 13.8.   Responses of a group of British adults (64 subjects) to synthetic voiced-voiceless stimuli shown in Figure 13.7.

cues were the relative onset time of laryngeal excitation after the consonant burst, referred to here as *voice onset time* (VOT) and the shape of the first formant onset, that is, the F_1 *transition*. These parameters were chosen because they are the two main cues used by adults to distinguish between voiced and voiceless initial stops. The pair of cognate stimuli was "coat" and "goat." VOT was varied in steps of 10 msec from 0 to 60 msec. The initial F_1 transition was either rising (the natural pattern for VOT values shorter than 30 msec) or level, that is, starting at the target frequency. The latter pattern is not found in natural speech with short VOT values. The stimuli were presented in varying random order through a loudspeaker at comfortable loudness level to British children between 2 and 14 years of age.

Normally hearing adults respond to these stimuli in a categorical fashion, as can be seen in Figure 13.8. Short VOT values gave rise to voiced labels "goat," and long VOT values gave rise to voiceless labels "coat." Around a VOT value of about 30 msec, listeners switched sharply from one label to the other. In other words, the physical continuum of VOT variations is not reflected in the labeling function. This phenomenon is often referred to as *categorical perception*. The use of the term *perception* in this context is, however, both vague and misleading for two reasons. First, we do not perceive categories: they are the result of our phonetic interpretation of sensory excitation of the auditory system. Second, *perception* may imply either discrimination or labeling. Discrimination abilities do not imply the existence of labeling strategies, but the ability to perform a labeling task necessarily requires the use of discrimination ability (Simon and Fourcin, 1978). For those reasons, we shall refer to the phenomenon mentioned above as *categorical labeling*.

In contrast with the adults, very young children do not demonstrate any evidence of categorical labeling as shown in Figure 13.9. This figure shows the responses of 2-, 3-, and 5-year-old children to stimuli similar to those shown in Figure 13.7, using exactly the same variables. The words used were different only in the case of 2-year-

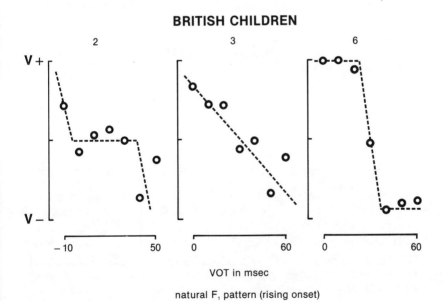

Figure 13.9.   Responses of British children to synthetic stimuli varying in the voicing dimension shown in Figure 13.7. There were 10 2-year-old, 17 3-year-old, and 22 6-year-old children. The top of the graph corresponds to 100% voiced labeling and the bottom to 100% voiceless labeling.

old children for reasons of vocabulary size: the words "Paul" and "ball" were used instead. These 2-year-old children do not reach very high consistency levels because of the large variability inherent in all results involving young children. The interesting feature about these results is that stimuli with extreme and more natural VOT values receive confident labeling, and all other intermediate stimuli receive virtually random labeling. Clearly, at the age of 2 children have not yet learned to label the physical continuum of auditory patterns in sharply defined categories. Rather, they seem to match their labeling on an absolute representation of naturally spoken patterns, and anything that does not fit the match is given a random response, that is, not identified. Three-year-old children, however, are beginning to sharpen the category boundary between the two extremes, but it is only when they reach the age of 6 that children exhibit adult-like categorical labeling behavior, at least for the stimuli with the natural rising F_1 onset.

The data obtained in Figures 13.8 and 13.9 were for the more natural case of a rising initial F_1 transition. Figure 13.10 shows the labels given by the children to stimuli with a level F_1 onset, that is, the unnatural F_1 pattern at short VOT values. A fascinating result ap-

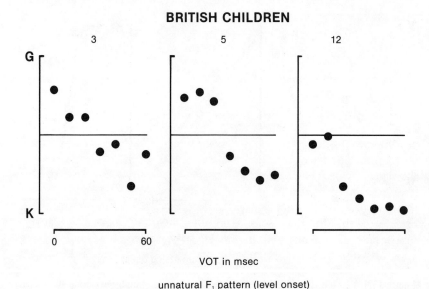

Figure 13.10.   Responses of British children to voiced-voiceless stimuli with a level F_1 onset. There were 17 3-year-old, 17 5-year-old, and 19 12-year-old children.

pears. Up to the age of 5, children do not utilize the presence or absence of an initial F_1 transition as a cue to their voiced-voiceless labeling. They only start to learn its distinguishing function after the age of 5, and make use of the cue in an adult fashion only after the age of 10. Only then do they reject the combination of short VOT and level F_1 onset as acceptable voicing cues. In other words, it takes them more than 10 years to learn the perceptual function of the F_1 transition pattern feature in this context, and about 6 years to learn the skill of reliable categorical labeling.

Although these experiments dealt only with two features of one manner dimension, similar trends of speech skill development may be found by using similar experimental techniques, both in production and perception. Moreover, these trends are probably symptomatic of much deeper and more general cognitive processes which underlie the development of children's perception and understanding of the world around them.

SOME CONCLUDING REMARKS

This chapter has emphasized the importance of auditory pattern processing in the general development of speech communication skills, not only in perceptual skills but also in productive skills. The auditory pattern approach has indeed proved useful in helping to understand normal processes of speech development. Of course there are other perceptual factors, and perhaps motor factors, that come into play, particularly in the visual domain. We may be encouraged to learn labials first because we can see them better. The data presented here show that the auditory pattern processing approach provides a powerful and fruitful tool for the interpretation of both productive and perceptual developmental data. In brief, if a baby has both motor and auditory systems in good working order, naturally he or she will use both. If the motor system is deficient, the auditory system will develop and be used essentially normally. If, however, the auditory system is deficient, this will often have catastrophic and permanent effects on the development of the motor system. Moreover, there is evidence suggesting that a lack of sensory stimulation of the auditory nerve actually prevents the normal development and maturation of the auditory system, at least in mice (Webster and Webster, 1976).

The crucial role of auditory pattern processing in the developmental period is of great consequence in the design of therapeutic strategies for hearing-impaired children. In other words, if a speech training sequence follows an order based on the natural sequence of development from simple to complex patterns, from temporal to frequential patterns and from low to high frequency patterns, and if one uses visual presentation of auditorily significant patterns, then the therapy has a much better chance of success (see, for example, Fisher et al., this volume) than if the sequence is aimed at improving intelligibility on the basis of broader and more subjective criteria.

ACKNOWLEDGMENTS

I would like to thank Professor Adrian Fourcin and Dr. Evelyn Abberton for their kind comments and suggestions during the preparation of the paper.

REFERENCES

Anthony, T., J. Bogle, D. Ingram, et al. 1971. Edinburgh Articulation Test. Livingstone, Edinburgh.

Eimas, P. D., E. R. Siqueland, J. Vigorito, and P. Jusczyk. 1971. Speech perception in infants. Science 171:303–306.

Fanz, R. L., J. R. Fagan, and S. B. Miranda. 1975. Early visual selectivity. In L. B. Cohen, and P. Salapatek (eds.), Infant Perception: From Sensation to Cognition. Academic Press, Inc., New York.

Fourcin, A. J. 1974. Speech perception in the absence of speech productive ability. In N. O'Connor (ed.), Language, Cognition Deficits and Retardation. Butterworth, London.

Fourcin, A. J. 1978, Acoustic patterns and speech acquisition. In N. Waterson and C. Snow (eds.), The Development of Communication. Wiley, New York.

Fourcin, A. J., and E. H. Lenneberg. 1973. Language development in the absence of expressive speech. In E. H. Lenneberg (ed.), Foundations of Language Development. IBRO-U.N.E.S.C.O.

Hall, M. E. 1938. Auditory factors in functional articulatory speech defects. J. Exp. Educ. 7:110–132.

Halle, M., G. W. Hughes, and J. P. A. Bradley. 1957. Acoustic properties of stop consonants. J. Acoust. Soc. Am. 29:107–116.

Jakobson, R. 1960. Why Papa and Mama? Mouton, The Hague.

Minifie, F. J., T. J. Hixon, and F. Williams. 1973. Normal Aspects of Speech, Hearing and Language. Williams & Wilkins Company, Baltimore.

Morley, E. M. 1965. The Development and Disorders of Speech in Childhood. Williams & Wilkins Company, Baltimore.

Roe, V., and R. Milsen. 1942. The effect of maturation upon defective articulation in elementary grades. J. Speech Disord. 7:37–45.

Simon, C. 1976. A development study of acoustic pattern production and perception in voiced-voiceless oppositions. Doctoral dissertation, University of London.

Simon, C., and A. J. Fourcin. 1978. Cross-language study of speech pattern learning. J. Acoust. Soc. Am. 63:925–935.
Tonkava-Yampolskaya, R. V. 1969. Development of intonation in children. Soviet Psychol. 7:48–54.
Webster, D. B., and M. Webster. 1976. Neonatal sound deprivation affects brain stem auditory stimuli. Arch. Otolaryngol. 103:392–396.
Weir, C. 1976. Auditory frequency selectivity in the neonate: A signal detection analysis. J. Exp. Child Psychol. 21:219–225.

CHAPTER 14

PHONATORY DEVELOPMENT IN YOUNG NORMALLY HEARING AND HEARING-IMPAIRED CHILDREN

Rachel E. Stark

CONTENTS

The most difficult practical issues in the educational management of young hearing-impaired children today center around decisions about the primary means of communication which they are to be taught. These decisions are hampered by the lack of appropriate assessment procedures. Although the hearing sensitivity, cognitive level, and communication skills of preschool deaf children can be assessed, adequate measures of the speech perception skills and prespeech vocal behaviors are not presently available. Such measures are needed not only for the initial assessment of hearing-impaired children, but also for evaluation of their progress in treatment. The need is especially great if an objective of the program they enter is to teach them to talk.

    This chapter is concerned with some measures of potential speech production abilities in young deaf children. These measures were derived by comparing the speech skills of hearing-impaired children who had not yet developed spoken language with those of much younger, normally hearing, prespeech infants. The purpose of the present study

This work was supported in part by NINCDS Grant No. 09628 and in part by an NINCDS Contract No. N01NS-2-2318.

in which these measures were developed was to compare the vocal output of normally hearing infants and preschool deaf children with respect to: 1) rate of vocal output, that is, the number of vocalizations produced per unit time; and 2) the developmental level of vocal output as determined by assessment of the types of vocalization produced.

It has been suggested that the spontaneous vocal behavior of the nonspeaking deaf child seems to resemble that of the younger normally hearing infant in at least some respects (Carr, 1953; Lach et al., 1970; Stark, 1967). If so, a comparison of the spontaneous speech behavior of the deaf child with that of the normal infant may provide a useful indication of speech production status before he or she is given amplification and/or treatment and of progress with respect to speech production after they are provided. It is also possible that the normal developmental sequence of vocal behavior may be useful in developing subgoals in treatment. These subgoals would be designed to render the deaf child's attempts to speak less effortful as well as more highly intelligible.

METHOD

Subjects

The subjects of the present study were:

1. Four infants who had normal hearing and whose speech and language development were entirely normal. These normally hearing infants were from middle-class families. They were recorded on a longitudinal basis throughout the first year of life.
2. Eleven hearing-impaired children, aged 15 to 24 months, who were recorded at the time when their hearing loss was first identified and before they were given a hearing aid. These children had hearing losses ranging from moderately severe to profound and were within the normal range of nonverbal intelligence. They were all from middle-class families and their parents wished to receive help in managing the child's problem.
3. Fourteen hearing-impaired children, age 2 years, 2 months to 3 years, 11 months, who were recorded on five different occasions (all within a 2-week period) after they had used a hearing aid for varying periods of time. These older hearing-impaired children were potential subjects in an experimental speech training program. They formed a more heterogenous group than the younger hearing-impaired children. They showed considerable variability

with respect to nonverbal intelligence, socioeconomic status of the family, and concern on the part of the parents. None of them, however, was able to produce single-word utterances intelligibly, and all were children of hearing parents.

Recording Procedures

Two of the normal infants were recorded in the home and two in the laboratory in a quiet room. During a portion of each recording session, the mother was asked to interact with the infant as she normally did. During the remainder of the recording, the infant was placed in front of toys or a visual display (mobile) and the mother withdrew from the child's immediate environment. At earlier ages, the infants were placed in an infant seat or were held by the mother. At later ages, they were seated in a playpen or on a play mat or were crawling and rolling on the play mat on the floor. Portions of each recording (approximately 20 to 30 minutes) that were relatively free of crying, fussing, or laughing were selected for the purpose of making the vocalization counts.

The 11 younger hearing-impaired children were recorded in a sound-treated room for a period of 1 hour. They were accompanied by their mothers or by both parents. The parents were asked to interact with the child for a portion of the hour as they would at home and to read a magazine and pretend to ignore the child for the remainder of the hour. Toys were available in the room and the child was free to move about as he or she wished. Portions of each recording (approximately 20 to 30 minutes) that were relatively free of crying, fussing, or laughing were again selected for the purpose of making vocalization counts for these children. The 14 older hearing-impaired children were recorded in the same circumstances as the 11 younger hearing-impaired children. However, the recordings were made over five different 20-minute baseline sessions in their case. One of the older children was accompanied by a social worker instead of his parents.

Rate of Vocal Output

Measures of the number of vocalizations produced per unit time were obtained for each of the above recordings. In order to derive a valid measure of vocalization rate, it was necessary first to make sure that a representative sample of vocal behavior had been obtained in a standard manner. Second, it was necessary to define a unit of vocalization which could be used reliably by more than one observer in arriving at a total count. It was found that reliable counts could not be obtained by listening to the audiotapes continuously and recording vocalizations by means of hand counter. Phonetic and acoustic criteria were considered in defining the vocal unit to be counted. It is probable that the most reliable and meaningful measures may be obtained by listening to the sounds produced and at the same time studying a visual representation in the form of a graphic level recording trace (intensity by time). In the present study, the counts were obtained by examining phonetic transcriptions of the children's vocal output. All of the sounds other than crying, laughing, and vegetative sounds, such as coughing and sneezing, which were produced by the normally hearing infants and the older hearing-impaired children had been transcribed by at least one listener in an initial cataloging of the data. In some cases, two listeners had performed this task. From these transcriptions, the number of syllabic units judged to be present were identified and counted. The percentage of agreement between two listeners for the total number of units identified (0.73) was consistently higher than the percentage of agreement between these listeners for the phonetic content of the syllables transcribed (0.56).

Level of Vocal Output

The level of vocal output was determined by examination of the different sound types recorded in the listeners' transcriptions. A number of investigators working independently (Oller, 1980; Stark, 1980; Zlatin-Laufer, 1975) have described a succession of stages of vocal development in preschool infants which occur in an invariant sequence. The concept of developmental stages derives from the work of Piaget (1952). It implies that clusters of vocal behaviors emerge within a given stage, that is, within the time period limited by the emergence of two successive levels. It has not yet been shown that vocal development does take place in all infants in a series of such stages, but there is agreement with respect to a set of milestone behaviors which are reported as characteristic of infants of different levels. These levels are shown below with their approximate age ranges in normal infants. They are characterized by the following vocal behaviors:

Level I: 0 to 8 weeks. Reflexive vocalization; crying, fussing, and vegetative sounds.
Level II: 8 to 20 weeks. Pleasure sounds; cooing and laughter.
Level III: 20 to 35 weeks. Vocal play; experimentation with squealing, growling, friction, and other noises (for example, "raspberries") which have a high frequency of occurrence and may be used in many different situational contexts.
Level IV: 6 to 10 months. Reduplicated babbling; production of series of consonant-vowel (CV) syllables, each one of which is perceived as having the same consonant and the same vowel.

Level V: 10 to 14 months. Protowords; phonetically consistent forms produced in relation to experiences which are constantly recurring. Nonreduplicated babbling, characterized by the use of different consonants and vowels within a series and also by vowel (V), vowel-consonant (VC), and CVC syllables, as well as CV syllables. A greater variety of stress pattern and intonational contour appears in this babbling, sometimes referred to as expressive jargon (Gesell and Thompson, 1934).

Level VI: 14 to 24 months. Production of single words, referring to specific objects or events. Initially these words may be used for a limited period of time only and then dropped. In a majority of infants there is a marked increase in the rate of acquisition of new words at 18 to 24 months of age, without subsequent loss of these words from the child's lexicon. This acceleration in growth of the lexicon probably coincides with emergence of representational thought in most infants, and thus marks the onset of language acquisition in a truly symbolic sense.

The catalog of each subject's vocalizations in the present study included descriptive comments and indications of the presence of grunts, squealing, laughter, and other nonspeech vocalizations as well as the phonetic transcriptions. Thus, the annotations and phonetic transcriptions combined provided a clear indication of the level of vocal development, according to the above definitions, which the child had attained.

RESULTS

Normal Infants

The number of vocalizations produced by the four normally hearing infants at each of five different age levels is shown in Table 14.1. First, it will be observed that two of the infants, V.W. and M.P.V., vocalized at a consistently lower rate than the remaining infants, J.S. and M. W. The first two infants were recorded in the home, not in the laboratory, so that they might have been expected to be more vocal than their peers, not less vocal. The differences may reflect true variation in rate of vocal output among normally hearing infants. In addition, it will be observed that the number of non-cry vocalizations produced increased with chronological age in all infants. The increase reflects an overall

Table 14.1 Mean number of vocalizations (voc) per minute produced at different age levels and in different developmental stages by four normally hearing infants

Age (in weeks)	J.S.		M.W.		V.W.		M.P.V.		Mean
	Stage of vocal development	No. voc per minute	Stage of vocal development	No. voc per minute	Stage of vocal development	No. voc per minute	Stage of vocal development	No. voc per minute	
9	II	4.74	II	3.47	II	0.55	II	2.00	2.69
15	II–III	7.85	II	4.89	II	1.43	II–III	1.50	3.92
22	III	5.35	III	5.86	III	3.00	III	3.21	4.36
30–36	IV	6.40	III–IV	3.65	III–IV	6.10	IV	7.78	5.98
46–48	IV–V	9.78	V	15.80	IV	4.50	IV	9.50	9.90
Mean		6.82		6.73		3.12		4.80	5.37

decrease in both frequency of crying and vegetative sounds, and a concomitant increase in the frequency of other sound types.

The level of vocal development which the infants were thought to have reached is also indicated in Table 14.1. In some cases, the infant was thought to be in a transition from one level to the next at the time of recording. For example, infant M. W. when recorded at 30 weeks of age produced elaborated vocal play in which a few single-stop consonant-vowel syllables were embedded. She was not yet babbling on these CV syllables, however. Individual differences between infants again have to be taken into account in evaluating level of development. Some infants may spend many weeks engaging in the use of expressive jargon and a relatively brief period of time in producing protowords (Dore et al., 1976). Other infants show the opposite effect, that is, their use of expressive jargon is limited to a very brief period of time but they may spend many weeks in the exercise of protowords. Infant M.W. at 46 weeks of age used a great deal of expressive jargon, pro- ducing long series of inflected nonsense syllables both when playing by herself and when looking at her mother. Her rate of vocal output (that is, number of vocal units per minute) showed a correspondingly high increase. Infant J.S., on the other hand, was beginning to produce word-like phonetically consistent forms in response to certain types of situations at 48 weeks of age, and did not use expressive jargon at all at this time. Thus, the number of vocal units per minute showed a more modest increase in his output at 48 weeks of age than in infant M.W.'s output at 46 weeks of age. Infants V.W. and M.P.V. were using dif- ferent CV syllables in their babbling at 46 to 47 weeks of age, but had not begun to use V, VC, or CVC syllables nor to employ a variety of stress patterns or intonational contours at this time.

Younger Hearing-Impaired Children

The number of vocalizations per minute which were produced by the 11 hearing-impaired children aged 15 to 24 months before they were given a hearing aid is shown in Table 14.2. Examination of this table indicates that there is no apparent relationship between the age of the child and the rate of vocal output in number of vocalizations per minute produced. The children have been grouped, however, according to the level of vocal development which they were judged to have attained at the time when they were first identified as hearing impaired. As in the case of the normal infants, the data suggest that there is an overall increase in rate of vocal output as increasingly higher levels of vocal development are attained. The means and ranges for the number of vocalizations per minute produced by the hearing-impaired children at

Table 14.2   Mean number of vocalizations (voc) per minute produced by 11 hearing-impaired preschool children before they were given a hearing aid

Child	Stage of vocal development	No. voc per minute	Age (in months)
J.McF.	II	3.1	18
N.C.		4.3	17
L.K.		1.8	17
B.P.		2.8	18
Mean		3.0	
T.K.	III	5.0	20
L.R.		5.6	18
C.D.		4.1	26
B.Q.		4.0	17
Mean		4.7	
R.J.	IV	9.8	15
S.G.		6.4	15
C.M.		14.3	24
Mean		10.2	
Grand Mean		5.58	

each of the levels shown corresponds quite well with the means and ranges obtained by the younger normally hearing infants judged to be at the same levels of vocal development.

The findings suggested that circular reasoning might have given rise to the judgment of similarity of vocal development in hearing-impaired and normally hearing children. In order words, knowledge of lower and higher vocalization rates might have influenced the author's judgment of the level of vocal development attained by individual hearing-impaired children. The catalogs of vocalization were therefore scanned a second time in order to make sure that this bias had not entered into the assignment of levels. When the vocalizations of these younger hearing-impaired children were transcribed, the listeners had prepared inventories of the vocalic and consonantal elements which they both believed to be in the child's repertoire (Stark, 1967). The inventories did not indicate point-by-point agreement as to the inventory of phonemes the child was capable of producing, but rather with respect to the overall vocal repertoire of the child. These inventories were also examined in reevaluation of the level of development the children might have attained at the time when their hearing impairment was first identified. Sample inventories are shown in Tables 14.3, 14.4, and 14.5.

Table 14.3. Inventory of sounds produced by an 18-month-old hearing-impaired child before he was provided with a hearing aid

Vowels	Consonants	Syllables	Emotional expression	Noises
æ	h		crying	grunt
ə	ʔ		laughing	sigh
a	x			heavy breathing
I	m̩			brief clicks
ɛ				
i				
e				

Subject: J.McF.—developmental stage, II; vocalization, 3.1 per minute

Table 14.3 describes the vocal repertoire of an 18-month-old hearing-impaired child judged to be at level II. This child was producing a number of brief isolated steady-state vowels which might be initiated or terminated by a voiceless portion indicated as /h/ or a glottal stop. He also produced, on two occasions only, a brief velar fricative /x/ and, considerably more often, a syllabic nasal consonant /m/. No consonant-vowel syllables were present in his repertoire and he showed no vocal play behaviors. Thus, he could not be judged to have attained levels III or IV. The presence of sustained laughter, however, indicated that he had reached level II. Unlike most normally hearing infants who are able to produce sustained laughter, however, J.McF. was not producing series of vowel-like sounds, but single vocalic elements only. In this sense, his vocal behavior was less well developed than might be expected. At the same time, however, the classes of vowel-like sounds which he was judged to be producing showed a greater variety

Table 14.4 Inventory of sounds produced by a 20-month-old hearing-impaired child before he was provided with a hearing aid

Vowels	Consonants	Syllables	Emotional expression	Noises
æ	m̩ p	mæ × 1	laughing	sigh
ǽ	ŋ ɡ	ɡI × 1	crying	nasal grunt
ə	n w̥		whining	sniff
e	ʔ ɓ			lip bubbling
a	ŋ̑ ŋ			tongue bubbling
	f			nasal humming
	b			
	h			

Subject: T.K.—developmental stage, III; vocalization rate, 5.0 per minute.

Table 14.5   Inventory of sounds produced by a 15-month-old hearing-impaired child before she was provided with a hearing aid

Vowels	Consonants	Syllables	Emotional expression	Noises
æ	m̩	mæ	crying	grunts
ə	m	mə	laughing	sighs
3	n	wæ		sniffs
ʊ	w	bæ		squeaking
	h	ðæ × 1		
	ʔ	jæ		coughing
	ð	h3		sneezing
	j	dæ × 1		
	d			

Subject: R.J.—developmental stage, IV; vocalization rate, 9.8.

than would be expected of a normally hearing infant at level II. Thus, this child's vocal repertoire was not similar in all respects to that of a normally hearing infant at the same level of vocal development. The similarity in rate of vocal output (in number of vocalizations per minute) which was observed may be related to the fact that J.McF., like young, normally hearing infants and also like many of his hearing-impaired peers, resorted to crying and fussing when he failed to communicate his intentions. Thus, he spent an inordinate amount of time in these vocal activities—as well as in laughing—and as a result the number of more speech-like vocalizations per minute was reduced.

The inventory of speech-like and nonspeech-like vocalizations produced by the hearing-impaired child T.K. (age 20 months) is shown in Table 14.4. This child produced an /h/-like sound and glottal stops both before and after vowel sounds. He also produced a large number of syllabic consonantal sounds, /n/, /m/, and /f/, and a variety of friction noises, some of them produced at the labial place of articulation and others at the velar. Many of these consonantal sounds were prolonged. They were produced when the child was playing by himself and when he was interacting with his mother. These behaviors, together with the "tongue bubbling" and "nasal humming" indicated in the "noise" category of the inventory, may be classed as vocal play behaviors and, thus, indicate that he had reached at least level III of vocal development. He was producing very few consonant-vowel syllables, however (a total of 2 for the entire recording session). It was therefore judged that he had not attained level IV. The rate of vocal output and the inventory of consonant sounds T.K. was producing were quite typical of a normally hearing infant in level III. The inventory of vocalic or vowel-like sounds with which he was credited, on the other hand, was more limited than would be expected for a normally hearing infant in level III.

The inventory of sounds produced by a third child, R.J. (aged 15 months), is shown in Table 14.5. This child was producing a glottal stop, nasal consonants (both a syllabic nasal consonant, /m/ and the syllabic initial consonants /n/ and /m/), glides, and the stop consonant /d/. She produced some of these consonants in CV syllables in babbling. Her babbling had progressed sufficiently for her to be capable of producing different CV syllables in a babbled series (for example, ahanae). Thus, she was judged to have attained level IV of vocal development. R.J.'s rate of vocal output was comparable to that of a normally hearing infant at the same level of vocal development. In spite of the advanced nature of her babbling, however, R.J. was credited with only a very small set of vowel-like sounds, many fewer than would be expected in a normally hearing infant at this stage of vocal development.

The level of vocal development attained by these 11 hearing-impaired children did not appear to show a significant relationship to age, nonverbal intelligence, or extent or type of hearing loss, except that none of the children with a profound loss had reached level IV. Other factors, such as the nature of mother-child interaction or time of onset or rapidity of onset of the hearing loss, may have influenced their level of vocal development. In addition, the level of vocal development attained by these children before they were given amplification did not appear to be predictive of their later progress in learning to speak. After he was provided with a hearing aid and placed in an appropriate treatment program, J.McF. was successful in learning to speak, whereas T.K., initially more advanced in vocal development than J.McF., was not able to do so. Longitudinal data obtained from these children after they were given a hearing aid suggests that some of them progressed quite rapidly to more advanced levels of vocal development, whereas others did not.

Older Hearing-Impaired Children

The children shown in Table 14.6 had all been provided with amplification. They had worn hearing aids for varying periods of time. Surprisingly, some of them were still judged to be at a very early level of vocal development. Of those still considered to be at level II, S.H. and M.K. were found to be multiply handicapped. S.H. was mildly retarded and mildly cerebral palsied, and M.K. was found to be severely retarded and to have some autistic behaviors. The third child in stage II had suffered lead intoxication. Yet another, not shown here, was visually impaired as well as hearing impaired.

Table 14.6   Mean number of vocalizations (voc) per minute produced by 14 hearing-impaired preschool children after they were given a hearing aid

Child	Stage of vocal development	No. voc per. minute	Age (in years, months)
S.H.	II	7.64	2, 7
G.H.		7.97	2, 5
M.K.		7.36	3, 11
Mean		7.67	
B.R.	III	11.80	3, 9
M.K.		12.15	3, 3
B.G.		20.40	2, 9
Mean		14.78	
T.B.	IV	5.92	3, 6
T.McL.		4.70	2, 2
T.C.		13.55	3, 10
R.F.		12.53	3, 7
S.E.		9.98	2, 8
A.S.		9.32	2, 6
T.W.		19.37	3, 6
C.W.		17.38	3, 4
Mean		11.59	
Grand mean		11.43	

Some of the remaining children in these older groups were difficult to assess in terms of level of vocal development. For example, the child A.S., who was deafened at 18 months of age as a result of meningitis, had produced a number of single words before her illness and would still attempt to do so upon request. She was unable to produce intelligible words, however, and showed no evidence of phonetic contrasts in her attempts at word production. Similarly, the child S.E. was proficient in sign language and, thus, had acquired word concepts and a considerable vocabulary in sign. Her attempts at spoken words, which were never spontaneous, were also unintelligible. Also, unlike normally hearing infants, some of the children in this group who were babbling used glottal stops inconsistently in the syllable-final position.

There does not appear to be a strong relationship between rate of vocal output and the level of vocal development attained by the children in this more heterogenous group. B.G., for example, was given a great deal of attention by his parents and encouraged to vocalize. He was an intelligent, profoundly deaf child who communicated well by means of vocalization and his own esoteric signs. He had not reached level IV (reduplicated babbling) at the time when the recordings were made, but he nevertheless showed the highest rate of vocal output of all of the older hearing-impaired children. T.McL. and T.B., on the other hand, who were capable of babbling, had a very low rate of vocal output. T.B. was a foster child who had been abused by his parents. T.McL. was the child of a school-aged mother. She would vocalize only for her grandmother who cared for her during the day. Both children appeared to withhold vocalizations in the laboratory setting even when rewards were made contingent upon their vocalizing.

SUMMARY AND DISCUSSION

The spontaneous vocalizations of young hearing-impaired children were found to resemble those of prespeech normally hearing infants in some respects and to differ from them in others. Of the three groups of children studied, the spontaneous vocalizations of normally hearing infants and of the younger hearing-impaired children resembled one another most closely, whereas the spontaneous vocalizations of the group of older hearing-impaired children appeared to be different from those of two younger groups. The spontaneous vocalizations of older hearing-impaired children who had some experience of hearing aid use were more numerous and generally more advanced than those of the younger hearing-impaired children, but they were also more variable with respect to level of vocal development attained. The older hearing-impaired children were a more heterogeneous group, showing a wider range of nonverbal intelligence, cultural background, and socioeconomic status than the two younger groups. The older children had also had a greater variety of educational experiences and in some cases had multiple handicaps, that is, handicaps in addition to the hearing loss. The results obtained suggest that vocalization rate increases with age and experience of hearing aid use, although adverse home circumstances may operate to inhibit spontaneous vocalization and thus reduce the rate of spontaneous vocal output. The level of vocal development which the child was judged to have attained appeared to increase after a period of hearing aid use and of exposure to treatment programs of various types in those children who were not multiply handicapped. It is noteworthy, however, that none of the children studied had attained stage V (protowords and expressive jargon) and only two were producing single words referentially. These two children never used these words spontaneously or intelligibly. This finding is not a function of subject selection procedures because level of vocal development was not a criterion for referral of children to the experimental training program referred to above.

Certain differences were observed between normally hearing infants and the hearing-impaired children judged to be at the same level of vocal development. These differences were in the inventory of vowel- or consonant-like sounds which were produced, rather than in the syllable shapes employed. Thus, the hearing-impaired child displayed the vocal behaviors and syllable shapes typical of a certain level of vocal development, but the total inventory of consonant-like and vowel-like sounds produced within his repertoire tended to be more limited than that of the normally hearing infant at the same level of vocal development. In addition, the rate of vocal output, that is, the number of vocalizations per minute produced by the hearing-impaired child after a period of hearing aid use, might be greater or less than would be found in a normally hearing infant at the same level of development.

These results may be thought of as supporting the findings reported in previous studies of the spontaneous vocalizations of deaf children. Such studies have suggested 1) that the spontaneous vocalizations of deaf children are more natural-sounding than their attempts at speech (Carr, 1953; Lach et al., 1970); and 2) that, at least after 6 months of age, the spontaneous vocalizations of deaf infants tend to be more stereotyped than those of normally hearing infants of the same age. The findings of the present study do not support the belief that the rate of vocal output declines in deaf children after 5 months of age and remains at a consistently low level, as suggested by Mavilya (1968).

What are the implications of the findings of this study for the speech and language training of hearing-impaired children? Is it possible for these children to learn to speak acceptably and intelligibly in a quite different sequence from that followed by the normal infant? Recent examination of teaching methods would suggest that it is not (Ling, 1976). Procedures by which the hearing-impaired child is taught single words before he or she can babble have resulted in unnatural speech and poor intelligibility. Programs in which the attempt has been made to follow a normal developmental sequence in training hearing-impaired children probably have been more successful in eliciting intelligible speech than those that have not (Ling, 1976; Osberger, this volume; Simmons, 1971).

The experimental training program in which some of the older hearing-impaired children discussed above were included, had as its primary aim facilitation of a normal developmental sequence. Two different approaches deriving from the measures proposed in the present study were employed. The first approach was designed to help the child develop more fully the inventory of vocal behaviors expected at the development level which he had already attained. Where this elaboration had not occurred spontaneously after the provision of a hearing aid, the child's vocal rate was frequently low (less than 7 to 8 vocalizations per minute). It was found to be of benefit to increase the vocalization rate of these children by means of operant conditioning procedures. Vocalization rate may be increased by a tangible food or toy reinforcement. In the above experimental program, room lights that had been off were turned on as a means of positive reinforcement (Goldstein and Stark, 1976; Stark, 1977). Such procedures may be most useful for children at lower developmental levels (levels II and III). In those children whose vocalization rate was higher (10 or more vocalizations per minute), it was found to be more effective to facilitate a variety of level-appropriate behaviors by means of imitation, modeling, and prompting. The child was then taught to combine these vocal behaviors with one another in a variety of ways and to produce them in longer sequences. Nonauditory aids were used as adjuncts to this training, but hearing aids might be used as effectively with some hearing-impaired children.

The stage process model upon which these procedures were based included the hypothesis that only after the hearing-impaired child's output has been elaborated and has become more characteristic of the developmental level which has already been attained will he or she begin to acquire the behaviors characteristic of the next highest developmental level. These new behaviors will be acquired in smaller and simpler units first and only gradually introduced in longer sequences or more complex combinations.

Experience with the training procedures outlined above suggests that they are likely to be effective whether or not the stage process model proves to be a viable one. These procedures together with effective use of nonauditory as well as auditory aids might benefit young hearing-impaired children to a greater extent than programs that begin training at too high a developmental level or progress too quickly to higher developmental levels. A better understanding of the processes of speech development in normally hearing infants will, however, be essential to the success of procedures based upon a normal developmental sequence. Such understanding would also make possible a more thorough and careful investigation of the effectiveness of existing speech training programs.

REFERENCES

Carr, J. 1953. An investigation of the spontaneous speech sounds of five-year-old deaf-born children. J. Speech Hear. Disord. 18:22–29.
Dore, J., M. B., Franklin, R. T. Miller, and A. L. H. Ramer. 1976. Transitional phenomena in early language acquisition. J. Child Lang. 3:1–28.

Gesell, A., and H. Thompson. 1934. Infant Behavior, Its Genesis and Growth. McGraw-Hill, New York.

Goldstein, Jr., M. H., and R. E. Stark. 1976. Modification of vocalization of preschool deaf children by vibrotactile and visual displays. J. Acoust. Soc. Am. 59:1477–1481.

Lach, R., D. Ling, A. H. Ling, and N. Ship. 1970. Early speech development in deaf infants. Am. Ann. Deaf 115:522–526.

Ling, D. 1976. Speech and the Hearing-Impaired Child: Theory and Practice. A. G. Bell Association for the Deaf, Washington, D.C.

Mavilya, M. 1968. Spontaneous vocalization and babbling in hearing impaired infants. In G. Fant (ed.), International Symposium on Speech Communication Abilities and Profound Deafness. A. G. Bell Association for the Deaf, Washington, D.C.

Oller, D. K. 1980. The emergence of the sounds of speech in infancy. In G. Yenikomshian, C. Ferguson, and J. Kavanagh (eds.), Child Phonology, Perception, Production and Deviation. MIT Press, Cambridge, Mass.

Piaget, J. 1952. The Origins of Intelligence in Children. International Universities Press, New York.

Simmons, A. A. 1971. Language and hearing. In L. E. Connor (ed.), Speech for the Deaf Child: Knowledge and Use. A. G. Bell Association for the Deaf, Washington, D.C.

Stark, R. E. 1967. Vocalization of the preschool deaf child. Annual Report No. 1, Neurocommunications Laboratory. The Johns Hopkins University School of Medicine, Department of Behavioral Sciences, Baltimore.

Stark, R. E. 1977. Measures of the effectiveness of nonauditory aids for preschool deaf children. J. Acoust. Soc. Am. 62(Suppl. 1):56.

Stark, R. E. 1980. Stages of speech development in the first year of life. In G. Yenikomshian, C. Ferguson, and J. Kavanagh (eds.), Child Phonology, Production, Perception and Deviation. MIT Press, Cambridge, Mass.

Zlatin-Laufer, M. 1975. Explorative mapping of the vocal tract and primitive syllabification in infancy: The first six months. Paper presented at the meeting of the American Speech and Hearing Association, November, Washington, D.C.

CHAPTER 15

THE ACQUISITION OF SEGMENTAL PHONOLOGY BY NORMAL AND HEARING-IMPAIRED CHILDREN

Carol Stoel-Gammon

CONTENTS

Most children acquire the phonological system of their mother tongue in a relatively short period of time. The first words typically appear early in the second year, and by the age of 6 or 7, the phonemic system is mastered (Sander, 1972; Templin, 1957). For children with a hearing loss, phonological acquisition is much slower, as would be expected. Studies of hearing-impaired children and adults indicate differences between "deaf" and normal speech on both the suprasegmental and the segmental level (Calvert, 1961; Dodd, 1976; Hudgins, 1937; Hudgins and Numbers, 1942; John and Howarth, 1965; Levitt and Stromberg, this volume; Levitt, et al., 1978; Smith, 1975; Stevens, Nickerson, and Rollins, this volume; Whitehead, this volume). Characteristic differences occurring on the phonemic level include omission of consonants, particularly in final position, confusion of the voicing distinction, substitution of stops for other classes of consonants, and substitution of centralized or diphthongized vowels for the target vowel (Dodd, 1976; Levitt et al., 1978; Levitt and Stromberg, this volume; Smith, 1975).

    Most previous research has involved children 8 years of age or older. By this age, articulatory patterns are usually well established,

This research was supported by the National Institutes of Health, Research Contract No. NO1-HD-3-2793-01.

267

and changing them requires a concerted effort on the part of the child, teachers, and parents. The study presented here focused on younger hearing-impaired children, 2 to 7 years old, many of whom were still in the developmental stages of language acquisition. The data on their productions is compared with those of young normal children, allowing examination of the similarities and differences in the patterns of phonological acquisition of the two groups.

METHOD

Subjects

The hearing-impaired group consisted of 21 subjects ranging in age from 2 years, 4 months (2;4) to 7 years, 3 months (7;3) with a median age of 4 years, 8 months (4;8). In general terms, the subjects were categorized as having a moderate to profound hearing loss in the unaided condition, and a mild to moderate loss when aided. For 16 of the 21 subjects, hearing loss was identified by the age of 15 months; for the others, age at time of identification ranged from 2;0 to 3;10. All the subjects were enrolled in total communication school programs in the state of Washington.

The normal subject group included 25 children ranging in age from 1;5 to 3;10 with a median age of 2;3. These subjects were assessed as having normal hearing, and intelligence within the normal range.

Data Collection

The data were collected using the picture-naming task of the Photo Articulation Test (Pendergast et al., 1965). The children's productions were recorded on a two-channel Teac A-2300 recorder. One channel recorded the subject's pronunciation of a given word, while the second was used for on-line commentary by an observer who noted visual details of the production (e.g., lip rounding, tongue protrusion, etc.). After each session, the audio tapes were transcribed phonetically by two trained transcribers using a system of fine phonetic transcription.

The analyses presented here are based on a subset of the data, namely, on the production of stop, fricative, affricate, and nasal phonemes.

An attempt was made to use only those words in which the target sounds were single consonants. In some cases, however, there were no such words, for example: medial /s/ in "pencil," medial and final /ʒ/ in "angels" and "orange." It should be noted that the classification of phonemes by position in the word was based on the adult form; there are a number of words in which the medial target phoneme was produced as the initial sound in the child's production, for example, banana occurs as [nænə], potato as [tedo].

At the time of data collection, the experimenter tried to have the children spontaneously produce the name of the picture on the card. In a majority of cases, the subjects complied. When they did not respond, or responded with the wrong word, the experimenter modeled the test word and asked the child to repeat it. The spontaneous productions were analyzed separately from the imitated ones and the two analyses were compared. Because there were no systematic differences between the two analyses, they were combined in the presentation of group results.

Data Analysis

The data were analyzed in two ways. First, the productions of all the hearing-impaired subjects, both cross-sectional and longitudinal, were compared with the productions of all the normal subjects. Second, the productions of six longitudinal subjects, three normal and three hearing impaired, were examined.

Group analysis of the hearing-impaired subjects was based on a total of 49 data collection sections. The number of sessions per child ranged from one to six, with 12 subjects involved in only one session and six subjects having four or more sessions. The group analysis of the normal subjects was based on 47 data collection sessions with the number of sessions per child ranging from one to six. Sixteen children were involved in only one session and five in four or more sessions.

RESULTS AND DISCUSSION

The productions of stop, fricative, affricate, and nasal phonemes were analyzed by position of the phoneme within the word. The percentage of correct responses and of certain error types for each group are presented in Table 15.1 (normal subjects) and Table 15.2 (hearing-impaired subjects). Responses were classified as distortions (percentage given in parentheses) if the place, manner, and voicing features were essentially correct but slightly off target, for example, the phoneme /s/ or /n/ produced with contact by the blade of the tongue, or /f/ produced as a bilabial fricative [ɸ]. The error types appearing on the tables are those which occurred in the data from both groups. Other substitutions were included only when they accounted for 5% (or more) of the responses for a given phoneme.

Table 15.1.   Normal subjects: percentage of correct productions and error types by phoneme in initial, medial, and final position

Target	No. tokens	Correct[a]	Voice error	Stop substitution[b]	Delete	Other substitution (≥ 5%)
p-	108	77	21	NA	0	
-p-	85	88	2	NA	1	
-p	73	92	0	NA	0	
b-	174	92(4)	6	NA	0	
-b-	74	77(4)	8	NA	5	
-b	32	25	62	NA	0	f 6
t-	153	67(7)	20	NA	0	
-t-	36	75(6)	14	NA	3	
-t	97	78(4)	0	NA	5	ʔ 6
d-	78	79(12)	6	NA	0	
-d-	61	56(2)	13	NA	20	
-d	36	42	50	NA	6	
k-	148	68(6)	20	NA	0	
-k-	73	88(6)	0	NA	0	
-k	80	85(4)	0	NA	5	ʔ 5
g-	65	83(5)	3	NA	0	t 5
-g-	39	81(8)	6	NA	3	
-g	77	40	54	NA	1	
f-	111	65(11)	0	5	0	pf 7
-f-	35	80(6)	0	3	3	
-f	41	80	0	0	0	
v-	27	7	0	81	0	
-v-	39	48(10)	13	7	7	
-v	30	23	43	3	13	
θ-	32	31	0	9	0	
-θ	31	39	0	6	0	f 26; s 23
ð-	33	0	6	82	0	s 9
-ð-	29	31	7	45	0	s 7
s-	103	45(24)	0	9	0	
-s-	34	44(17)	0	35	0	
-s	41	51(26)	0	5	5	θ 10
z-	28	29(7)	43	3	0	dz 14
-z-	37	30	62	2	0	
ʃ-	39	23(21)	0	18	0	tʃ / ts 18; s 18
-ʃ-	28	36(14)	0	4	14	s 32
-ʃ	74	23(16)	0	3	0	s 50; θ 5
tʃ-	38	47	0	26	0	ts 11
-tʃ-	25	36	0	32	0	s 12; ts 8
-tʃ	29	34	0	21	0	ts 21; ʃ 7
dʒ-	31	0	48	42	0	ts 6
-dʒ-	29	21	41	28	7	
-dʒ	28	4	26	4	4	ts 21; s 14
m-	77	92	0	0	0	

Table 15.1.   (*Continued*)

Target	No. tokens	Correct[a]	Voice error	Stop substitution[b]	Delete	Other substitution (≥ 5%)
-m-	36	86	0	3	3	
-m	69	90	0	3	4	
n-	64	87(5)	0	0	0	
-n-	36	83(8)	0	0	3	p/b 6
-n	73	81	0	4	12	
-ŋ-	33	54	0	6	6	ŋk/ŋg 6
-ŋ	35	89	0	0	0	n 6

[a] Parentheses indicate percent responses classified as distortions; these were *not* included in percent correct response.

[b] Only homorganic stops (i.e., stops produced at the same place of articulation as the target phoneme) were classified as a *stop substitution*. NA, not applicable.

Examination of the tables revealed regular patterns of correct productions and error types for both groups. Looking first at the similarities between the two subject populations the authors found the following: 1) the class of stop consonants had the highest percentage of correct responses, followed by nasals, fricatives, and affricates; 2) within each sound class, labial consonants were produced correctly more often than nonlabials (except /v/); 3) voiceless stops in the initial position tended to be voiced, whereas voiced stops, fricatives, and affricates in the final position were devoiced; 4) homorganic stops were substituted for fricatives and affricates, particularly in the initial position; 5) nonlabial fricatives and affricates were often substituted for by other fricatives (or affricates), for example, [f, s] for /θ/; [ʃ, ts] for /tʃ/; and 6) deletions occurred primarily in the final position.

Moving on to examine the differences between the two groups, we found that these fell into two categories; response patterns which were common to both subject populations, but which differed in the degree to which they occurred, and patterns which were unique to a single group. The first category includes the following: 1) deletions occurred primarily in final position for both groups but not to the same extent: final consonants were deleted in 35% of the responses of the hearing-impaired subjects, compared with 3% of the normals; 2) the pattern of substituting a homorganic stop for a fricative or affricate was common to both groups, and for both occurred more frequently in the initial position. This response pattern was substantially greater among the hearing impaired, occurring in 30% of the productions of fricatives and affricates in all positions, and 48% in the initial position;

Table 15.2.   Hearing impaired subjects: percentage of correct productions and error types by phoneme in intial, medial, and final position

Target	No. tokens	Correct[a]	Voice error	Stop substitution[b]	Delete	Other substitutions (≥ 5%)
p-	109	62	30	NA	1	
-p-	72	87	7	NA	0	
-p	69	78	0	NA	9	ʔ 7
b-	150	91(3)	3	NA	0	
-b-	75	77(2)	9	NA	5	
-b	26	19	27	NA	35	m 11
t-	109	42(7)	20	NA	3	p/b 11; h 7
-t-	30	56(17)	0	NA	13	h 10
-t	91	62(12)	0	NA	37	ʔ 21
d-	72	62(6)	0	NA	3	g/k 10
-d-	59	49	7	NA	20	
-d	32	25	19	NA	44	n 6
k-	134	38(7)	16	NA	6	h 18; ʔ 9
-k-	62	54(19)	0	NA	8	p/b 6
-k	70	37(1)	0	NA	37	ʔ 16
g-	53	51(8)	0	NA	11	h 15; t 8
-g-	25	49(3)	11	NA	5	
-g	62	11(3)	16	NA	50	ʔ 11; ŋ 5
f-	108	29(6)	0	42	2	
-f-	31	29(6)	0	26	19	k 10; ʔ 6
-f	30	33(10)	0	13	23	ʔ 10
v-	29	0	0	90	0	d/t 10
-v-	32	22(9)	9	48	9	
-v	25	12	8	6	44	
θ-	25	12(4)	0	60	0	s 8
-θ	27	15(7)	0	0	41	s 22; f 22
ð-	27	7	4	70	4	
-ð-	32	22	9	41	6	p 6; ʔ 6
s-	86	14(10)	0	44	0	p/b 7; h 6
-s-	35	11(3)	0	40	20	k/g 11; p/b 6
-s	36	19(8)	0	6	42	θ 8; f 6
z-	25	8	12	36	12	dz 8, n 8
-z-	25	8	20	24	12	θ/ð 12
ʃ-	32	28(6)	0	6	9	j 16; tʃ 12; h 9; s 6
-ʃ-	21	19(29)	0	14	14	ts/tʃ 10; s 10; k 5
-ʃ	70	23(16)	0	3	0	ʔ 18
tʃ-	33	15(3)	0	33	9	h 15; k/g 6; tɬ 6; ʃ 6
-tʃ-	26	27(12)	0	19	4	ʔ 12; k/g 8
-tʃ	29	17	0	3	21	ʃ 17; ʔ 14; s 10
dʒ-	30	3	23	50	3	k 6

Table 15.2.   (*Continued*)

Target	No. tokens	Correct[a]	Voice error	Stop substitution[b]	Delete	Other substitutions ($\geq 5\%$)
-dʒ-	27	3	26	30	19	
-dʒ	33	0	15	0	39	ɬ 15; ʔ 12; ʃ 9; s 6
m-	66	74	0	24	1	
-m-	38	53	0	32	3	f 5
m-	65	57	0	8	25	
n-	60	53(8)	0	0	0	l 12; m 7; p/b 7; n 5
-n-	32	47	0	6	12	m 19
n-	65	37	0	0	52	ŋ 5
-ŋ-	35	29(3)	0	3	14	ŋk/ŋg 17; n 9
-ŋ	28	39	0	0	32	m 7; ʔ 7

[a] Parentheses indicate percent responses classified as distortions; these were *not* included in percent correct responses.

[b] Only homorganic stops (i.e., stops produced at the same place of articulation as the target phoneme) were classified as a *stop substitution*. NA, not applicable.

the comparable figures for the normal subjects were 6% overall and 31% in the initial position. In addition, the hearing-impaired subjects used a similar pattern of substitution in productions of nasal phonemes, maintaining place of articulation but changing manner from nasal to oral, particularly for the phoneme /m/ (see Table 15.2); and 3) although both groups evidenced a pattern of intraclass substitutions in the production of fricatives, for example, [f] for /θ/, [s] for /ʃ/, [ʃ] for /z/, this pattern accounted for a greater proportion of the responses of the normal subjects than of the hearing impaired (cf. productions of /v, θ, s, ʃ/, Tables 15.1 and 15.2).

In addition to the response patterns, which were common—to a greater or lesser degree—to subjects in both groups, there were a few patterns that were unique to a given group. On the whole, these accounted for a relatively small proportion of the data. For the hearing impaired, the author found evidence of the following patterns: 1) substitution of a glottal stop for target consonants, particularly in the final position (Table 15.2 shows this substitution pattern comprising 10% to 21% of the productions of final /t, k, g, f, θ, ʃ, tʃ/), 2) substitution of the palatal fricative [ʃ] for the affricates /tʃ, dʒ/; and 3) substitution of the back consonants [h, k, g] for other nonlabial consonants. The pattern of substitution is not well defined, varying from phoneme to phoneme position to position. For example, [h] was produced for target /-t-, k-, g-, t-/ in 10% to 18% of the responses, and for /t-, ʃ-, s-, n-/

in 5% to 9%; whereas [k] or [g] served as substitutes for /d-, -f-, -s-, -ʃ-, tʃ-, -tʃ-, dʒ-/ in 5% to 11% of the responses for each target sound. The only substitution pattern present in the normal data, but not in data for the hearing impaired, was that of depalatalization of /ʃ, tʃ, dʒ/, so that [s] was substituted for /ʃ/ and [s] or [ts] for /tʃ, dʒ/. (This error type also occurred in the responses of the hearing-impaired subjects, but not to any significant degree.)

In sum, certain patterns were present in both sets of data analyzed. Basically, the patterns of substitutions present in the productions of the normal subjects were also found in the responses of the hearing impaired, although the distribution may have been different. In contrast, however, a number of response patterns observed in the data for hearing-impaired subjects did not occur, or occurred only rarely, in the productions of the normally hearing children. The substitution of a glottal stop for final stops, fricatives, and affricates serves as one example of this difference.

A basic difference in the two data sets lies in the range of substitution types in terms of place and manner of articulation. In general, the errors of the normal subjects differed from the target phoneme by one or two features. Thus, for the initial affricate /tʃ/ we had substitutions of an alveolar stop and an alveolar affricate in the normal data (Table 15.1), whereas the substitutions of the hearing impaired ranged from an alveolar stop to a palatal fricative to a velar stop to a lateral fricative to [h] (Table 15.2). In other words, the substitutions of the hearing-impaired subjects were greater in number and tended to deviate further from the target phoneme.

One reason for the greater range of responses was undoubtedly the nature of the data base. As noted earlier, the group data included responses of both longitudinal and cross-sectional subjects. Given the differences in degree of hearing loss, age at the time the loss was identified, and educational programs, we would expect to find a greater variation in the responses of hearing-impaired subjects. By comparison, the normal subjects constituted a relatively homogeneous group. Analysis of the responses of individual subjects will allow us to determine if the observed differences are merely a consequence of pooling the data across subjects, or if, in fact, they represent differences in the developing phonological systems of the two populations.

Tables 15.3 and 15.4 present longitudinal data from three normally hearing (Table 15.3) and three hearing-impaired (Table 15.4) subjects. The normal subjects range in age from 1;7 to 2;1 at the beginning of data collection to 3;0 to 3;2 at the end. The hearing-impaired subjects range in age from 3;2 to 5;4 at the first session to 5;3 to 7;0 at the final

Table 15.3. Longitudinal normal subjects: productions of initial /p,f,t,s/

Subject	Age	/p-/ pencil[a]	pig	pipe	/f-/ fork	feather	fish	/t-/ TV	toothbrush	table	/s-/ saw	scissors	sandwich
N 1	1;7	(pf)[a]	(p)	(p)	s	(ɸ)	(f)	(t)	(t)	(tʰ)	(s)	t	s*
	1;10	pʰ	p	(p)	pf	(pf)	(h)	tʰ	t	tʰ		(s)	s
	2;2	pʰ	pʰ	pʰ	f	f	f	tʰ	tʰ	tʰ	t	s*	s
	2;5	(pʰ)	pʰ	pʰ	f	f	pf	tʰ	tʰ	(tʰ)	ts	s	(s)
	2;9	pʰ	pʰ	pʰ	f	p	θ	tʰ	tʰ	tʰ	s	(s)	s
	3;0	(pʰ)	pʰ	pʰ	f	f	f	tʰ	tʰ	tʰ			
N 2	1;8	p	p	(b)	tʃ	(ɸ)	(p)	(c)	tʰ*	k	t	t	(j)
	2;0	kʰ	p	(pʰ)	p	f	(w)	tʰ	(tʰ)	d	s*	s*	(s)
	2;3	(pʰ)	pʰ	(pʰ)	p	ɸ	ɸ	tʰ	tʰ	tʰ	s	s	(h)
	2;8	(pʰ)	pʰ	pʰ	f	f	f	tʰ	tʰ	tʰ	s	ts	s
	2;11	pʰ	pʰ	p	f	ɸ	f	tʰ	tʰ	tʰ	s	s	s
	3;1	p	pʰ		f		pf	tʰ	tʰ	tʰ			ʃ
N 3	2;1	(p)	pʰ	(t)	(f)	(t)	(f)	(t)		t	(s)	s*	(t)
	2;4	pʰ	pʰ	(pʰ)	ɸ	(f)	f	tʰ		tʰ	s	s*	(s)
	2;6	p	pʰ	(pʰ)	f	(f)	f	tʰ		tʰ	θ	s	
	2;8	p	pʰ		f	(f)	f	tʰ	(tʰ)	t	θ	(s*)	s
	2;11	p	pʰ	pʰ	f	pf		tʰ	p	tʰ	s*	s*	ts
	3;2	p	pʰ	pʰ	pf	f	f	tʰ	(tʰ)	tʰ	s*	s*	s*

[a] Parentheses indicate response was imitated; *, distorted (produced by blade rather than tip of tongue).

Table 15.4. Longitudinal hearing-impaired subjects: productions of initial /p,f,t,s/

Subject	Age	/p-/			/f-/			/t-/			/s-/		
		pencil	pig	pipe	fork	feather	fish	TV	toothbrush	table	saw	scissors	sandwich
H 1	3;2		(b)ᵃ	(ɸ)	(pw)	(v)	(0)	m	(h)	0			t
	4;5		m			(p)	p	m	h	t	ħ	m	t
	4;9	(pʰ)	0	(ɸ)	β	(p)		0		0	p	s*	t
	5;0	pʰ	pʰ	(p)	(f)	(pf)	ɸ	0		ħ	(l)	(t)	t
	5;3		pʰ	(pʰ)	p			pʰ		ħ	(t)	t	t
	5;6	b	(pʰ)	(p)	p	(w)	(p)	ħ	(h)	ħ	(t)	t	t
H 2	3;5	pʰ	pʰ	(pʰ)		(p)	p	pʰ	(t)	tʰ	t	s*	(j)
	3;10	tʰ	pʰ	(pʰ)		(f)	(p)	tʰ	tʰ	tʰ	(t*)	t	s
	4;4	ɸ	pʰ	pʰ	ɸ	p	b	tʰ	(tʰ)	tʰ	(tʰ)	s	b
	4;8	pʰ	pʰ	pʰ	f	f	f	tʰ	tʰ	k	s*	θ	t*
	5;0	pʰ	pʰ	pʰ	f	f	f	tʰ	tʰ	c	s*		s
	5;3	pʰ	pʰ	pʰ	f	f	f	t	tʰ		f		ts
H 3	5;4	(h)		(pʰ)	pʰ	(h)	ħ	ħ	(h)	ħ	(t)	ħ	dʒ
	6;0	h	h	(pʰ)	(pʰ)	p	p	b	(tʰ)	ħ	t*	tʰ	p
	6;4	(pʰ)	pʰ	(pʰ)	pʰ	(p)	p	pʰ	(tʰ)	ħ	t*	d	b
	6;8	t	pʰ	(pʰ)	pʰ	p	ɸ	b	(tʰ)	tʰ	s*	t*	t
	7;0	pʰ	pʰ	(pʰ)	pʰ	p	t	t	(tʰ)	tʰ	t*	ts	t

ᵃ Parentheses indicate response was imitated; *, distorted (produced by blade rather than tip of tongue); 0, deleted.

session. All three hearing-impaired subjects were male, each classified as having a severe to profound hearing loss unaided and mild to moderate loss aided. The loss was identified at age 2;0 for subject H1, 0;7 for H2, and 3;9 for H3. All three subjects attended total communication preschools and were subsequently enrolled in total communication programs in the public schools.

The responses shown in Tables 15.3 and 15.4 represent renditions of initial /p, f, t, s/ as they were pronounced in certain test words from the Photo Articulation Test (Pendergast et al., 1965). Studies of phonological acquisition of normally hearing children indicate that all four of these sounds are usually acquired by the age of 4;0, although correct articulation of /s-/ may be achieved later (Olmsted, 1971; Sander, 1972; Templin, 1957). Table 15.3 shows that the three normal subjects under study produced /p-/ and /t-/ correctly by age 2;6 whereas /f-/ and /s-/ were still not consistently produced correctly at around age 3;0.

The range and variation[1] of renditions of a given phoneme were found to be quite narrow. For /p-/ and /t-/, responses typically varied between aspirated and unaspirated stops with place and manner class remaining correct. Variation in productions of the two fricatives was somewhat greater, particularly in the early stages. Even here, however, the range was small, with common substitutes being homorganic stops, that is, [t] for /s/, [p] for /f/, or fricatives produced at nearby places of articulation, for example, [θ] for /f/, [ʃ] or [θ] for /s/.

In comparison, the responses of the hearing-impaired subjects (Table 15.4) revealed a much slower progression toward correct production and much greater range and variation of response types, both within and across subjects. Whereas correct production of /p-/ appeared to be mastered by all three subjects, only subject H2 had acquired /f-/ and possibly /t-/, and none of the three produced /s/ correctly with any consistency. As with the normal subjects, the variation of responses was greatest in the early sessions and decreased over time. The range of responses was much broader, however; for example, renditions of /t-/ varied from a glottal fricative [h] to labial stops [p, b] to unaspirated [t] to omission. (The frequent substitution of a labial for /t/ in "TV" seemed to be due to regression assimilation whereby the word was pronounced as [bibi].)

---

[1] The term *range* refers to how far substitutions deviate from the target sound in terms of place and manner of articulation; for example substitutions of [k, d, m, r] for /f/ represent a wide range of responses, whereas [s, θ, p, v] for /f/ represent a narrow one. The term *variation* refers to the number of different substitutions produced for a target phoneme.

The question of variation is an important one because it relates directly to the success or failure of a communicative act. It is, of course, easiest to understand a person whose pronunciation of a word (or sentence) is correct. If, however, the pronunciation is incorrect, but the correspondences between the phonemes of the speaker's form and the standard form are systematic and predictable, the listeners can "decode" the message after a bit of practice. Understanding the message is extremely difficult, on the other hand, when the relationship between the two forms is not constant, but varies from one production to the next. Returning to Table 15.4, we can see that the responses of all three subjects became more stable over time. The trend was particularly striking in subject H1, who produced a wide variety of substitutes for each phoneme at ages 3;2 and 4;5 but relatively few at 5;6.

For speech to be intelligible, productions of target phonemes should not only be systematically related to the correct form, they should be distinct from one another (see Fisher et al., this volume). The child who produced /p-/ correctly as [pʰ] and consistently substitutes [pʰ] for /f-/loses the phonemic distinction between /p-/ and /f-/, even though the relationship between the target and the substituted form is constant. In contrast, the child who substitutes [ɓ] for /b/ and [b] for /p/ maintains the /b/-/p/ distinction, though neither target is produced correctly. Returning to Table 15.4, we see that, on the whole, the subjects maintained the contrasts between the four phonemes analyzed therein. For subject H2, the distinctions were not only maintained, they were essentially correct by the final session, except for renditions of /s-/. For subject H1, the distinction between /t-/ and /s-/ was clearly present in the final session, although neither phoneme was articulated correctly. Renditions of /p-/ and /f-/ overlapped somewhat, but remained distinct in a majority of productions. Systematic differences in the responses of H3 were more difficult to determine because of variation within productions of the target phonemes, even at the last session; but on the whole it appears that phonemic differences were maintained in spite of the variation.

The responses in Table 15.4 revealed a pattern of acquisition that can be divided into three stages. In the first stage, the child produced a wide variety of substitutions for the target phoneme; some of the substitution patterns were also found in the speech of young normally hearing children, for example, [t] for /s/, [p] for /f/; whereas others were not, for example, [h] for /t/. In the second stage, the range of substitutions narrowed and eventually stabilized to a single sound. Finally, in stage 3, the child produced the phoneme correctly. Given the small number of subjects and the limited set of data, this pattern of development can only be hypothesized, not stated as fact. Research based on longitudinal data from a larger sample size and on the full range of phonemes is needed before it can be substantiated or refuted.

CONCLUSION

This chapter presents a comparison of aspects of phonological acquisition of normal and hearing-impaired children, based on analyses of group and individual data. In large part, the patterns of development were similar, although the rate of development was considerably slower for the hearing impaired. Group analysis of incorrect productions of stops, fricatives, affricates, and nasals revealed a set of substitution types common to both populations, for example, voicing of initial stops, devoicing of final stops, fricatives, and affricates, and substituting homorganic stops for fricatives. The longitudinal data indicated that these error types were present in the early stages of development of normal children, but were overcome by the age of 3 or so. They remained longer in the phonological systems of the hearing impaired and, according to studies of older hearing-impaired children (Levitt et al., 1978; Smith, 1975) may never be overcome.

Although the patterns of development of the two groups were similar in many ways, there were important differences. First, there was a set of response types which occurred frequently in the data of hearing-impaired subjects but rarely or not at all in the data of normal subjects. The substitution of a glottal stop and of [h] for a variety of target phonemes and the deletion of final consonants are typical examples of this set. Second, the range of response types in terms of place and manner of articulation was much greater among the hearing-impaired subjects than the normal subjects. The longitudinal data indicated that the range for any one subject narrowed as the phonological system developed, although the range across subjects may remain wide. Finally, on the individual level, the variation of responses for each target phoneme was greater for the hearing-impaired subjects.

REFERENCES

Calvert, D. R. 1961. Some acoustic characteristics of the speech of profoundly deaf individuals. Doctoral dissertation, Stanford University, Stanford, Calif.

Dodd, B. 1976. The phonological systems of deaf children. J. Speech Hear. Disord. 41:185–198.

Hudgins, C. V. 1937. Voice production and breath control in the speech of the deaf. Am. Ann. Deaf 82:338–363.

Hudgins, C. V., and F. C. Numbers. 1942. An investigation of the intelligibility of the speech of the deaf. Genet. Psychol. Monogr. 25:289–392.

John, J. E. J., and J. N. Howarth. 1965. The effect of time distortions on the intelligibility of deaf children's speech. Lang. Speech 8:127–134.

Levitt, H., H. Stromberg, C. Smith, and T. Gold. 1978. The structure of segmental errors in the speech of deaf children. In D. L. McPherson (ed.), Advances in Prosthetic Devices for the Deaf.: A Technical Workshop. National Technical Institute for the Deaf, Rochester, N.Y.

Olmsted, D. 1971. Out of the Mouth of Babes. Mouton, The Hague.

Pendergast, R., S. Dickey, J. Selmar, and A. Soder. 1965. Photo Articulation Test. King, Chicago.

Sander, E. K. 1972. When are speech sounds learned? J. Speech Hear. Disord. 37:55–63.

Smith, C. R. 1975. Residual hearing and speech production in deaf children. J. Speech Hear. Res. 18:795–811.

Templin, M. 1957. Certain Language Skills in Children: Their Development and Interrelationships. University of Minnesota Press, Minneapolis.

SENSORY AIDS AND SPEECH TRAINING

CHAPTER 16

INDEPENDENT DRILL: A ROLE FOR SPEECH TRAINING AIDS IN THE SPEECH DEVELOPMENT OF THE DEAF

Robert A. Houde and Judith L. Braeges

CONTENTS

The majority of profoundly deaf children finish their education without intelligible speech (Jensema, Karchmer, and Trybus, 1978). Although the reasons for this failure are not well understood, there is general agreement that the quantity of highly skilled individual teaching required to develop speech in the profoundly deaf child is extremely large—larger than can currently be provided for the majority of deaf students. The prospects for speech would be greatly improved if a more efficient means of training could be devised.

SPEECH TRAINING AIDS

For the past few decades considerable effort has been devoted to the development of electronic speech training aids with the hope that they might provide a significant improvement in the effectiveness of speech training for the deaf. This effort has resulted in a number of devices which could be called successful from the point of view that they correctly displayed certain phonetic distinctions and characteristics in speech (see Strong, 1975, for a comprehensive survey). These devices, however, were not successful in improving the effectiveness of speech training. None came into widespread clinical use, and the few formal evaluations indicated approximately equal results for training with and without the aids (Boothroyd, 1973; Kopp and Kopp, 1963; Stratton, 1974). These results suggested a reexamination of the speech training process and of the role that might be played by electronic aids. Can they be of value? Are we asking them to do the right things?

SPEECH TRAINING

In order to identify where a speech display might serve, we examined speech training in detail. Although the practice of speech training varies greatly, most programs can be factored into the following three elementary activities:

1. *Activities in which the general* use *of speech is encouraged and reinforced, but specific errors are not identified or corrected* The feedback provided to the student is limited to indications that his or her utterance was or was not understood. This "training" may be provided by all individuals in contact with the student—not just speech teachers.
2. *Correction and reinforcement of specific speech skills in the* natural *communication utterances of the student* Particular errors are identified and analyzed, corrective directions are provided, and another attempt is elicited. This speech training activity requires knowledge of articulatory phonetics and skills in communicating with the student. Thus it can usually be provided only by trained individuals.
3. *Correction and reinforcement of specific speech skills in* structured, *directed utterances of the student* Each utterance is analyzed, errors are identified, and corrective directions are communicated to the student. The activity is very structured. This training is usually provided by speech teachers in individual, one-on-one settings.

   Individual structured training can be further partitioned into two components:

1. *Initial development of speech skills* A great deal of teacher skill is involved in assessing the student's utterances, apprising the stu-

dent of the degree of correctness of each attempt, and in directing
his or her next attempt.

2. *Reinforcing drill* As the student's skill improves, the teacher's
   activity changes from individualized instructions to simpler communications of correct or incorrect. This drill activity is characterized by a great deal of repetition.

What function might a speech display perform in these activities?
The basic function of a speech display is to exhibit the characteristics
of speech in such a way that phonetic differences in production are
clearly and consistently displayed in an easily interpreted form, that
is, the basic function of a speech display is to provide a phonetic analysis and to feed back or present the results of that analysis.

It is difficult to see how a speech display could serve the first
speech training activity. The encouragement and reinforcement of
speech involves interpreting the meaning of an utterance and making
an appropriate response, functions which are beyond the present capabilities of speech displays.

In the second speech training activity, corrections are made in
utterances that occur naturally in meaningful communications. Correction involves phonetic analysis and feedback which theoretically
could be assisted by an instrument; however, this activity is usually
carried out in an unstructured classroom setting in which one teacher
is instructing several students and speech corrections are not the primary objective. Under these conditions it would be difficult to use a
speech training aid without disrupting the normal flow of the classroom.[1]

In the third activity (structured speech training), phonetic analysis
and feedback of the student's performance are carried out in a one-on-
one, systematic manner. In this case, a speech display would appear
to have a direct role. There are two ways in which a speech display
might serve this activity:

1. The speech display might assist the teacher in the phonetic assessment of the student's production and in the communication of
   the results of the assessment to the student (feedback).

2. The speech display might provide the student with the means of
   independently assessing and reinforcing his or her own utterances.

---

[1] We are concerned here with speech training aids, relatively large devices which
cannot be "worn" or used continuously in natural settings. Speech reception aids, which
are wearable and which permit much more powerful training procedures, are not considered in this paper. With the exception of the conventional hearing aid, an effective
speech reception aid is yet to be realized.

The Assistance Role

In order to be of value in the role of assisting the teacher in structured speech training, the instrument must perform the phonetic analysis and communication function better than the teacher. If the instrument is simply as good as the teacher, then the information it provides is entirely redundant and of no value. To be of some benefit it must provide something which is not provided by the teacher alone. Can an instrument provide either a more accurate phonetic analysis or more clear feedback than a teacher?

In general, the phonetic analysis of an instrument is not more accurate than that of a good teacher (exception: voice onset time). The instrument, however, does not fatigue and may be more consistent than the teacher.

In the case of the feedback function, the instrument may be more direct and less ambiguous than the teacher. For example, the difference between /s/ and its error /st/ is directly communicated in a spectrographic display, but is quite difficult to describe in language. ("You closed your /s/; you stopped the air.")

Thus, there is a basis for expecting some increase in the effectiveness of a teacher assisted by a speech training aid that provides clear consistent feedback of performance. The value of the instrument in assistance may be significant; however, it is not likely to be dramatic. The difference in the clarity of feedback provided by a good teacher and that provided by a good instrument is not large enough to account for a great change in effectiveness. Good teachers can be very good speech display instruments.

The Independent Work Role

In the role of providing the student with the means of working independently, the value of the speech display can be very direct. It may permit the delivery of individual structured speech training services beyond the limits that can be provided by the speech teacher, that is, the delivery of a much larger quantity of individual speech training.

What portion of individual structured speech training might be served by independent work with a speech display? As was discussed earlier, structured speech training can be partitioned into two components of activity: 1) the initial instructional component, and 2) the drill component.

The design of a system which delivers the initial instructional component through independent work is beyond the present capabilities of technology. The availability of low-cost computers has encouraged this possibility, however, and a number of laboratories are currently planning work in this direction.

The second type of structured speech training activity, drill, in which the tasks are repetitious and the feedback is simple (correct-incorrect) would appear to be very well suited for independent work with a speech display.

The Role of Speech Training Aids

An analysis of the requirements of speech training and of the general capabilities of speech training aids suggests two roles in which aids might significantly affect speech training for the deaf:

1. *In assisting the teacher in individual structured training by providing phonetic analysis and feedback to the student* In this role, the speech training aid might be expected to realize a modest but significant increase in the teacher's effectiveness.
2. *In providing the student with the means of independently judging the correctness of his or her utterance* In this role, the speech training aid can be expected to provide a major increase in the speech teacher's effectiveness by allowing the teacher to deliver individual structured training to a number of students simultaneously. In this role an aid may function as a teacher multiplier.

**A SYSTEM OF INDEPENDENT DRILL
IN STRUCTURED SPEECH TRAINING**

In a conventional structured speech training program, the student whose development of a speech skill reaches the point at which he or she can occasionally perform it correctly is provided with articulation practice to raise the performance to the automatic level.

The authors have developed a program in which the practice portion of structured training is carried out by the student working independently with a speech display. The display used in this program is the Speech Spectrographic Display (SSD), which was reported by Stewart, Larkin, and Houde (1976). The SSD displays speech as an instantaneous broadband spectrogram on a television screen.

The student uses the spectrographic display to independently judge the correctness of each attempt. At first glance this would appear to involve the difficult task of "reading" spectrograms. The student's task, however, is considerably less difficult than that. He must simply distinguish his correct production of the phoneme from his particular error, and this distinction may be made on the basis of a few relatively

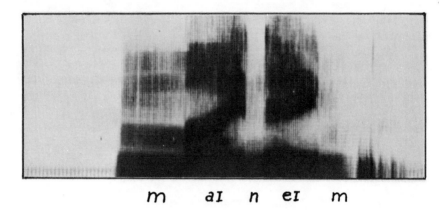

m   aɪ   n   eɪ   m

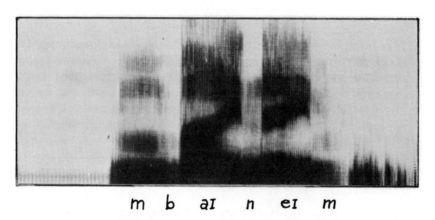

m   b   aɪ   n   eɪ   m

Figure 16.1.   Student criterion for distinguishing the /mb/ error of /m/: correct /m/ has
no white space before the vowel. *Top*; correct /m/ in "my name"; *bottom*; error /mb/
for /m/ in "my name."

simple spectrographic characteristics. Figures 16.1 and 16.2 show the
criteria that distinguish two of the common errors encountered in deaf
speech: /mb/ for /m/, and /t/ for /d/.

The teacher prepares the student for independent drill by teaching
the criterion by which he or she can distinguish the error from the
target phoneme. In most cases the student's error of a phoneme is
predominantly of one type, and only one criterion is necessary. In those
cases in which the student produces different errors of one phoneme,
the criteria for all the errors are taught to him if the teacher feels he
can handle this more complex situation. If not, the criteria for only the

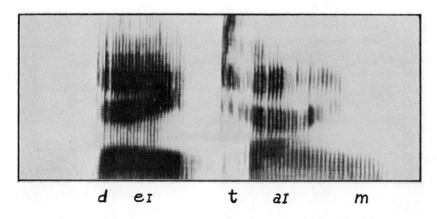

d   eɪ   t   aɪ   m

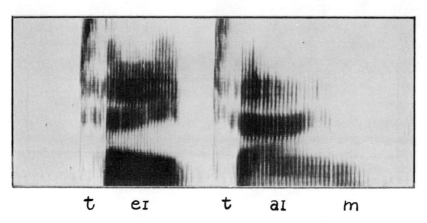

t   eɪ   t   aɪ   m

Figure 16.2.   Student criterion for distinguishing the /t/ error of /d/: correct /d/ has no long light space after the line. A template is provided for the student to show the maximum voice onset time permitted. *Top*; correct /d/ in "daytime"; *bottom*; error /t/ for /d/ in "daytime."

dominant error is taught and the others are corrected during drill by the teacher/drill supervisor.

To assist the teacher in this task of identifying the error criteria, catalogs have been prepared for each phoneme showing the spectrographic and articulatory characteristics of the phoneme and its common errors.

Armed with knowledge of how to tell right from wrong spectrographically, the student practices the target phoneme in a set of utterances prepared for him by the teacher. Practice is guided by a worksheet on which the student checks off a box for each correct production

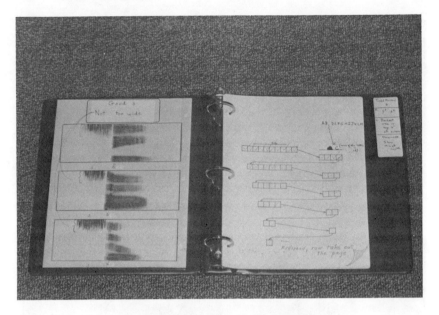

Figure 16.3.   The individual workbook.

of the target. Two different target words are assigned on each work-sheet to vary the drill. Completing this worksheet requires 44 correct productions of the target phoneme.

The student's worksheets are assembled in a looseleaf binder which constitutes his or her individualized program of drill—the personal workbook (see Figure 16.3). The workbook contains a set of spectrographic models and the appropriate judgment criterion on the left side and corresponding worksheets on the right side.

The student works independently under the supervision of the speech teacher in 20-minute work sessions. When the student has completed three worksheets independently, he or she is directed (by the next worksheet) to call the teacher for a test. The test (15 productions of the target words) provides a measure of both production and judgment. The results of the test determine whether the student continues to work at the same task, advances to a more difficult task, or drops back to a less difficult task.

Tasks are graded in five levels of difficulty,[2] beginning with the target phoneme (a consonant) in simple CV syllables and ending with

[2] This program's basic structure of subskills, ordered in increasing difficulty, owes its origins to the system of speech training developed by Ling (1976).

the target consonant in an abutting position. The five levels of difficulty are shown in Table 16.1.

The teacher assigns words and short phrases to be drilled at each level. The assignment is individualized for each student on the basis of the phonemes which he or she can produce successfully. Words are assigned in which only one phoneme is produced in error—the target phoneme. For this purpose, word lists were organized for each level of difficulty, grouped by target phoneme and nontarget phonemes.

The procedure described above permits a teacher to supervise the independent work of three or four students simultaneously (see also Houde, 1980). In this supervision, the teacher encourages diligent work, administers performance tests, directs the pronunciation of assigned words, explains their meanings, and listens for the introduction of new errors. This latter function is essential to prevent the student from drilling new errors, those which he or she has not been prepared to identify on the spectrogram. In addition to supervising drill, the teacher's role includes preparing the student's drill program.

At this time, procedures have been detailed only for initial and final consonants; however, in principle this procedure can be extended to include any speech skill the error of which can be distinguished independently by the student.

EVALUATION

The independent drill procedure described above was evaluated with children at the Rochester School for the Deaf. The 51 children of the first nine classes (ages 6 to 13) were assigned to two experimental groups: the independent-drill group and the drilled-by-teacher group. The groups were defined by dividing each class into two equal parts on a random basis. In addition, a control group was defined consisting of 17 students from the next three classes adjacent to the oldest experimental class.

Table 16.1.   Levels of difficulty

Level	Phonetic context	Examples (target /t/)
1	(C) V	tea
2	(C) V C	top
3	(C) V C V	tuba
4	V (C) V C	attack
5	V C (C) V	tiptoe

Both experimental groups were provided with 20 minutes of drill per day, 4 days per week, in addition to their regular speech training within the school's program. In the independent-drill group, students drilled in groups of three or four at a time using a spectrographic display in the procedure outlined above. In the drilled-by-teacher group, each student received individual drill, equal in quantity and within the same general procedure as was provided by the independent-drill group. The control group received no special drill, only the conventional training provided by the school.

The target phonemes assigned to the students in both experimental groups were not balanced. They were selected by the student's speech teacher on the same basis normally used in planning a student's program, but within the constraints that the task had to be an initial or final consonant, and that certain target errors could not be assigned because they were not clearly distinguishable on the spectrographic display (for example, /l/ versus /n/).

The articulation skills of all students were measured at the beginning and at the end of the 5-month evaluation period (one semester).

RESULTS

On the 27 students assigned to the independent-drill group, all but one[3] learned to operate the SSD, to use the work procedures, and to judge the spectrographic characteristics of their utterances independently. The number of sessions required to learn to operate the SSD ranged from one to four with an average of 2.1. The number of sessions required to learn to discriminate errors from correct production ranged from one to five with an average of 1.1.

Consonant articulation skill was measured before and after the experimental training period. The consonant articulation test determined the percentage of correct production of each consonant in a CV or VC context, in imitation. A measure of articulation gain was defined as the difference between the pre- and post-training articulation skills. The articulation gains resulting from the various test conditions are shown in Table 16.2.

The differences between the independent-drill group and the drilled-by-teacher group are not significant; however, all differences in articulation gain between the phonemes that were drilled and those that were not drilled are significant at the 0.01 level. It is clear that

---

[3] The one exception simply refused (for the entire semester) to take instruction beyond the basic operation of the display.

Table 16.2.   Average articulation gain

Group	Phonemes drilled (%)	Phonemes not drilled (%)
Independent drill by SSD	30.7	3.2
Drilled-by-teacher	24.7	3.3
Control group		6.5

articulation skill was significantly affected by drill, but not by the manner in which it was delivered. For this procedure, the effectiveness of independent drill was equal to that of individual teacher drill.

Another aspect of the difference between the SSD-drilled group and the teacher-drilled group is seen in Figure 16.4, which shows the average learning rates of students in each group. Learning rate was measured as the number of phoneme levels completed per training session. The phoneme levels are those levels of difficulty as shown in Table 16.1. Again, no significant difference was found in the average performance of the two groups, both being approximately 0.1 phoneme levels per day (SSD drilled: 0.097; teacher drilled: 0.109). As seen in Figure 16.4 the ranges of learning rates of the two groups were found

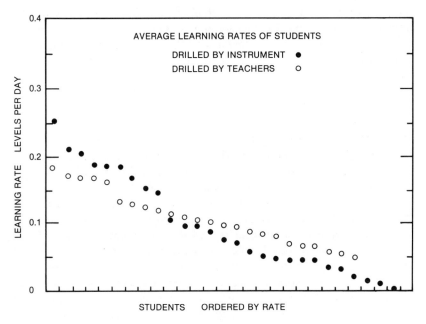

Figure 16.4.   Average learning rate of students.

to be significantly different. The independent-drill (drilled by SSD) group exhibited a wider range of learning rates than the drilled-by-teacher group. The above-average SSD-drilled students have higher rates than above-average teacher-drilled students, whereas below-average SSD-drilled students had lower rates than the below-average teacher-drilled students. Apparently, the instrument permits students to work at their own pace, whereas the effect of a teacher is to control the pace of work—not too slow, but also not too fast.

DISCUSSION

Can a deaf child work independently and effectively with an electronic speech training aid? The answer is a most definite yes. In this study all of the children were able to carry out independent work with the instrument. This is considered to be the most important finding of this study. A related finding is that speech teachers were also able to work effectively with the speech display instrument. An important factor in this teacher acceptance is that this drill program is viewed as an extension of the teacher's present program rather than as a disruptive replacement for the present program.

How general is this finding? It is clearly specific to this procedure, but it may generalize to other speech display instruments. In principle, any speech instrument that consistently and clearly displays a phonetic difference (and is simple to operate) can be used to train the production of that difference. One important factor, however, in the use of an instrument in this procedure is the range of phonetic differences that it can handle, that is, the number of different training problems it can address. Instruments with much less phonetic range than the spectrographic display, although clear, consistent, and simple in operation, could not be used in this general procedure.

The value of independent drill with a speech display can be considered in terms of cost effectiveness or time effectiveness. The cost of drill delivered by this system is less than half of that delivered by teachers alone. More importantly, however, the quantity of individual drill that can be delivered by a teacher through independent work is four times greater than that deliverable by the teacher alone.

The independent drill system is not considered to be a complete speech training program in itself. The system was intended to serve as an extension of the speech teacher's activities, without disrupting the existing speech training program. The independent drill provided by this system is a component of structured speech training, which in turn is a component of a complete speech training system that develops the use of speech in natural communication.

REFERENCES

Boothroyd, A. 1973. Some experiments on the control of voice in the profoundly deaf using a pitch extractor and storage oscilloscope display. IEEE Trans. on Audio and Electroacoust., AU-21, pp. 274–278.

Houde, R. A. 1980. Evaluation of independent drill with visual aids for speech training. In J. D. Subtelny (ed.), Speech assessment and speech improvement for the hearing impaired. A. G. Bell Association for the Deaf, Washington, D.C.

Jensema, C. J., M. A. Karchmer, and R. J. Trybus. 1978. The rated speech intelligibility of hearing impaired children: Basic relationships and a detailed analysis. Office of Demographic Studies, Series R, No. 6. Gallaudet College, Washington, D.C.

Kopp, G., and H. Kopp. 1963. Visible speech for the deaf. Final Report, Grant RD-526, Vocational Rehabilitation Agency (SRS), Washington, D.C.

Ling, D. 1976. Speech and the Hearing Impaired Child: Theory and Practice. A. G. Bell Association for the Deaf, Washington, D.C.

Stewart, L. C., W. D. Larkin, and R. A. Houde. 1976. A real time spectrograph with implications for speech training for the deaf. Proceedings of the International Conference on Acoustics, Speech, and Signal Processing, pp. 590–593.

Stratton, W. D. 1974. Intonation feedback for the deaf through a tactile display. Volta Rev. 76:26–35.

Strong, W. J. 1975. Speech aids for the profoundly/severely hearing impaired: Requirements, overview, and projections. Volta Rev. 77:536–556.

CHAPTER 17

APPLICATION OF THE SPEECH SPECTROGRAPHIC DISPLAY IN DEVELOPING ARTICULATORY SKILLS IN HEARING-IMPAIRED ADULTS

Jean E. Maki

CONTENTS

In the development of speech production skills, it may be assumed that the hearing-impaired adult would need to understand the production characteristics of the intended target, learn control of the speech mechanism to achieve the target, and develop appropriate use of the target within the English language. It is possible that speech training aids can facilitate learning in each of these areas by providing visual feedback which is displayed immediately and can be used to associate articu-

---

This work was conducted at the National Technical Institute for the Deaf in the course of an agreement with the U.S. Department of Education.

latory movement with the related acoustic features. Instruments are currently available that convert the acoustic signal into a visible form. In the use of these instruments, visual patterns serve to supplement information received through distorted auditory cues, incomplete speech-reading cues, or confusing orthographic cues.

Efforts to present speech in a visible form have led to the development of instruments that are capable of displaying frequency and intensity changes over time. Considerable information exists concerning the underlying principles of visible speech, the display characteristics, and research and clinical applications (House, Goldstein, and Hughes, 1968; Koenig, Dunn, and Lacy, 1946; Kopp and Green, 1946; Potter, Kopp, and Kopp, 1966; Riesz and Schott, 1946; Stark, Cullen, and Chase, 1968; Steinberg and French, 1946). The focus of this chapter is on one instrument, the Speech Spectrographic Display (SSD) (Stewart, Larkin, and Houde, 1976), and its use with hearing-impaired adults.

The Speech Spectrographic Display presents frequency information between 100 and 5000 Hz on the vertical axis and time on the horizontal axis. Intensity variations over a 30-dB range are reflected in the relative darkness of the trace. The visual characteristics of the SSD suggest application of the instrument in at least three areas of instruction. The first relates to learning the articulatory features of speech, that is, identifying characteristics of sounds with respect to voicing, manner of production, and place of production. The second area of instruction involves associating the acoustic features of speech with the appropriate articulatory movements. The third area of instruction involves learning appropriate use of the target within the language.

APPLICATION OF THE SSD IN
LEARNING ARTICULATORY FEATURES

When learning about the articulatory features of speech, a major concern is whether a speech training aid provides sufficient information to distinguish speech sound characteristics. The potential application of any visual feedback device would logically depend on the variety of articulatory features which can be differentiated using the visual patterns.

In an effort to evaluate distinctiveness of speech sound patterns on the SSD, a same/different discrimination task and a pattern identification task were administered to separate groups of severely hearing-impaired adults (Maki, 1978). Results of the two tasks demonstrated that hearing-impaired adults could use visual patterns from the SSD to distinguish several important features of speech production. Relatively distinctive patterns result from voiced-voiceless contrasts, differences in manner of production, differences in tongue positioning for vowels, changes in tongue placement over time, and durational differences. Pattern confusions occurred for short central vowels and place of production features for consonants.

Given the above information, there is a variety of contrasts which could be illustrated using the visual display. These include: 1) contrasting a single feature such as voicing; 2) contrasting two features simultaneously; 3) demonstrating a combination of features important to production, such as correct tongue placement, change in tongue placement, and appropriate timing for diphthongs; 4) illustrating independence of voicing and articulatory movements; and 5) demonstrating the effect of context on sound production. All of the above are relatively abstract articulatory concepts which the hearing-impaired speaker must understand to achieve correct production. In this regard, any visual training aid is valuable to the extent that, by providing a concrete display, it circumvents the difficulty of describing and/or understanding the characteristics of speech production.

When considering use of a display to teach articulatory skills, a three-way association must be made between the articulatory target, such as /s/, the related visual feature(s) on the display, and the articulatory movements required to achieve the target. Although data from the identification task mentioned earlier showed rapid improvement in identifying visual sound patterns, it can only be assumed that subjects were basing their identifications on the appropriate visual features.

In order to assess whether hearing-impaired subjects could associate visual characteristics with the appropriate articulatory targets, a display interpretation task was administered to 10 severely hearing-impaired adults (Maki et al., 1981). The subjects, trained during therapy to use the SSD in evaluating their own speech, were asked to evaluate the speech production of other severely hearing-impaired speakers using only the visual patterns from the SSD. Those visual characteristics which were used accurately to evaluate speech production included: low-frequency periodic energy to signal presence or absence of voicing; relative position of the first three formants to indicate accurate vowel production; changes in formant position for diphthongs; high-frequency random energy for fricative and plosive production; vowel duration; continuous energy to indicate blending; and extraneous low-frequency information to signal intrusive voicing.

Thus, pattern interpretation data has shown that hearing-impaired adults can discriminate and identify visual differences for many aspects of speech production. And further, trained subjects can relate SSD visual features with speech production characteristics in order to evaluate production accuracy. These findings provide strong support for using the SSD in teaching the articulatory features of speech.

APPLICATION OF THE SSD IN ASSOCIATING
TARGET FEATURES WITH ARTICULATORY MOVEMENTS

It would seem that for a target, for example, voice onset time, a difference would exist between conceptually understanding the production characteristics of a target and learning control of the mechanism to achieve correct production. Application of a visual training aid, such as the SSD, might prove useful in learning how the articulatory mechanism achieves a specific target. Although this application has not been studied directly, it is a possible factor to consider in those studies in which improved articulatory skills resulted through use of visual training aids (Maki and Streff Gustafson, 1978; Stark, 1971; Stark et al., 1968).

In one study conducted with the SSD, it was found that the vowel production of hearing-impaired adults who used the display improved significantly, whereas non-SSD subjects showed little improvement (Maki and Streff Gustafson, 1978). When speculating as to why this occurred, it is conceivable that SSD subjects had several advantages that were not available to non-SSD subjects. The feedback relative to production accuracy which SSD subjects received was immediate, more objective, and was presented via concrete visual displays. In contrast, non-SSD subjects received slightly delayed feedback based on a subjective perceptual judgment and delivered via abstract linguistic explanations. In addition, SSD subjects could evaluate their own speech in a more analytical manner, whereas non-SSD subjects received a more general evaluation of the entire production based on another's judgment. As a result, it is suggested that feedback from the SSD is more concrete, more consistent, permits immediate feedback which the student can analyze, and is more specific than feedback based solely on the instructor's perceptual judgment.

To prevent an overly enthusiastic response concerning the advantages of using visual feedback, it is equally important to recognize the limitations of this or any visual training aid. With respect to the SSD, display characteristics do not provide distinctive contrasts for all phonetic differences. For example, visual cues on the SSD are not distinctive enough to allow hearing-impaired subjects to discriminate differences in place of production for consonants. As a result, the potential exists for place of production errors to be interpreted as correct when using only the display for feedback. Secondly, the display has a 30-dB dynamic range; and depending on instrument settings, low-intensity plosives and fricatives may not appear on the trace. Therefore, correct approximations with relatively low intensity may be interpreted as incorrect. And finally, it must be considered that an analytic, visual approach may not be appropriate for all learners.

APPLICATION OF THE SSD IN
LEARNING APPROPRIATE USE OF THE TARGET

In the study by Maki et al. (1981), subjects evaluated speech production using only SSD visual patterns. An analysis of the errors in that study showed that several errors in interpretation resulted when subjects inappropriately related orthographic symbols with the acoustic features of speech. To illustrate, a "silent" letter was assigned acoustic features, a sound represented by a double letter (e.g., "mm" in *hammer*) was evaluated as longer, and an acoustic feature of /ɪ/ was assigned to /aɪ/. It is assumed that the last error occurred because both /ɪ/ and /aɪ/ are represented by the same orthographic symbol. These errors suggest that the SSD, which reflects the spoken characteristics of language, might be applied in teaching the hearing impaired to relate the spoken and written forms of English appropriately.

APPLICATION OF THE SSD DURING SEMI-INDEPENDENT PRACTICE

Because hearing-impaired adults were able to evaluate accuracy of production using a selected set of SSD patterns, a study was designed to assess whether subjects could use the visual patterns to evaluate their own speech during ongoing analysis. The study was designed to evaluate the SSD by comparing subjects' judgments of accuracy and their speech production skills with and without use of visual feedback. Secondly, it was designed to observe whether any changes would occur during the session, either in speech production or in identifying correct and incorrect productions. If changes in either area did occur, the major question was whether improvement would occur only while using the SSD or would be observed for the non-SSD condition as well.

Method

Subjects The group consisted of 10 hearing-impaired adults with varying degrees of hearing loss. The mean age of the group was 20 years, 11 months, and the mean pure tone average for the better ear was 88.2 dB hearing threshold level (HTL) (re ANSI, 1969) with a standard deviation of 16.3 dB. With respect to auditory discrimination of speech, performance ranged from limited skills in discriminating spondee words to demonstrated ability in identifying words within sentences. Using a profiling system (Johnson, 1976), speech intelligibility for the group was 3.4, indicating that when subjects read a standard paragraph, more than half of the words were intelligible to trained listeners. The only criterion for subject selection was that they demonstrate difficulty in producing one or more articulatory targets within a word, yet be stimulable for the target sound(s).

Instrumentation In order to obtain necessary data, the following instrumentation was used: a Spectraphonics Speech Spectrographic Display; a number encoding and decoding unit (Silver, 1979b); a Wollensak cassette tape recorder (Model 2590); a control unit (Silver, 1979a); and an Electrovoice 651 microphone. During each test session, the following information was recorded onto cassette tape: 1) the subjects' productions of the target words; 2) digitally encoded numbers to identify each production; 3) synchronization signals to permit automatic operation of the SSD; and 4) the subjects' judgments of accuracy.

Data Collection A multisyllabic utterance was selected for each subject. The selected utterance contained one or more targets which were difficult for the subject, but which could be produced. Different utterances were used because of the varying skills of the subjects. The target sounds included: /s/, /s/, and /t/ in *sister* (3 subjects); /m/ in *hammer* (2 subjects); /st/ in *Stephen*; /sp/ in *special*; /s/ and /s/ in *processing*; /z/ in *easy*; and /t/ and /t/ in /ti di ti/. During a 30-minute individual session, each subject produced the utterance 200 times, separated into blocks of 25 trials. Visual feedback from the SSD was used during even-numbered blocks. After each production, the subject was required to judge the accuracy of production.

After the subject completed the first block of 25 trials, data collection was interrupted. At this point, the experimenter taught the subject to identify visual characteristics of the target sound(s) and to differentiate correct and incorrect productions spoken by the experimenter. When the subject could distinguish correct from incorrect visual patterns, data collection was resumed for block 2, in which visual feedback from the SSD was used to judge accuracy of production. Blocks 3 and 4 were recorded next, interrupting only to adjust equipment for non-SSD and SSD conditions, respectively.

After block 4, approximately 5 minutes of instruction was provided to improve production of the target(s) or increase subjects' skills in relating the visual information to their own speech production. Blocks

5 through 8 were recorded without further instruction and with alternated use of visual feedback. Thus, with this procedure, subjects used visual feedback during even-numbered blocks, but had to rely on internal monitoring to judge accuracy of production during odd-numbered blocks.

Data Analysis   Three individuals listened to the taped recordings and independently judged accuracy of production for the target sound(s). Two of the auditors were speech pathologists trained in evaluating hearing-impaired speech, and the third was an untrained listener who was instructed to listen for correct productions of the various targets. An utterance was judged correct when two or three listeners agreed on accuracy. The percentage of correct productions was calculated for each block of 25 trials.

The subjects' judgments of accuracy were obtained from the tape recordings. During the test sessions, when subjects judged a production as correct and pressed a response button, a 1000-Hz signal was recorded onto the tape. On playback, this signal stopped the recorder, allowing the experimenter to identify those productions which the subjects judged as correct. The percentage of agreement between subjects and auditors was calculated for each block. Separate calculations were made for those productions judged by auditors to be correct and for those judged to be incorrect. In addition, percentage agreement between subjects and auditors was calculated for each block. Separate calculations were made for those productions judged by auditors to be correct and for those judged to be incorrect.

Results

In general, results of this study showed that when subjects used the SSD they were better able to judge the accuracy of their speech production. In addition, speech production skills and subjects' ability to identify correct productions improved during the session. For both areas, improvement was noted for SSD and non-SSD conditions.

Judging Speech Production Accuracy   Figure 17.1 shows the percentage of agreement between auditors' and subjects' judgments of accuracy. When comparing SSD blocks 2, 4, 6, and 8 with non-SSD blocks 1, 3, 5, and 7, it was found that subjects were better at judging accuracy of production when using the SSD. Although this was generally true, group performance differed somewhat when looking at judgments of incorrect and correct productions separately.

For incorrect productions that occurred during block 1, subjects correctly identified 53.6% of the incorrect productions; that is, subjects performed at chance level. Performance on subsequent non-SSD

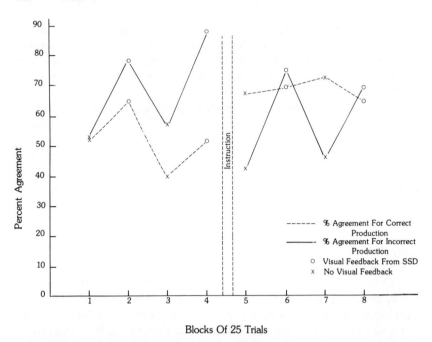

Blocks Of 25 Trials

Figure 17.1.   Using separate graphs for correct and incorrect productions, percentage of agreement is shown between auditors' and subjects' judgments of production accuracy. Auditors' judgments were obtained from an auditory analysis of the productions conducted after the test sessions; subjects' judgments were recorded during the test sessions with subjects using visual feedback from the SSD during even-numbered blocks only.

blocks was approximately the same or poorer. In contrast, subsequent SSD blocks showed 25% to 30% greater accuracy when identifying incorrect productions. The highest average scores, 78.5% (block 2) and 86.4% (block 4), resulted when subjects were using the SSD and identifying incorrect productions.

When identifying correct productions during the first 4 blocks, subjects were 10% to 12% more accurate during SSD blocks 2 and 4 when compared with non-SSD blocks 1 and 3. Although subjects were more accurate when using the SSD, it should be noted that the higher average score was 65.9% (block 2) which then decreased to 51.2% for block 4. Thus, subjects were poorer at identifying correct productions than incorrect. For blocks 5 through 8, a change in performance occurred. As shown, subjects' ability to identify correct productions improved for both SSD and non-SSD blocks. With or without the SSD, subjects were able to identify correct productions with approximately 70% accuracy.

Speech Production Performance   Figure 17.2 shows the percentage of correct productions for each of the 8 blocks. As seen in the figure, speech production scores increased from 21.6% correct for block 1 to approximately 70% correct for block 8. The largest improvements in speech production accuracy occurred for blocks 2 (16.1% increase) and 5 (23.5%). A plateau was observed during blocks 3 and 4, and some degree of improvement occurred for SSD blocks that followed block 5.

Discussion

Results of this study provide answers to some basic questions concerning semi-independent use of the SSD during speech practice sessions. In general, results support application of the SSD for semi-independent practice. In addition, results can be used to establish certain guidelines relative to clinical application of the Speech Spectrographic Display.

Judging Speech Production Accuracy   There are three major aspects that should be discussed with respect to the data collected on judging speech production accuracy. These involve: 1) judgment of accuracy with and without visual feedback; 2) use of the SSD to judge

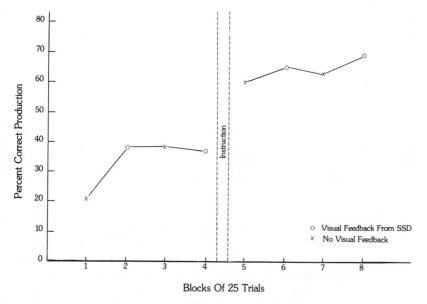

Figure 17.2.   Percentage of correct productions of target sounds for each of 8 blocks. Subjects used visual feedback from the SSD during even-numbered blocks only.

correct and incorrect productions; and 3) improved ability to judge accuracy of production without visual feedback.

Results of this study are clear with respect to using the SSD in judging speech production accuracy. In Figure 17.1, comparisons of block 1 with 2, 3 with 4, 5 with 6, and 7 with 8 demonstrate that subjects evaluated speech with greater accuracy when using visual feedback. In order to perform better with the SSD, subjects had to understand the visual characteristics of the patterns and whether those characteristics reflected correct or incorrect productions. Of nearly equal importance is that subjects completed the task of producing and evaluating 200 productions within 20 to 30 minutes. Thus, each judgment required an approximate decision time of 4 to 6 seconds.

Comparison of the graphs in Figure 17.1 shows that when using the SSD, subjects were better at identifying incorrect productions than correct productions. This was most evident for blocks 2 and 4. Within block 4, an average score of 51.2% for identifying correct productions indicates that subjects were guessing; however, the score of 86.4% for incorrect productions indicates otherwise. It is suspected that subjects were being very critical of their speech when using the instrument initially. As a result, their identification of errors was highly accurate and their identification of correct productions was poor. For this investigation, listeners were instructed to judge close approximations as correct, that is, to ignore minor sound distortions and timing errors. Similarly, subjects were instructed to look for major clues in the visual patterns and were not taught to identify cues which related to minor variations. Although subjects received no instruction concerning interpretation of these subtle differences, it is believed that subjects began to detect minor variations in the patterns, proceeding to identify those productions as incorrect. For example, a low-intensity fricative perceived as /s/ would be judged as correct by listeners. The same production, however, might not satisfy the subject who had previously produced a "darker" (i.e., better) production. As a result, listeners and subjects did not initially achieve a high degree of agreement for correct productions.

When comparing performance before and after instruction, it is interesting to note that subjects' identification of correct and incorrect productions was about equal after instruction. It can be seen in Figure 17.1 that this has happened because subjects became poorer at identifying incorrect productions and more accurate in identifying correct productions. The two most obvious reasons for this change in performance relate to the instructional segment and the subsequent improvement in speech production.

It is believed that instruction on display interpretation encouraged a less critical evaluation of the patterns resulting in improved identification of correct productions. In a similar manner, the instructional segment might have influenced subjects' ability to identify incorrect productions. Because subjects were encouraged to be less critical of correct patterns, it is possible that they were also less critical with incorrect productions. If true, this would result in decreased accuracy when identifying incorrect productions.

Another reason for poorer identification of errors relates to improved speech production which occurred after instruction. As speech production improved from 20% correct (Figure 17.2, block 1) to approximately 60% correct (block 5), a plausible assumption is that existing errors came closer to the target sound(s). For example, as errors changed from sound omissions to sound substitutions, the interpretation task would become more difficult.

The above results indicate that intermittent instruction is needed to assist subjects in refining pattern interpretation skills. Two points should be emphasized. First, the SSD provides sufficient information to allow critical evaluation of speech. It may be necessary, however, to instruct students to interpret the patterns in a general way and to ignore minor variations. Secondly, the criteria for judging a production as correct will change as the student improves production. As a result, there is a need for continual assessment of speech and the related visual features in the patterns. Therapy objectives and student capabilities should be used to determine which visual features reflect successful achievement of the goal and which visual features should be ignored.

Results of this study showed that improvement in identifying correct productions was not restricted to those blocks in which visual feedback was used. This suggests that while students were using the SSD to evaluate their speech, they simultaneously developed some use of internal feedback, that is, auditory, tactile, or kinesthetic awareness. This finding is of major importance because a skill that exists only when using a visual display would be of questionable value. For the optimal situation to occur, the visual monitoring of speech must lead to awareness and development of internal feedback mechanisms.

It is interesting that judgment skills improved only for those productions which were correct. This suggest that subjects' self-monitoring skills were not finely developed. As a result, they were missing the less obvious feedback related to incorrect productions. It is important to remember that the test sessions lasted 30 to 45 minutes. Of that time, subjects used the SSD for approximately 10 to 15 minutes. It is believed that increased exposure to the visual patterns would improve subjects' ability to identify incorrect as well as correct productions. This question awaits further research with the SSD to study the response of control and experimental groups over an extended period of time.

Improvement of Speech Production Skills   Speech production data, shown in Figure 17.2, indicate that subjects were able to use the SSD to effect a change in speech production. It was also observed, however, that productions improved considerably after additional instruction was provided. During the instructional segment after block 4, subjects were permitted to produce the target word, receiving clarification concerning analysis of the visual patterns. At that time, the instructor corrected misconceptions relative to pattern interpretation and offered suggestions as to how speech production might be improved. It is felt that during blocks 2 and 4 subjects had the opportunity to experiment with speech production and receive immediate feedback concerning the acoustic results of various articulatory gestures. It is further believed that this experimenting allowed subjects to discover the range of patterns which could be produced by altering articulatory features. At the point of instruction, all that subjects required was confirmation that they were interpreting the visual patterns correctly. This could account for the fact that subjects improved their production by approximately 25% immediately after instruction.

With respect to speech production data, there were two major findings which provide some direction when utilizing the SSD for independent practice. The first point is that subjects could evaluate their own speech independently with the SSD and effect a change in their speech production. Assuming that certain requirements are met relative to use of the SSD, it is clear that the instructor need not be present at all times. The second point is that intermittent instruction is needed to facilitate learning. This conclusion is supported by the increase in production accuracy immediately following the instructional segment. It is felt that the instructional segment was needed to assist subjects in identifying those features that were insignificant and those that were critical to speech production accuracy.

Summary of Clinical Considerations

Results of this investigation provide support for use of the SSD for independent practice. The procedures, although designed for research, specify some areas of concern when considering clinical application of the SSD.

The first concern is to choose therapy goals that reflect the capabilities of the instrument. The target utterances selected for this study were distinctive on the SSD patterns. The second concern involves evaluation of the student. Subjects in this study were taught to identify the visual features for their target sounds. If the student cannot consistently and accurately identify correct and incorrect productions, there is little chance that the instrument can facilitate learning.

The time factor is also a concern. In this study, 5 to 15 minutes were needed to teach each subject to identify the important visual features and to assess the subjects' ability to distinguish correct from incorrect. In addition, it should not take more than 10 seconds to make a decision concerning accuracy of production. This, of course, depends on the difficulty of the task. For example, the number of visual features that must be identified and evaluated will alter the time needed for interpretation. In general, however, limited amounts of time should be required for teaching the visual contrasts or for actual display interpretation during the practice sessions.

Because subjects in this study were not 100% accurate in evaluating the displays, it is recommended that some form of monitoring be provided. This task might be performed by a person or through recording techniques such as those used in this study. Regardless of the method used, some form of monitoring is recommended to ensure accurate interpretation of visual patterns.

The last concern relates to dependence on visual feedback. Results of this study showed that skills in speech production and judging correct productions improved; and furthermore, that the improvement was observed during both SSD and non-SSD blocks. Thus, because subjects showed improvement during non-SSD blocks, it is clear that some of the skills they learned were not confined to use of visual feedback. The design of this study required that subjects use the SSD during alternate blocks. It is possible that this requirement forced subjects to develop some awareness of internal feedback, an awareness that might have been left unchanged had subjects used visual feedback during the entire practice session. This question awaits further research which will define optimal techniques for use of the SSD. Until that time, the instructor should be aware of the potential dependence on instrumentation.

CONCLUSION

Results to date support use of the SSD with hearing-impaired adults. The instrument provides visual patterns which distinguish a variety of articulatory features. Hearing-impaired adults can interpret the patterns with a high degree of accuracy and can use the instrument to improve articulation and develop self-monitoring skills.

There are many aspects of speech communication that a clinician needs to consider. Results with the SSD demonstrate that instrumentation can be used effectively in the development of articulation skills. This would free the clinician to concentrate on conversational skills, counseling, and other critical areas of therapy. The client, the instrument, and the clinician all have important roles in defining and/or achieving therapy objectives. With respect to the role of instrumentation, it is hoped that this chapter provides sufficient information to aid in appropriate clinical application of the Speech Spectrographic Display.

REFERENCES

American National Standards Institute. 1970. American National Standard. Specifications for Audiometers, ANSI-S3.6-1969. New York: American National Standards Institute, New York.

House, A., D. Goldstein, and G. Hughes. 1968. Perception of visual transforms of speech stimuli: Learning simple syllables. Am. Ann. Deaf 113:215–221.

Johnson, D. 1976. Communication characteristics of a young deaf adult population: Techniques for evaluating their communication skills. Am. Ann. Deaf 121:409–424.

Koenig, W., H. Dunn, and L. Lacy. 1946. The sound spectrograph. J. Acoust. Soc. Am. 17:19–49.

Kopp, G., and H. Green. 1946. Basic phonetic principles of visible speech. J. Acoust. Soc. Am. 18:74–89.

Maki, J. 1978. Visual discrimination and identification of spectrographic patterns by hearing-impaired adults. Paper presented at the meeting of the American Speech and Hearing Association, November, San Francisco.

Maki, J., and M. Streff Gustafson. 1978. Clinical evaluation of the Speech Spectrographic Display with hearing-impaired adults. Paper presented at the meeting of the American Speech and Hearing Association, November, San Francisco.

Maki, J., M. Streff Gustafson, J. Conklin, and B. Humphrey Whitehead. 1981. The Speech Spectrographic Display: Interpretation of visual patterns by hearing-impaired adults. J. Speech Hear. Disord. 46:379–387.

Potter, R., G. Kopp, and H. Kopp. 1966. Visible Speech. Dover Publications, New York.

Riesz, R., and L. Schott. 1946. The visible speech cathode-ray translator. J. Acoust. Soc. Am. 18:50–61.

Silver, G. 1979a. Automated control of the Spectraphonics Speech Spectrographic Display using a Wollensak 2590 A-V cassette recorder and logic interface. Unpublished technical report. National Technical Institute for the Deaf, Rochester, N.Y.

Silver, G. 1979b. Digital encoding and decoding of stimulus/trial identification numbers using a 2-channel audio tape recorder. Unpublished technical report. National Technical Institute for the Deaf, Rochester, N.Y.

Stark, R. 1971. The use of real-time visual displays of speech in the training of a profoundly deaf, non-speaking child: A case report. J. Speech Hear. Disord. 36:397–409.

Stark, R., J. Cullen, and R. Chase. 1968. Preliminary work with the new Bell Telephone Visible Speech Translator. Am. Ann. Deaf 113:205–214.

Steinberg, J., and N. French. 1946. The portrayal of visible speech. J. Acoust. Soc. Am. 18:4–18.

Stewart, L., W. Larkin, and R. Houde. 1976. A real-time sound spectrograph with implications for speech training for the deaf. Paper presented at the IEEE International Conference on Acoustics, Speech and Signal Processing, Philadelphia.

CHAPTER 18

COMPUTERS AND SPEECH AIDS

Raymond S. Nickerson, Kenneth N. Stevens, Ann M. Rollins, and Victor W. Zue

CONTENTS

In 1971, the authors began exploring the development of a computer-based system of speech training aids for deaf children (see Nickerson, Stevens, and Rollins, 1979). Although there were no illusions about solving the problem of teaching speech to deaf children simply by involving a computer, the authors were impressed by the fact that with a computer one can analyze speech and speech-related signals in many different ways, and one can represent the results of those analyses either visually or tactually in a wide variety of display formats.

There are additional concerns to be addressed, however, about practicality and accessibility, both physically and financially, to the average deaf child. Even a child who happens to attend a school that has a computer, and who happens to be selected for a program involving its use, is not likely to see it for more than a few minutes a day, a few days a week for a few weeks. That is not much time in which to have a significant impact on speech that has been grossly defective every day for several years.

With respect to these concerns, the attitude of the authors was—and is—that with the rapidity of advancement of computer technology, it is not too early to begin learning how to apply this technology to the problem of teaching speech. Before discussing what has been learned as a result of the initial efforts, it will be useful to consider briefly the assumption that these impediments are likely to be only temporary.

TRENDS IN COMPUTER TECHNOLOGY

Several major trends have characterized advances in the design of computer components since computers first became commercially available about 30 years ago: decreasing size, decreasing power requirements, increasing speed, increasing reliability, and decreasing costs. Perhaps the fact that progress has been characterized by these types of changes should not be surprising; however, the speed of the progression from vacuum tubes to transistors to integrated circuits to large-scale integration (LSI), and now to very-large-scale integration (VLSI) has been nothing short of incredible. Who, 30 years ago, could have anticipated the rapidity of these developments?

On the basis of performance measures that take speed, word size, instruction set, and a variety of other factors into account, the conclusion has been drawn that the performance/price ratio, that is, the amount of performance per unit price, has increased at the rate of about 50% per year for medium-sized computers and minicomputers since the early 1960s.

What is perhaps even more astonishing than the rapidity of developments in computer technology is the way the rate of change itself has accelerated over time. The advent of LSI and the resulting "computer on a chip" contributed significantly to this acceleration. Although the term "revolution" is greatly overworked these days, there is no more accurate way to describe what has happened in the area of microprocessor technology since the introduction of the first commercially available microprocessor, the INTEL 4004, in 1970. By 1977, some 20 U.S. companies were manufacturing microprocessor chips (Toong, 1977). The microprocessors that are being produced are appearing everywhere, not only in sophisticated military and industrial systems, but in automobiles, office equipment, home appliances, and children's games.

The effect of this innovation, like that of all the others, can be measured in terms of cost. Noyce (1977) pointed out that as a result of the development and volume production of microelectronic components, the cost of hand-held calculators decreased by a factor of 100 over the course of a decade. Perhaps one of the most striking examples of the effect of the development of integrated circuitry on computer component costs is seen in the following comparison: in 1959 the price of a single high-quality transistor was $20.00; in 1979, the price of a transistor that was part of a high-density integrated memory circuit was about ½₀th of one cent (Rosen, 1979). This represents a price reduction of five orders of magnitude in 20 years.

What is going to happen in computer technology during the next 20 or 30 years is anybody's guess. One thing, however, is clear: the trends that have characterized progress in the past can be expected to continue into the immediate future at least. In 1978 Mead and Conway noted that LSI technology was then capable of putting tens of thousands of transistors on a single silicone chip and that achievable circuit density is approximately doubling every year. Given that the linear dimensions of transistors can be reduced to less than 1/10th of their current size before some fundamental physical or chemical limitations are encountered, chips containing over a million transistors seem likely to be produced relatively soon. Kahn (1978) estimated that systems containing digital components with submicron dimensions will be achievable by the mid-1980s, and that the implementation on a single chip of a processor with computational capability exceeding that of large 1978-vintage machines by one or two orders of magnitude should be possible within the same time frame. Dhaka (1975) made the startling prediction that by the mid-1980s, it will be possible to build on a single chip a 32-bit microcomputer with a million bits of memory for about $20.00.[1]

The realization of these possibilities will depend on the development and refinement of nonoptical methods of circuit production such as x-ray or electron-beam lithography. But such techniques are being developed, and one or more of them undoubtedly will be brought to the point of practical applicability.

In terms of developing communication aids for deaf people, these trends indicate that computing resources which will be available to be applied to this problem will far outdistance our knowledge of how to make effective use of those resources. Kay (1977) predicted that during the 1980s, "both adults and children will be able to have as a personal possession a computer about the size of a large notebook with the power to handle virtually all their information-related needs" (p. 231). Will we have the knowledge by then that will be required to realize the potential represented by this technology for improving speech and other communication skills of the deaf? (For details regarding expected developments in microelectronics during the next few years, see Nickerson, 1982).

---

[1] Since this chapter was written, Bell Laboratories has developed a microprocessor (the MAC-32) that has over 100,000 components on a single chip, and Hewlett-Packard has developed one with over 450,000 (Johnson, 1981).

THE ORIGINAL BBN SYSTEM OF SPEECH TRAINING AIDS

The system of speech training aids built in 1971 was modeled on an earlier system developed to facilitate the teaching of certain aspects of pronunciation to people learning a second language (Kalikow and Swets, 1972; Nickerson and Stevens, 1973; Nickerson, Kalikow, and Stevens, 1976). The system was built around a Digital Computer Corporation PDP 8E, a minicomputer representative of the state of the art in the late 1960s and early 1970s. The complete system included the PDP-8E computer with 8000 words of core memory, analog circuits for measuring pitch and nasalization, a filter bank to analyze the speech spectrum, tape recorders including a tape-loop playback device, a set of push buttons and control knobs, and a visual display.

Speech information was obtained not only from a voice microphone but also from a miniature accelerometer attached by two-way adhesive tape either to the child's throat or to the surface of the nose. When attached to the throat, the accelerometer was used to determine the glottal waveform and, hence, the fundamental frequency of voiced speech sounds. When attached to the nose, it provided a measure of the amount of sound energy emitted through the nostrils, which could be used to infer the degree of nasalization. Although some preliminary work was done with vibrotactile displays, the main emphasis in the project was on visual representations of various aspects of speech. The display was a Hewlett-Packard 1300A point-plotting scope, with 1024 × 1024 resolution, a P31 phosphor, and a nonglare filter.

Several independent programs were written for the system to produce a number of visual displays. Some of the displays were gamelike in character and were intended to provide the child with a situation in which interesting things could be made to happen by doing certain voice exercises. Other displays involved more straightforward representations of various speech parameters (fundamental frequency, speech amplitude, voicing, nasalization) as functions of time, and were used more often in training sessions. Additional programs were written to perform various types of analyses on recorded speech. Only one program was resident within core memory at any given time; programs not in use were stored on a magnetic tape device.

Two systems were built and installed in schools for the deaf, one at the Clarke School for the Deaf in Northampton, Massachusetts, and the other at the Lexington School for the Deaf in New York City. The most common use of the systems in speech training was as an aid for a teacher interacting with a student in a one-to-one tutorial situation. Additional uses included: 1) independent unsupervised drill; 2) diagnostic measurements of children's speech; and 3) demonstrations for teachers in training.

Training typically was focused on one specific speech problem at any given time. Among the problems that have received attention are the following: timing, velopharyngeal control, pitch control, and voice quality (especially breathiness). Relatively little attention was given to articulatory problems, which, in retrospect, was unfortunate; but the displays that were developed were not well suited in most cases for articulatory training.

Most students who were trained with the help of the system showed improvements in those attributes of their speech on which the training was focused:

> . . . (a) reduced incidence of nasalization in vowels, (b) shifting of average fundamental frequency into a more appropriate range, (c) reduced incidence of inadvertent changes in fundamental frequency in phrases and sentences, (d) reduced number of inadvertent pauses between words, and (e) improved spectrum of glottal output (Nickerson et al., 1979; p. 99).

However, such improvements were not consistently accompanied by increases in overall speech intelligibility. One possible reason is that training was concentrated on aspects of speech that are less important for intelligibility than are some others (Nickerson et al., 1979).

We concluded that training involving the use of such computer-generated displays can indeed be effective in modifying speech in specific objectively measurable ways. We also concluded, however, that better understanding is needed of how any particular sample of defective speech would have to be changed in order to improve its intelligibility (Nickerson and Stevens, 1980). One of the functions that any successor to our system should be designed to serve is that of facilitating the acquisition of such information. If that kind of knowledge were available, speech training—with or without computer systems—could be far more effective than it currently is.

WHAT WE THINK WE HAVE LEARNED

Computer technology is a potentially powerful resource to apply to the problem of teaching speech to deaf children, and this potential should be developed. The proper preparation of teachers who are to use this kind of technology is essential. This preparation is not needed to acquaint teachers with computer technology per se, but to acquaint them with the relationships among the acoustics of speech, the physiology of its production, and the various displays the system can produce. This teacher preparation could be done in the context of a regular inservice training program with both teachers and researchers working together to consider the speech training problems of individual children.

There is a great need for a much better understanding of the relationship between intelligibility and the physical properties of speech. Research on this question is necessary to provide the basis for adequate diagnosis, setting of training objectives, and evaluation. The full potential of computer technology, or any other resource that may be applied to the speech teaching problem, is unlikely to be realized until this better understanding is achieved.

Although prosodics are undoubtedly very important to the production of natural sounding speech, we have come to believe that adequate articulatory skills are probably the sine qua non of intelligibility. If this belief is valid, then a system of displays that is to be maximally effective should probably include a spectrographic display.

The problem of carryover is fundamental. It is one thing to teach a child to do certain things with his or her voice in a speech training laboratory; it is another to make sure that what the child learns to do in the laboratory carries over into everyday speech. In this regard, a distinction should be made between speech that is produced for the sake of practicing speech skills and speech that is produced for the purpose of communicating. Too little thought has been given to the possibility that these may be qualitatively different activities in terms of their cognitive demands. What one thinks about when practicing speech skills is the speech production process. What one thinks about when communicating is what one is saying or, perhaps more accurately, the meaning of what one is saying, and not the process of saying it. For this reason, it is important that the training procedures that are defined for use in the speech laboratory provide for the elicitation of spontaneous speech and for the evaluation and remediation of problems in the context of speech that is produced for the sake of communicating.

Ultimately, for a speech training aid to be maximally effective it will probably have to be wearable. This follows in part from the belief that the teaching of speech is probably a much less effective approach to the problem than helping a child to learn it spontaneously. That is to say, we think the most effective approach to this problem would be to provide a child continuously with a visual and/or tactual display that is sufficiently rich to provide the missing auditory feedback suitably coded in some other modality. This is probably not technically feasible at the present time, although beginning efforts in this direction are being made (Goldstein et al., this volume). Already computers can effectively turn the home television screen into a terminal, however. It seems reasonable to assume, then, that the future holds the technology that will make it possible to give a child more powerful training devices than the 10 to 20 minutes per day that has been practical up to the present time.

It is important that the activities in the speech laboratory be coordinated with the speech training that is done in the classroom and elsewhere. To this end, the establishment of policies and procedures that will assure continuing communication between laboratory and classroom teachers is critical.

Among the features of the original Bolt Beranek and Newman (BBN) system that we believe to be worth preserving in future systems of this sort are the following: 1) flow mode display capability; 2) freeze and capture capability, which, when coupled with flow mode capability, provides the important option of monitoring continuous speech and capturing the contents of the display (the last 2 seconds of speech) for careful inspection at any time; 3) auditory capture and replay; 4) data analysis capability to make measurements of duration, amplitude, and frequency directly from a display; and 5) flexibility. Perhaps the single most important feature of a computer-based system is the flexibility it provides and the opportunity to experiment with different displays and display formats and to evolve an effective system through use.

Our system's limitations include the following: 1) lack of the ability to store and retrieve prerecorded samples of speech and speech-like stimuli for use in auditory testing and training; 2) lack of a spectrographic display; 3) lack of ability to provide language training; and 4) lack of a carefully designed user interface. It is not possible, for example, to load user programs from the training stations; and no attempt was made to integrate the system software components and provide access to them through a simple command language.

FUNCTIONAL SPECIFICATION OF A CURRENTLY FEASIBLE SYSTEM

The system described in preceding sections of this paper was built using computer technology that was state of the art over 10 years ago. As noted, much has happened in computer technology during this time with implications for the design of future computer-based speech training systems. Given the current state of the art of computer technology and what was learned from the authors' first effort to build and use a computer-based system of speech training aids for the deaf, how would one design a new system today? A tentative answer to that question will be given in a list of desirable functional capabilities and characteristics of the system, and then by discussing the technical feasibility of realizing these capabilities and characteristics with currently available technology. The functional capabilities such a system should have include the following:

1. The ability to display in real time a variety of aspects of a speech signal including amplitude envelope, fundamental frequency, formant frequencies (especially the second formant frequency), nasalization, and spectrographic information
2. Sufficient buffer storage to hold and display 2-second segments of speech for both teacher and student
3. Instantaneous and continuous display capability
4. Freeze and capture capability
5. Provision for the user to change display parameters (e.g., time scale)
6. Auditory record and playback capability, with playback of precisely the segment of speech represented on the display. Audio playback should be synchronized with regeneration of the display
7. Editing capabilities to permit isolation and replay of specific portions of an utterance
8. A simple command language through which the user can access the various display programs, change display parameters, and so on
9. Capability to prestore digitally and to access randomly a few hundred to a thousand utterances or other auditory stimuli of up to 5 seconds duration each—these stimuli should be designed for use in auditory testing and training
10. Capability to make quantitative measurements directly from the display (e.g, amplitude, frequency, duration), and to perform statistical analyses on such measurements
11. Ability to store and display alphanumeric text
12. Totally digital circuitry

One of the more significant ways in which this system would differ from the one that the authors originally built involves inclusion of spectrographic display capability. Several points should be made regarding this addition.

First, although sound spectrograms have been used extensively in speech research over the past few decades, it was not until very recently that speech researchers began to understand fully the relationship between such a visual representation and the underlying articulatory gestures responsible for the production of speech sounds. Research conducted by Cole et al. (1979) and Cole and Zue (1979) has shown that a great deal of information regarding the phonetic content, and hence the underlying articulatory gestures, of an utterance can be determined from a visual examination of a spectrogram. These results are directly relevant to the problem of speech training for deaf children. If underlying articulatory gestures can be inferred from a spectrographic display, such a display should be useful in diagnosing and correcting poor speech articulation.

Second, focusing on a spectrographic display as a key part of a second-generation speech training system is indicative of a significant modification in our view of how speech training should proceed. The original effort attempted to improve speech by providing training of individual speech skills separately. Although these individual skills are undoubtedly important for proper articulation, speech production probably must be treated as an integrated skill, involving coordinated interactions among the various articulators, which can best be represented by a spectrographic display.

Third, the technology to generate real-time spectrographic displays did not exist during the period of earlier projects. It was not until 1977 that real-time displays appropriate for speech training became commercially available (Stewart, Larkin, and Houde, 1976).

Figure 18.1 shows the basic configuration of a computer-based speech training system that contains most of the desirable features outlined above and is technologically feasible at the present time. The

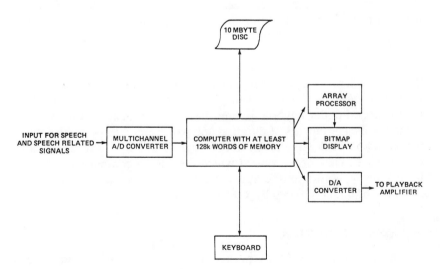

Figure 18.1. Possible configuration of a computer-based speech training system. Characteristics of individual components are discussed in the text.

computer could be any of several minicomputers. The speech wave-form would be digitized and stored in the computer memory and in a secondary storage device. Digital storage (rather than analog, as on a tape recorder) allows immediate access for playback. In order to save 2 seconds of a speech at a sampling rate of 10 kHz, the system should have at least 128,000 words of directly addressable primary memory. This amount of memory would also allow the development of adequate display and data management programs. A secondary storage device, probably a set of removable discs, should have a storage capacity of at least 10M bytes. This memory would allow approximately 500 2-second utterances, sampled at 10 kHz, to be stored and available for playback.

Data base management programs should be included, such that any one of the utterances could be retrieved instantaneously for display and listening purposes. Data acquisition would be accomplished through a multichannel analog-to-digital converter. Channel selection would be under program control. Playback of digital waveforms would make use of the digital-to-analog converter. The analog output could be used for listening by the speech teacher, and could also be fed to a master hearing aid amplifier into which deaf students would be able to plug their hearing aids during speech training.

An array processor is needed to perform signal processing tasks such as spectrum analysis and formant and pitch extraction in real time. Computed spectra and speech parameters could be displayed in flow mode in many forms, including the spectrographic form, and could be frozen for detailed inspection.

The configuration shown in Figure 18.1, with the characteristics just described, has sufficient processing and storage capacity to permit the development of a command language that would give the user easy keyboard access to the various display capabilities. Cursors could also be positioned under keyboard command so as to facilitate the making of simple measurements of duration and parameter values. Such a sys-tem could be built with current technology for a few tens of thousands of dollars. In view of the rate at which the cost of computer hardware is decreasing, a system of comparable capability should be producible at a cost of under $10,000 by 1985.

PERSONAL COMPUTERS

One of the more noteworthy events in computer technology in recent years is the appearance on the market of an assortment of "personal" or "home" computers. These are relatively inexpensive ($500 to $1500) general-purpose machines that are designed for use in the home or individual office. In terms of processing speed, memory capacity, and general performance capabilities, they are comparable or superior to computers that would have cost several tens of thousands of dollars a decade ago. Examples of these machines are the Apple II, the Pet, the Sorcerer, the TRS-80, and the TI-99/4. They are widely advertised in both trade journals and popular magazines. Typically, standard peripheral equipment includes a keyboard data-entry device and a visual (often color) display. All of these machines can be programmed in one or more of several common languages (e.g., BASIC, FORTRAN, COBOL). Vendors also typically offer a library of programs addressing a variety of interests, for example, personal data management, education, or entertainment. These programs usually are stored on tape cassettes and can be purchased for nominal cost.

Personal computers are attractive for many reasons. They are relatively inexpensive—their cost in many cases is less than that of a terminal for a time-shared system—and their operating costs are negligible. (Even including purchase price of both hardware and software, if a machine is used heavily, the cost per hour of usage is very small.) Personal computers are usually compact, portable, and easily maintained or, if necessary, replaced. They require no special facilities, nor are they subject to some of the fluctuations in performance resulting from the load that other users are putting on the machine, as is the case with time-sharing systems.

The personal machines that are currently available probably have fairly limited potential for application to the problem of speech training; although their potential for providing training (either explicitly or implicitly, via recreational programs) in other language and language-related skills would seem to be great, albeit virtually unexplored. What will be generally available as low-cost personal machines a relatively few (e.g., 5, 10, or 15) years from now, however, will undoubtedly represent much greater capacity than our first system, which is another compelling reason for trying to learn how to apply computer technology to the speech training problem now.

REFERENCES

Cole, R. A., A. Rudnicky, V. W. Zue, and D. R. Reddy. 1979. Speech as patterns on paper. In R. A. Cole (ed.), Perception and Production of Fluent Speech. Lawrence Erlbaum Associates, Hillsdale, N.J.

Cole, R. A., and V. W. Zue. 1979. Speech as eyes see it. In R. S. Nickerson (ed.), Attention and Performance. VIII. Lawrence Erlbaum Associates, Hillsdale, N.J.

Dhaka, V. A. 1975. Evolution of new hardware technology. Natl. Comput. Conf. 47:1061–1062.

Johnson, R. C. 1981. Thirty-two bit microprocessers inherit mainframe features. Electronics, Feb. 24:138–141.

Kahn, R. E. 1978. Submicron digital technology. Unpublished memorandum, Defense Advanced Research Projects Agency, Arlington, VA 22209.

Kalikow, D. N., and J. A. Swets. 1972. Experiments with computer-controlled displays in second-language learning. IEEE Trans. Audio Electroacoust. AU-20:23–28.

Kay, A. C. 1977. Microelectronics and the personal computer. Sci. Am. 237(3):231–244.

Mead, C., and L. Conway. 1978. Introduction to VLSI systems. Addison-Wesley, Reading, Mass.

Nickerson, R. S. 1982. Information technology and psychology—A retrospective look at some views of the future. In R. A. Kasschau, R. Lachman, and K. R. Langhery (eds.), Information Technology and Psychology: Prospects for the Future. Praeger Publishers, New York.

Nickerson, R. S., D. N. Kalikow, and K. N. Stevens. 1976. Computer-aided speech training for the deaf. J. Speech Hear. Disord. 41:120–132.

Nickerson, R. S., and K. N. Stevens. 1973. Teaching speech to the deaf: Can a computer help? IEEE Trans. Audio. Electroacoust. AU-21:445–455.

Nickerson, R. S., and K. N. Stevens. 1980. Approaches to the study of the relationship between intelligibility and physical properties of speech. In J. D. Subtelny (ed.), Speech Assessment and Speech Improvement for the Hearing Impaired. A. G. Bell Association for the Deaf, Washington, D.C.

Nickerson, R. S., K. N. Stevens, and A. M. Rollins. 1979. Research on computer based speech diagnosis and speech training aids for the deaf. Final Report on Contract No. 300-76-0116, BBN Report No. 4029.

Noyce, R. N. 1977. Microelectronics. Sci. Am. 237(3):63–69.

Rosen, B. M. 1979. Morgan Stanley Electronics Letter. September 28.

Stewart, L. C., W. P. Larkin, and R. A. Houde. 1976. A real-time sound spectrograph with implications for speech training for the deaf. Conference Record, International Conference on Acoustics, Speech and Signal Processing, Philadelphia, pp. 590–593.

Toong, H-M. D. 1977. Microprocessors. Sci. Am. 237(3):146–161.

RECENT DEVELOPMENTS IN SPEECH AND AUDITORY TRAINING

CHAPTER 19

TRAINING STRATEGIES IN FUNCTIONAL SPEECH ROUTINES

Peter M. Blackwell

CONTENTS

This chapter deals with those issues of speech and auditory training of the hearing impaired that have to do not so much with the mechanics of speech but rather the functions of speech acts and other contextual factors that motivate or modify speech interaction. Knowledge of the acoustic nature of speech or the issues in the perception of the speech signal is critical in establishing a meaningful developmental sequence for a speech and auditory training curriculum, but a sufficient and efficient program also must address the pragmatic aspects of speech acquisition.

Keenan (1974) noted that the young child is involved not only in a mastery of the linguistic code but also a code of conduct. Bruner (1975) added that

> Whatever the grammatical structure of the utterance, it is encoding a convention . . . that the speaker must understand in some simpler, NON-LINGUISTIC way before he is likely to comprehend or to use such utterances appropriately. The relation between the instrumental . . . function of an utterance and its grammatical structure is . . . crucial to language acquisition. (p. 3)

Although it is not unusual for speech training programs to include orientation to some of the types of utterances that Gleason and Weintraub (1976) called *routines*, the focus is generally a practice of the utterance in a limited and often unrealistic contextual reference. A list of routines would include greetings, thanks, warnings, commands, requests, insults, promises, rhymes, incantations, jokes, riddles, celebrations, and rituals. The suggestion here is that routines, conversational speech activities, or "functional speech" must be seen not as some add-on to the speech curriculum, as "worthy goals," nor even as ends in themselves, but as an integral part of the speech acquisition and mastery process, in which the dynamics of the speech act are utilized as a powerful motivation and facilitator of communication.

Before identifying some strategies for the use of functional speech routines in a school program it will be useful to discuss some aspects of the nature of the routines and how they are perceived by adults, as identified by Gleason and Weintraub (1978).

1. Parents act differently depending on whether the interaction is that of reference or routine. "When the input language functions primarily to aid the acquisition of referentiality, parents are concerned with children's competence, with their understanding of concepts" (p. 204). They are concerned that the child understands rather than produces. For instance if a parent asks, "Where's the light, Johnny?" he or she is satisfied if there is a glance or look in the right direction. With routines, however, performance is a critical issue and parents are concerned that the child says the right thing at the right time.
2. Adults mark routines as if to distinguish them from other linguistic behavior. The most common marker is *say*, as in "Say 'thank you' Jeremy"; "Say 'hello' to Mrs. Spencer"; or later, "What do you say?"
3. Routines are often empty or almost empty of meaning and certainly parents do not elaborate on or explain them. It is the learning of the code of conduct that seems to be the primary goal.
4. Although there is little explanation of the content of the routine itself, there is considerable and explicit teaching as to appropriateness and timing with verbal reinforcement, such as "good" or "right" for correct performance.
5. The grammatical structure of the routine is simple with little restructuring from production to production, allowing routines to become highly ritualized and therefore predictable.

APPLICATION TO A TRAINING PROGRAM

To be effective, a training program for hearing-impaired children should involve the variety of opportunities for speech interaction at appropriate stages, such as with parents, grandparents, other relatives, neighbors, community contacts, or authority figures. The utilization of functional speech routines in the speech curriculum will provide opportunities for facilitation of the speech act, enhancement of effective relationships, a set of structures that can be generalized to new social situations, and a set of structures that enhances fluency.

Facilitation of the Speech Act

Some of the essential features of the speech act include: awareness of intent, anticipation, productive response, turn taking, and initiation. The activity "pat-a-cake" provides an example of the process involved at the early level (parent-infant program or preschool).

Awareness of Intent   This skill usually develops from a ritualization of interaction through looming or mock threats. The activity includes more and more verbalization until the recitation of a rhyme triggers readiness to enter into the interaction on the part of the child. Of the essence here is that the ritual is often performed at predictable times, such as changing diapers, feeding, or putting to bed. If there is no awareness of intent on the part of the hearing-impaired child, the focus on ritualization of speech acts is an important starting point.

Anticipation   Ritualization leads to anticipation, which involves the recognition of familiar linguistic patterns (not always meaningful, but familiar), at which stage children begin to focus on the internal phonological structure of the routine, especially the rhyming or stressed aspects.

Productive Response   It is not unusual for parents to capitalize on anticipation of pausing before the last word of lines of rhymes to encourage production of those salient words.

Turn Taking   Verbal production quickly leads to verbal turn taking between parent and child. This may not be very meaningful in content but is powerful in its interaction process.

Initiation   Having developed some mastery over the verbal structure, the child is able to initiate the interaction process at will.

At a later stage (through high school), it is important to note if the student can identify the *questioning* intent of a teacher or another adult. This is an important skill to develop prior to even understanding the question. One skill utilized at the secondary level of the Rhode Island School for the Deaf is to encourage an immediate response to a teacher's question by means of several alternatives: "Excuse me, was that a question you asked?" or "I know you asked a question; would you repeat it?" or "I know you asked me a question, but I don't know the answer."

This response strategy has reduced awkward moments of silence as well as inappropriate question formation adaptations on the part of teachers. Anticipation, response, turn taking, and initiation can be built effectively into the question interaction.

Enhancement of Affective Relationships

The late development of speech in any child produces anxiety in the parents, and in the case of the hearing-impaired child the problems seem greatly magnified and they extend over many years. Encouragement to wait soon becomes hollow, and parents often begin to ask for more speech work, or they add the services of a speech-language pathologist or other private practitioner to the educational program.

The utilization of routines opens the possibility of more immediate verbal production, certainly within a more manageable time frame. Parents are not so much concerned about articulation ability at the early stages as they are concerned about appropriate and timely production. In response to this, the Rhode Island School for the Deaf piloted an activity that involved the cooperation and commitment of five families. The role of routines in language acquisition was explained and a trial example was chosen (Parent: "Have a nice day!" Child: "Thank you, you too!"). The idea was that the speech personnel at school would work on the "mechanics" of the speech while the parents would concentrate on the content for use. The children ranged from 5 through 14 years of age and were severely to profoundly hearing impaired.

The first activity involved explaining the routine to the children, thereby establishing intent and anticipation. Some of the children seemed to have little sense for routine interaction: one 5-year-old, after the first input of "Have a nice day!," went to the window and looked out, saying, "No, raining!"

Day 1 required a parent to be at the door to initiate the routine when the child was about to leave for school. Most of the children remembered that they were to respond but could not remember the words. On day 2 the children were obviously more aware of the responsibility and said things such as, "I forget; what I say?"

By the end of the first week all families had success and, in some cases, by the fifth day the older students initiated "Have a nice day!," requiring the parent to shift roles.

A Set of Structures That Can Be Generalized to New Social Situations

Routines are very portable in that this kind of interaction occurs throughout a culture and the format is highly predictable. This was demonstrated by the next phase of the program in which parents asked a neighbor or grandparent to initiate the routine to establish an awareness that this routine did not belong merely to the parent-child interchange. Consequently, bus drivers, teachers, and the principal reported that these children initiated this routine during the following weeks. A further generalizing skill is to develop modifications or new routines for similar functional settings.

A Set of Structures That Enhances Fluency

The predictable and portable nature of the routine structure enhances fluency in that the attention is not on meaning or generation but on performance. This level of speech play and speech interaction continues to be highly predictive and involved with phonological sequences rather than grammatical or semantic units.

If hearing children use the routines of social interaction and speech play to enhance their speech fluency, how important it is that we utilize them in the speech program for hearing-impaired children. Some of the results observed in the program in Rhode Island have been: 1) growing confidence on the part of the children to handle speech routines and social situations; 2) growing confidence on the part of parents, in that success can be realized earlier; 3) generalization on the part of parents to help their children cope with new social situations by identifying the routines that will be required; and 4) changes in perceptions and attitudes on the part of bus drivers and others toward the children.

As more and more information becomes available through the adult-child interaction studies it is imperative that schools and speech programs evaluate the curriculum in the light of that knowledge so that speech for the hearing-impaired child is a process of power in social situations rather than an experience of anxiety, dependency, and failure.

REFERENCES

Bruner, J. S. 1975. The ontogenesis of speech acts. J. Child Lang. 2:1–19.
Gleason, J. B., and S. Weintraub. 1976. The acquisition of routines in child language. Lang. Soc. 5:126–136.
Gleason, J. B., and S. Weintraub. 1978. Input language and the acquisition of communicative competence. In K. Nelson (ed.), Children's Language. Vol. 1. Gardner Press, New York.
Keenan, E. O. 1974. Conversational competence in children. J. Child Lang. 1:163–183.

CHAPTER 20

DEVELOPMENT AND EVALUATION OF SOME SPEECH TRAINING PROCEDURES FOR HEARING-IMPAIRED CHILDREN

Mary Joe Osberger

CONTENTS

The teaching of speech generally has been considered an essential part of the hearing-impaired child's educational curriculum. Unfortunately, the data that have been reported over the years indicate that teachers have been largely unsuccessful in helping these children develop adequate speech production skills. For example, investigators have consistently found that, on the average, only about 20% of the speech produced by children with profound hearing losses is intelligible to their listeners (Brannon, 1964; John and Howarth, 1965; Markides, 1970; Smith, 1975).

Numerous reasons have been offered by educators and researchers for the apparent lack of success in developing satisfactory oral communication skills in this population. The majority appear to attribute this failure to poor and inefficient teaching, but few studies have gathered quantitative data to support this notion. As a consequence, new training strategies are continually being developed in the hope that they

This project was supported by private funds from the Lexington School for the Deaf. The analysis of the data was supported by Public Health Service Grant No. 09252 and the F. V. Hunt Postdoctoral Fellowship from the Acoustical Society of America.

will be more successful than the previous ones in helping hearing-impaired children develop intelligible speech. Typically, the programs are descriptive in nature, lacking empirical data which demonstrate the effectiveness of the proposed procedures. Today, there is little, if any, quantitative data to demonstrate the relative effectiveness of the various speech training procedures.

The approach taken to this problem has involved the use of systematic speech training procedures, structured to permit a detailed quantitative mapping of each child's progress in the development of specific speech skills. The advantage of such an approach is that modifications and refinements in the training program can be based on repeated objective measurements rather than simply on clinical intuition. Another advantage is that systematic speech training procedures can be easily transmitted from one teacher to the next, avoiding the common situation in which good results are obtained only by a gifted teacher.

For the past several years, speech training procedures for hearing-impaired children have been evaluated. There are three major goals of this research:

1. To obtain baseline data which quantify the length of time required by hearing-impaired children to develop certain speech skills, correct certain errors, or both
2. To determine, through repeated evaluations of the training strategies, those procedures that are effective in developing (or correcting) speech skills and those in need of modification
3. To identify at an early stage those children who are not showing satisfactory progress with the applied training procedures and who may require special intervention strategies

This chapter is a progress report on this evaluation of nonsegmental and segmental training strategies. The data have been collected over a 2-year period as part of a research and demonstration project at the Lexington School for the Deaf in New York.

THE SPEECH TRAINING PROGRAM

The speech training procedures, an adaptation of Ling's (1976) system, included training on nonsegmental voice patterns and the segmental aspects of speech using an auditory-oral approach. A major goal of the program was to train speech production to a high level of automaticity so that the skills would carry-over to a variety of phonetic environments and linguistic materials. The program included several drill techniques designed to promote automaticity and to assist in the child's development of an auditory-kinesthetic feedback loop.

Production on an Imitative Basis   The child was required to produce correctly the target speech pattern on the basis of auditory cues only. The child had to perceive and produce the speech pattern correctly to achieve successful performance on this level.

Production on Demand   The child was required to produce the target speech pattern without the aid of the teacher's model. The productions were elicited by visual cuing (picture or written word). No auditory processing was required of the child with these tasks, and, thus, successful performance on this level was dependent only on the child's ability to produce the desired pattern (and his or her ability to decode the visual cuing system). These tasks, which represented a slight departure from a strictly auditory-oral approach, were incorporated into the training scheme for the following reasons: (1) to provide the child with additional practice in producing the various speech targets; (2) to assess the child's ability to produce the various patterns without the teacher's model; and (3) to help the child develop those skills necessary for the successful carry-over of the various patterns to spontaneous speech.

Discrimination   The discrimination tasks also employed the visual cuing system. For these tasks, the teacher first produced a particular pattern; the child was required to imitate the teacher's model and then point to the symbol corresponding to the teacher's production. Successful performance on this level was dependent upon the child's ability to perceive and discriminate patterns through audition alone.

The three groups of tasks (production on an imitative basis, production on demand, and discrimination) were not necessarily hierarchical, and training was generally performed in these areas simultaneously. If the severity of a child's hearing loss precluded successful performance on the imitation or discrimination tasks, training was continued on the production-on-demand tasks.

The children's performance in the speech training program was monitored by means of a checklist system throughout the school year. The checklists, which corresponded to the various levels of the program, specified the speech tasks to be taught to the children. The children were then required to meet predetermined criteria for acceptable performance before a check was given for a particular task. The checklist data were collected during each child's individual speech tutoring session, 15 minutes per day, 4 days a week.

Nonsegmental Voice Patterns

During the first evaluation period, procedures designed to improve nonsegmental voice patterns (duration, intensity, pitch) were employed with a group of 20 severely and profoundly hearing-impaired children, ranging in age from 7 to 10 years. Because one of the goals was and still is to evaluate a speech training system with children typically found in schools for the deaf, children were not excluded from participating in the program if they were suspected to have problems in addition to a hearing handicap.

At the end of the school year, the children's performance was analyzed using the checklist data. The results will be summarized only briefly, because they have been presented in detail in a previous report (Osberger et al., 1978). Perhaps the most significant, although not surprising finding was that the children progressed through the stages of the training program at very different rates. Based on their rate of progress, the children were divided into three groups, post hoc. Group 1, consisting of seven children, developed the new speech skills at a very rapid rate. Group 2, consisting of six children, showed a steady but slower rate of progress. The progress of the children in group 3, consisting of seven children, was inordinately slow. On the average, the rate of progress shown by the children in group 3 was twice as slow as the progress shown by the children in group 2 and roughly four times as slow as the rate of progress shown by the children in group 1. Examination of background and other important variables indicated that degree of hearing loss, the presence of additional handicapping conditions, or both, were the most closely linked to the children's performance in the speech training program.

Modification of the Training Strategies

After the initial evaluation, the training program was analyzed to identify those procedures in need of modification. Our data suggested that drill work on strings of nonsense syllables produced with differing voice patterns (duration, intensity, pitch), as recommended by Ling (1976), did not adequately train the children to produce the suprasegmental patterns of English. For example, a child might be able to produce a syllable with a low, mid, and high pitched voice, but this skill in and of itself did not guarantee that the child would be able to produce the subtle changes in fundamental frequency (F_0) typical of spoken English. Also, there is no direct evidence to indicate that the production of these differing voice patterns is a prerequisite skill for the production of the suprasegmental features of English. Therefore, procedures that were geared more toward the development of some of the suprasegmental aspects of speech than those suggested by Ling (1976) were developed. The modified procedures include training on duration and pitch. Work on intensity, which will not be discussed, was restricted to teaching the child to use socially-appropriate voice levels (e.g., a *whisper* when someone else is trying to sleep; a *shout* when cheering at a football game, etc.).

Table 20.1 summarizes the duration level of the program. Note that only two different durations were included—a long duration and a short duration. These durations were chosen to represent the durations of stressed and unstressed syllables, respectively. Emphasis was placed on achieving the correct durational relationship between stressed and unstressed syllables for several reasons. First, it has been empirically demonstrated that duration is a predominant cue for the perception of stress by normally hearing listeners (Fry, 1955). Secondly, the speech of hearing-impaired children often contains distortions of the temporal relationships between stressed and unstressed syllables (Boothroyd, Nickerson, and Stevens, 1974; Nickerson et al., 1974; Osberger and Levitt, 1979). Thirdly, recent research indicates that when the durational relationship between stressed and unstressed syllables is corrected in the speech of hearing-impaired children, significant improvements in intelligibility may result (Osberger and Levitt, 1979).

The duration patterns were first taught with nonsense syllables in a phrase structure. After these were mastered by the child, the same patterns were applied to meaningful units (i.e., words) in phrases. When this stage was reached, the teachers were encouraged to use phrases that contained language familiar to the children, while still maintaining the correct duration patterns. The first tasks on this level involved work on strings of syllables of the same duration (i.e., all short or all long), progressing to three-, four-, and five-syllable strings

Table 20.1.   A summary of the duration level of the speech training program

	Nonsense syllables		Phrases	
Fixed durations	1—3 long	1—3 short	1—3 long	1—3 short
Example	3 long	3 short	3 long	3 short
	baaa baaa baaa	ba ba ba	come here now	six fat cats
Varied durations	3—5 syllables		3—5 syllables	
Example	biii bi biii	(L-S-L)	close the door	
	fu fu fuu	(S-S-L)	it's a dog	
	mo mooo mo	(S-L-S)	that's not it	

of varied durations (i.e., long-short-long). Although the initial tasks involved one-syllable utterances, the emphasis was on the production of the desired duration patterns within a phrase structure. Single-syllable productions were employed primarily to orient the children to the nature of the training tasks and to provide a manageable task for those preschool children who had never received structured speech training.

Table 20.2 summarizes the pitch level of the speech training program. Rather than focus on the production of syllables on discrete pitch levels, emphasis was placed on the production of different intonation contours, which are often found to be improperly produced in the speech of the hearing impaired (Green, 1956; Mártony, 1968; Smith, 1975; Stewart, 1968). The children were first taught to produce the terminal fall. Work was then initiated on pitch peak, which is produced as a rise followed by a fall in fundamental frequency. This particular contour is used by normal speakers to cue word emphasis (Lieberman, 1968). In normal speech, a rise in F_0 is usually accompanied by an increase in intensity. Although no attempt was made to isolate these two events in the speech training program, the child was required to produce a perceptible change in pitch on these tasks. Once the child mastered the peak in the final position, the location of the peak was moved within the utterance. This technique has been very useful in teaching the children that changes in pitch can convey changes in the linguistic content of a message.

A contour with a final rise in fundamental frequency, which is produced by normal-hearing speakers to signal a yes-no question (Lie-

Table 20.2. A summary of the pitch-intonation level of the speech training program

	Nonsense syllables		Phrases (3 syllables)
Terminal fall			
Example	buuu bu buuu	(L-S-L)	John is home
	la la laaa	(S-S-L)	eat the cake
Peak (final)			
Example	wooo wo <u>wooo</u>	(L-S-L)	we're at <u>school</u>
	mi mi <u>miii</u>	(S-S-L)	the big <u>boy</u>
Peak (shift)			
Example	du <u>duuu</u> du	(S-L-S)	give <u>me</u> some
	fa <u>faaa</u> faaa	(S-L-L)	the <u>big</u> boy

The underlined syllable denotes the syllable that is produced with a rise in F_0, followed by a fall in F_0.

berman, 1968), was not included in the program. Previous data have shown this to be an extremely difficult contour to produce for most children with profound losses (McGarr, 1976). Furthermore, most questions in conversational English appear to be cued by linguistic structure, rather than changes in fundamental frequency.

As in the original version of the training program, the revised set of procedures required the children to perform the three groups of tasks (production on an imitative basis, production on demand, and discrimination) for the training levels involving duration and pitch.

Evaluation of the Modified Procedures

The modified procedures were evaluated with a group of 21 preschool children, ranging in age from 2;11 years to 6;3 years, with a mean age of 4;4 years. Three of the children were severely hearing impaired; the remainder had profound hearing losses. As in the previous study, the data were taken directly from the checklists which the teachers filled out during each child's speech tutoring session (15 minutes a day, 4 days a week).

The largest body of data was gathered for the first two sections of the duration level (one and two syllables of fixed durations; three, four, and five syllables of varied durations). Therefore, the following sections are limited to a presentation of some of the major findings of the children's performance on these aspects of the training program.

First, it should be noted that the younger group of children showed the same pattern of performance with respect to rate of learning as did the older children in the previous study. That is, some children acquired the skills at a very rapid rate and others displayed a steady, but slower rate of progress, whereas other children showed very slow or negligible progress. In order to evaluate more precisely the revised training procedures, this stage of the data analysis focused upon the length of time required by the children to learn the specific speech skills.

Table 20.3 summarizes the length of time required by the children to complete the first section of the duration level. A total of 15 children began training on this level but, as shown in the table, some of the children failed to acquire all of the speech skills before the end of the school year. Therefore, complete data are not available for all children. The data show that the children learned the production-on-demand tasks in the shortest period of time. Recall that these tasks required the child only to produce correctly the duration pattern; successful performance was not dependent on any auditory processing. It took the children roughly two times longer to learn the imitation and discrimination tasks than the production-on-demand tasks, with three of the children failing to complete the second discrimination task (long versus short). This pattern of performance is consistent with earlier findings (Osberger et al., 1978).

The above data were subjected to two separate two-way analyses of variance to determine if number of syllables (one versus two) or duration of syllables (long versus short) significantly affected rate of learning. The results revealed no significant difference in the length of time required by the children to learn the tasks as a function of syllable number or syllable duration.

Figure 20.1 shows the performance of five children who advanced to the next training level. The children were required to produce, through audition, phrases consisting of nonsense syllables or phrases with meaningful units (words), with three, four, or five syllables of varied durations.

The data show several rather interesting interactions between syllable number, phrases with words, and phrases consisting of nonsense syllables. First, the three-syllable durational patterns were more quickly learned when they were produced in the context of phrases with words than when they were produced as phrases with nonsense syllables. For the four-syllable utterances, it took the children essentially the same amount of time to learn to produce the durational patterns with nonsense syllables as with words. For the five-syllable utterances, there is a reversal of the pattern observed for the three-syllable utterances. That is, it took the children a longer period of time to produce the five-syllable durational patterns in the phrase context with words than as a phrase with nonsense syllables. A two-way (time × syllable number) analysis of variance revealed that the difference

Table 20.3. Summary of the length of time (days) required by a group of children to learn to produce, imitate, and discriminate nonsense syllables of fixed durations

	1 Short	1 Long	2 Short	2 Long	Voice/ no voice	Long/ short
Production on demand						
No. days	5.8	5.2	5.8	6.2		
No. subjects	15	15	15	15		
Imitation						
No. days	12.0	10.2	12.0	16.8		
No. subjects	15	15	14	14		
Discrimination						
No. days					10.5	8.0
No. subjects					15	12

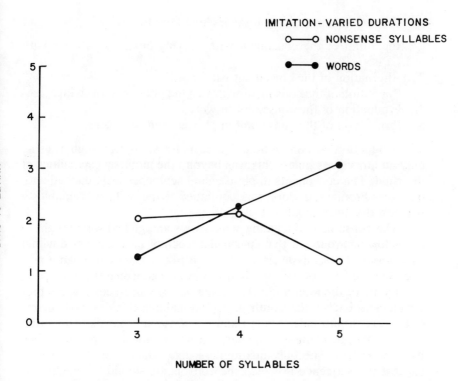

Figure 20.1.   The mean length of time required by the children ($N = 5$) to learn how to imitate through audition varied duration patterns in nonsense syllables and words.

in the length of time required to learn the five-syllable patterns for words and nonsense syllables was statistically significant (F = 10.16; $P < 0.01$). There was no significant difference in the amount of time required to learn words and nonsense syllables for the three and four syllable utterances.

Segmental Speech Patterns

Training procedures in this area were also adapted from Ling's (1976) system. These procedures were evaluated with the older (7 to 10 years old) children during the first year of the project. Although vowels and consonants were included in training, discussion will be limited to the data obtained on consonant production because many of the children who advanced to this level of the program had a fairly well-developed vowel system.

The consonant training tasks included the following:

1. Repetition of the consonant with varying intensity patterns with /i,a,u/
2. Alternation of the consonant with /i,a,u/
3. Repetition of the consonant with varying pitch patterns with /i,a,u/
4. Production of the consonant in words
5. Production of the consonant in phrases and sentences

Production was on an imitative basis for steps 1 through 4, using only auditory cues unless this was beyond the auditory capabilities of the child. The consonants in phrases and sentences were elicited with pictures. Production work was continued if the child was unable to perform the discrimination tasks.

The consonants (including semivowels and glides) were taught in the following groups, with no particular teaching order specified within each group: (1) semivowels /w,j/ and /h/; (2) voiced consonants produced in the front of the mouth /b,m,v,ð/; (3) consonants produced in the middle of the mouth /d,n,ʃ,s/, glide /l/; (4) voiced consonants produced in the back of the mouth /g,ŋ/; (5) remaining voiceless consonants /p,t,k,f,θ/; (6) affricates /dʒ,tʃ/; and (7) consonant blends. This order of consonant teaching was similar, but not identical to that described by Ling (1976). The only quantitative data which were available to suggest the sequence in which the consonants should be taught was the pattern of errors in deaf children's speech (Smith, 1975). These data, plus Ling's (1976) program, and the previous experiences of the project teachers, were used to develop the above teaching order.

Nine of the 20 children progressed to consonant training during the first year of the project. Tasks were completed for 14 of the consonants. A two-way analysis of variance (consonant × time) revealed a significant difference in the length of time taken to learn the different consonants ($F = 2.20$; $P < 0.05$). When the consonants were grouped by manner of production (plosive, fricative, nasal) or voicing (voiced or voiceless), there was no significant difference in the rate of learning. The only significant difference ($F = 7.21$; $P < 0.01$) between the consonants in learning time was based on the place of production (front, mid, back). This finding is illustrated in Figure 20.2. As the data show, the sounds produced in the front of the mouth required the least amount of time to learn, followed by sounds produced in the back of the mouth. The sounds that required the longest period of time to learn were the sounds produced in the middle of the mouth. Also, the difference in learning time between the front sounds and the back sounds is much

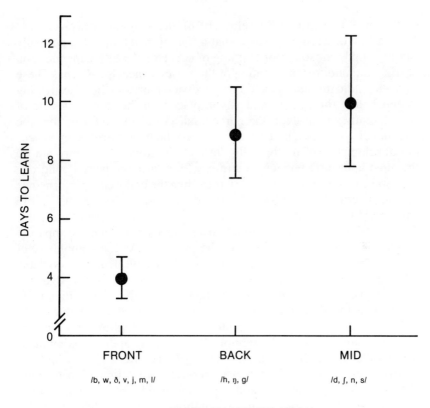

Figure 20.2.   The mean length of time required by the children ($N = 9$) to complete the tasks for 14 consonants. The *bars* represent the standard error of the mean. The data are plotted as a function of place of articulation for the consonants.

greater than the difference between the back sounds and the middle sounds.

Discussion

First, an important finding in this study, as well as in the previous study (Osberger et al., 1978), is that, on the average, the children learned to produce the speech patterns with a visual prompt before they could imitate (through audition alone) or discriminate these same patterns. This finding suggests that the ability to produce a speech pattern may precede and assist in the hearing-impaired child's perceptual decoding of the corresponding auditory signal. A similar finding has been reported by Lieberth and Subtelny (1978) and Subtelny (this volume). This pattern of learning is somewhat different than that of the normally hearing child whose motor learning of speech is largely dependent on hearing and auditory perception of the various speech patterns. These data also indicate that the auditory-feedback loop may be more readily established if the initial emphasis is placed on the motor aspects of speech, rather than upon the perceptual. Given this information, the "acoupedic" approach (Pollack, 1970), which primarily emphasizes the development of motor skills through auditory input, may not be the most appropriate teaching strategy for hearing-impaired children.

Some discussion is necessary regarding the children's performance on the discrimination tasks. As the data show in Table 20.3, more children failed to complete this type of task than the imitation tasks. The difficulty with the discrimination tasks became even more apparent during the subsequent sections of the program. As the complexity of the task increased (e.g., discrimination of syllable length or syllable number in three, four, and five syllable utterances), very few of the children were able to perform the tasks correctly. The difficulty in performing the discrimination tasks did not appear to be due to an inability to hear the speech stimuli because the children could imitate the same patterns through audition. Provided the auditory stimulus is perceptible to the child, an imitation task requires the child only to "parrot" or "mimic" the target pattern. The discrimination task apparently places greater demands upon the child's processing abilities and short-term memory than an imitation task. The child must, for example, be able to associate an auditory stimulus with its visual representation, compare what he or she has heard with the alternatives (a task which requires auditory memory and sequencing abilities), and finally, the child must have developed the concept of "choice making." Thus, what is generally assumed to be an easy task for an adult (i.e., a closed-set discrimination task), may prove to be quite complex for a young hearing-impaired child. This is not to suggest that a discrimination task is an inappropriate activity in a speech (or auditory) training program. In fact, this type of activity may be an important adjunct to the development of the auditory-kinesthetic feedback loop. However, our data suggest that introduction of the discrimination tasks might be more appropriate after the preschool age.

Another point that deserves discussion is the pattern of learning for the duration tasks involving nonsense syllables and words in a phrase context. The data indicate that training with nonsense syllables did not always facilitate production of the target speech pattern in words. Similar findings have been reported for normally hearing children by Costello and Onstine (1976), who observed that it took the children longer to learn to produce a target speech pattern in nonsense syllables than in meaningful words. The use of nonsense syllables may be a very useful teaching strategy for some children, but production of the speech target in the context of nonsense syllables does not seem to be a prerequisite skill for intelligible production of that same target in words.

The data obtained on the consonants are interesting for several reasons. First, the order of rate of learning, based on place of production, is in agreement with the order of sounds prone to the fewest errors in the speech of the hearing impaired (Gold, 1978; Smith, 1975). That is, an analysis of the frequency of errors based on place of production in the speech of the hearing impaired has shown that sounds produced in the front of the mouth are most often produced correctly, followed by the back sounds, and then sounds with a more medial place of production. One reason why the alveolar sounds may be more difficult to produce than the velar sounds may involve the fact that more sounds are produced in the middle of the mouth than the back of the mouth. Because of this, precise positioning of the articulators is necessary in order to correctly differentiate all the sounds with a medial place of articulation. Greater variability in articulatory placement can be tolerated before the velar sounds are misperceived by the listener.

The rank ordering of consonants by place of articulation (i.e., front, back, mid) has important implications for the development of speech training procedures. If an approach is adopted to initiate training with the easiest sounds, progressing to the more difficult ones, then training would begin with the labial sounds, irrespective of the manner of production. After these sounds are mastered, the velar sounds would be taught, followed by the alveolar sounds. Additional data are needed, however, in order to further substantiate this pattern of learning.

SUMMARY AND CONCLUSIONS

From the data collected, the following conclusions are drawn:

1. The rate of progress in the development of the various speech skills varies across children. Children who show little or no progress after a specified period of time may require more individualized training procedures to meet their needs. Our data do indicate that a strictly auditory-oral approach may not be entirely appropriate for all children. However, there is no indication whether any of the children would have attained a higher level of performance if other approaches to speech training had been employed.

2.   Many children, even those with severe and profound hearing losses, can learn to imitate and discriminate a variety of speech patterns through audition alone. The ability to perform these tasks is not always reliably predicted from their audiograms. In addition, successful performance on auditory tasks may not be evident until after the child has received a substantial amount of systematic training.

3.   Many children with severe and profound hearing losses require a very systematic and structured program in order to develop the auditory-kinesthetic (or tactile-kinesthetic) feedback loop. Some feedback mechanism is essential if the speech production skills are to be carried over and incorporated into the child's spontaneous productions.

4.   For many children with severe and profound hearing losses, the ability to produce a speech pattern precedes and facilitates the perception of that same pattern.

5.   Auditory discrimination tasks, even with a closed-set response format, may be too complex for young (below 5 years) hearing-impaired children, particularly those children who have a limited amount of hearing. Because the ability to discriminate a speech pattern does not appear to be a prerequisite to the production of that pattern, training time may be more effectively used if discrimination tasks are not introduced until later in the training program.

6.   The use of nonsense syllables may not always facilitate the transfer of motor speech skills to meaningful, linguistic units. In some cases, the production of speech targets in nonsense syllables may be more difficult than the production of these same targets in words in phrases.

7.   Quantitative measurement of the time required by hearing-impaired children to acquire the various aspects of speech may provide information essential to the development of systematic speech training strategies.

The studies conducted here represent only a small portion of the work needed in this area. The training sequence focused on those skills which, unless correctly developed, can lead to some of the errors which are so perceptually prominent in the speech of the hearing impaired (e.g., poor timing, pitch problems). The training procedures are not viewed as all inclusive. Other aspects of speech production such as those involving the correct posture of the laryngeal and articulatory mechanisms as described by Stevens, Nickerson, and Rollins (this volume) should not be overlooked in the training sequence.

An issue that has direct effect on the development of speech training procedures concerns the aspirations that parents, educators, and researchers have for hearing-impaired children's speech production skills. Although professionals in this field have all met hearing-impaired people who have developed intelligible and normal-sounding speech, it is perhaps unrealistic to expect this level of performance from the majority of profoundly hearing-impaired children. Rather, it is important to begin to define and describe a hierarchy of speech intelligibility goals. For example, the first level of the hierarchy might consist of the following description:

> Child's message is understood by parents when it is produced in familiar situations with an abundance of contextual cues present.

One of the more advanced levels might contain this description:

> Child's message is understood by persons unfamiliar with his or her speech (or the speech of any hearing-impaired person) in a situation with minimal contextual cues.

Once these goals have been determined, speech training procedures can be developed to help hearing-impaired children achieve the goals.

Perhaps the most important conclusion reached here is that speech training programs should not be presumed to be effective until their effectiveness is substantiated by quantitative measurements. Emphasis should be placed on isolating the strengths and weaknesses attributable to the training strategies themselves, the skills of the teacher, child-related variables, and so on. This approach will facilitate the development of procedures which can be implemented by a variety of teachers which, in turn, will eliminate the mysticism of the master teacher. These evaluations have also been concerned with the children's performance in a structured speech training session. This has been used as a starting point for the studies, but it is recognized that the true test of the effectiveness of the training rests in the spontaneous use of the speech skills in everyday communication situations.

ACKNOWLEDGMENTS

The author is indebted to Dr. Harry Levitt, City University of New York, and to Janet Head, Margot Cusack and Eileen Swarts, Lexington School for the Deaf, for their advice and guidance during the course of the project and the preparation of this manuscript. The assistance of Dr. Kenneth Stevens, MIT, and Dr. Claude Ruffin-Simon, University College London, in the revision of some of the training procedures is greatly appreciated.

REFERENCES

Boothroyd, A., R. Nickerson, and K. Stevens. 1974. Temporal patterns in the speech of the deaf—A study in remedial training. S.A.R.P. Report #15, Clarke School for the Deaf, Northampton, Mass.

Brannon, J. B. 1964. Visual feedback of glossal motions and its influence on the speech of deaf children. Doctoral dissertation, Northwestern University, Evanston, Ill.

Costello, J., and J. Onstine. 1976. Modification of multiple articulation errors based on distinctive feature theory. J. Speech Hear. Disord. 41:199–215.

Fry, D. 1955. Duration and intensity as physical correlates of linguistic stress. J. Acoust. Soc. Am. 32:765–768.

Gold, T. 1978. Speech and hearing skills: A comparison between hard-of-hearing and deaf children. Doctoral dissertation, City University of New York, New York.

Green, D. S. 1956. Fundamental frequency of the speech of profoundly deaf individuals. Doctoral dissertation, Purdue University, Lafayette, Ind.

John, J. E., and J. N. Howarth. 1965. The effect of time distortion on the intelligibility of deaf children's speech. Lang. Speech 8:127–134.

Lieberman, P. 1968. Intonation, Perception and Language. MIT Press, Cambridge, Mass.

Lieberth, A., and J. Subtelny. 1978. The effect of speech training on auditory phoneme identification. Volta Rev. 80:410–417.

Ling, D. 1976. Speech and the Hearing-Impaired Child: Theory and Practice. A. G. Bell Association for the Deaf, Washington, D. C.

Markides, A. 1970. The speech of deaf and partially hearing children with special reference to factors affecting intelligibility. Br. J. Disord. Commun. 5:126–140.

Mártony, J. 1968. On the correction of the voice pitch level for severely hard of hearing subjects. Am. Ann. Deaf 113:195–202.

McGarr, N. 1976. The production and reception of prosodic features. Paper presented at the meeting of the A. G. Bell Association for the Deaf, June, Boston.

Nickerson, R., K. N. Stevens, A. Boothroyd, and A. Rollins. 1974. Some observations on timing in the speech of deaf and hearing speakers. BBN Report No. 2905, Cambridge, Mass.

Osberger, M. J., A. Johnstone, E. Swarts, and H. Levitt. 1978. The evaluation of a model speech training program for deaf children. J. Commun. Disord. 11:293–313.

Osberger, M. J., and H. Levitt. 1979. The effect of timing errors on the intelligibility of deaf children's speech. J. Acoust. Soc. Am. 66:1316–1324.

Pollack, D. 1970. Educational audiology for the limited hearing infant. Charles C Thomas, Springfield, Ill.

Smith, C. R. 1975. Residual hearing and speech production in deaf children. J. Speech Hear. Res. 18:795–811.

Stewart, R. B. 1968. By ear alone. Am. Ann. Deaf 113:147–155.

CHAPTER 21

DEVELOPMENT AND IMPLEMENTATION OF THE AUDITORY SKILLS INSTRUCTIONAL PLANNING SYSTEM

Terry L. Thies and Jane L. Trammell

CONTENTS

The use of audition is the easiest, most direct avenue for development of functional communication skills. Because development of these skills is a major goal in the education of hearing-impaired pupils, and because these skills are directly related to all academic achievement, it is essential that this avenue for learning be fully utilized.

The aim of auditory training is to enable the pupil to develop strategies for the perception of auditory patterns. This is accomplished through auditory experiences that provide frequent repetition of the message together with the immediate opportunity to make the correct association. These learned associations can, with practice, become automatic and available for retrieval, utilization, and integration into the gestalt of communication. Most, if not all, hearing-impaired children have some facility for hearing spoken communication. The development of auditory skills is essential, not only for perception, but for production of speech as well. This chapter describes the Auditory Skills Instructional Planning System (ASIPS), which is designed to 1) improve comprehension of spoken language, and 2) increase linguistic fluency and speech intelligibility.

DEVELOPMENT

The initial development of the project began in 1973 with approval of a 3-year grant from the Bureau of Education for the Handicapped. In order to capitalize on the experience and expertise of both teachers and audiologists, a team approach was devised. The project staff was composed of six audiologists working 1 day a week, 12 teachers working after school hours, and an instructional technologist as project coordinator. Teacher-audiologist teams met weekly and conferences were held with many national consultants.

A review of existing auditory training programs and materials revealed a need for an instructional system applicable to a broad age range of peripherally hearing-impaired children. Such a system should include: 1) objectives written in performance terms and arranged as sequentially as possible; 2) sample mediated activities for the objectives; and 3) an assessment tool which could be used as a placement guide and which would evaluate a student's abilities and progress.

As the teams continued to work, a philosophy evolved centering on the concept of the redundancy of language. Because of peripheral hearing loss, the hearing-impaired child has to reach closure on information that is only partially received. The child learns to predict the message through practice in utilizing the available redundant cues in language. One provides auditory training by manipulating the redundancy level of messages in specific training sessions, as well as in communication situations throughout the instructional day. In effect, through auditory training, the hearing-impaired child acquires sharper tools so that when other visual and contextual information is minimal, he or she can make maximum use of auditory cues.

DESCRIPTION

The nucleus of the Auditory Skills Instructional Planning System is the *Auditory Skills Curriculum* (Office of the Los Angeles County Superintendent of Schools, 1979a), which includes four areas of ability: Discrimination, Memory-Sequencing, Auditory Feedback, and Figure-Ground. Terminal performance objectives (TPOs) were written for each of the four areas. These TPOs are broad statements covering categories of abilities included under each of the areas. A total of 64 intermediate performance objectives (IPOs) were written, stating specific behaviors related to the broader TPOs, including assessment procedure, pupil behavior, and assessment criterion. The objectives are assessed by using language related to the academic and social needs of the individual. The exact language is not specified purposely, in order that auditory training be an integral part of language development. A minimum of three sample activities were created for each IPO, describing the instructional procedures and required materials. Also included in the curriculum are a guidelines section, which presents the rationale and philosophy of auditory training, and an appendix, which contains operational definitions and other resource materials.

A second component of the system is the *Test of Auditory Comprehension* (TAC) (Office of the Los Angeles County Superintendent of Schools, 1979b). The TAC was developed parallel to the sequence of objectives in the Auditory Skills Curriculum in the areas of: 1) Discrimination—differentiation among messages; 2) Memory-Sequencing—recall of messages in proper sequence; and 3) Figure-Ground—demonstration of selected abilities under various listening conditions.

Realizing that auditory skills do not always develop in an absolute sequence, and that it is virtually impossible and unrealistic to isolate specific skills, 10 subtests were developed and ordered in a general hierarchy of complexity. Audiologists worked closely with teachers of the hearing impaired in designing test content to reflect everyday listening experiences.

Subtests I through III assess suprasegmental discrimination, proceeding from gross differentiation between speech and nonspeech stimuli to discrimination among various speech phrases differing in rhythm, stress, and intonational pattern.

Subtests IV through VI assess discrimination and memory-sequencing abilities for messages containing one, two, and four critical elements.

Subtests VII and VIII assess comprehension abilities requiring a higher level of auditory-cognitive integration. Subtest VII measures comprehension of simple stories by sequencing events, and subtest VIII measures comprehension of complex stories by recalling details.

Subtests IX and X assess auditory figure-ground abilities. Simple and complex stories are presented in a background of competing speech messages at a signal-to-noise (S/N) ratio of 0 dB. The competing speech background was produced by simultaneously recording two female speakers reading prose material. The level of the competing message was selected on the basis of S/N measurements reported in the literature for school classrooms, and on the results of pilot studies with young normally hearing school children. This competing message provides meaningful intermittent vocal distractions simulating one of the more difficult listening tasks confronting the hearing-impaired pupil in the regular classroom.

Final revision of test items and ordering of subtests were made based on the results of pilot testing with normally-hearing children, ages two through six, and field testing with pupils with varying degrees of hearing loss, ages 3 through 12. A standardization study was carried out in 1976–1977, wherein the TAC was administered by audiologists to 750 hearing-impaired pupils at 28 schools and programs across the country. Ages of the pupils ranged from 4 through 12 years, with moderate through profound hearing loss. The sample represented a variety of educational settings, from most restrictive (self-contained special classes or schools for the deaf) to least restrictive (pupils mainstreamed into regular public schools, with and without supportive services). A second normative study was carried out with 195 secondary school pupils 13 through 17 years of age.

Results of analyses with the data obtained on the standardization sample indicated that the TAC is a valid instrument: it differentiates among levels of auditory functioning, yields predictive information about the use of a pupil's residual hearing, and is appropriate to the population for which it was designed. The TAC has a higher degree of reliability as determined by measures of internal consistency as well as correlation of test-retest scores. Inter-examiner consistency was also demonstrated.

Like the TAC, the *Audio Worksheets* (Office of the Los Angeles County Superintendent of Schools, 1980) are tied closely to the Auditory Skills Curriculum. These materials include worksheets and accompanying programmed cassettes for use with a program-stop recorder. "Assessment activities" were designed according to the specifications of intermediate performance objectives. "Learning activities" were designed to provide programmed training leading to mastery of the objectives. Both assessment and learning activities include three listening conditions: 1) clear (with no competing message); 2) competing message at +6 dB S/N; and 3) competing message at 0 dB S/N. Like the activities in the Auditory Skills Curriculum, the mediated activities are presented as models from which similar activities can be generated.

Inservice materials constitute the fourth component of the system. Four filmstrips with accompanying cassettes and three videotapes are currently being used in our programs. These materials provide overview information on the total system, the TAC, and general concepts related to the rationale and philosophy of auditory training.

IMPLEMENTATION

After completion of the first draft of the Auditory Skills Curriculum (ASC) in 1976, field study began in selected classes in Los Angeles County and also at Lexington School for the Deaf in New York. Several revisions were made as field studies extended to larger numbers of classrooms. One to three hours of audiology time per week was available to each classroom participating in the early field study efforts. By the 1978–1979 school year, the curriculum was in use in all hearing-impaired elementary and intermediate classrooms operated by the Office of the Los Angeles County Superintendent of Schools. More recently the office has extended use of the system to secondary students (Trammell and Owens, 1981) and has been involved in widespread inservice efforts.

ASIPS Implementation Model

ASIPS Inservice Successful implementation of the system depends, initially, on the scope and methods of inservice. Effective inservice education requires strong administrative support and commitments from teachers and audiologists.

TAC Administration The TAC is individually administered to pupils while they are wearing their usual classroom amplification. Once the starting point for testing has been determined with the screening task, subtests are administered sequentially until two successive subtests are failed.

Performance Profile The data gained from the standardization study provides for both criterion-referenced and norm-referenced interpretation. When raw scores are plotted on a profile graph, a pupil's performance on a continuum of auditory abilities can be seen. Transformation of raw scores to *t* scores provides a means for comparing a pupil's performance to others of similar age and degree of loss.

IPO Assessment TAC results enable the audiologist and teacher to place the pupil on the curriculum in one or more TPO areas. Specific IPOs are then selected for assessment.

Selection of ASC Objectives Based on the results of IPO testing, specific objectives are selected from the Auditory Skills Curriculum and included in the pupil's Individual Educational Plan (IEP).

Auditory Training   Auditory training is begun with activities from the ASC, sample mediated activities (worksheets and filmstrips with accompanying cassettes), or teacher-made activities.

Often, IPOs from one or more areas of the curriculum are chosen for training. A pupil may be working on suprasegmental tasks in the discrimination strand (such as pitch, intonation) as well as working on similar tasks in the auditory feedback strand (such as imitating or modifying pitch and intonation).

Reassessment   After training, reassessment of a pupil's auditory skills is accomplished at the IPO level and/or by readministration of the TAC.

Record Keeping   Just as inservice is the key to initiation of the program, consistent record keeping is essential to flow of the model. A record of testing and training provides a means for charting growth in the acquisition of auditory skills for an individual pupil as well as an evaluation of the effectiveness of the system.

Successful implementation involves close cooperation among teacher, audiologist, and administration. The following describes the respective roles of personnel as they have evolved in the authors' program.

The Teacher's Role

1. Projects a positive attitude toward the use of audition as an important avenue for learning and makes optimal use of personal and classroom amplification systems.
2. Develops, in conjunction with the audiologist, individual pupil assessment plans and assesses selected Intermediate Performance Objectives.
3. Selects performance objectives and instructional strategies according to group and individual needs, and implements auditory training activities designed to meet selected objectives.
4. Incorporates principles of auditory training into *all* school activities.
5. Confers weekly with audiologist regarding pupil progress on specific objectives and the effectiveness of instructional strategies, and maintains a record of individual pupil assessment and training activities.

The Audiologist's Role

1. Evaluates the suitability and effectiveness of personal and classroom amplification and inservices teachers and aides on daily monitoring procedures.

2. Administers and interprets the Test of Auditory Comprehension and assists teacher in selection, development, and administration of IPO assessment.
3. Observes pupil's auditory functioning in various classroom situations and participates in selection of performance objectives and instructional strategies.
4. Serves as a resource in use of instructional equipment, and participates in instructional activities for purposes of demonstration and/or evaluation of specific pupil performance.

The Administrator's Role
1. Establishes the development of auditory skills as an integral part of the school's total curriculum and evaluates the effectiveness of the auditory skills program through classroom observation and review of pupil progress records.
2. Encourages innovation and exploration of varied methods and materials and secures funds for purchase and maintenance of amplification and specialized equipment for auditory training.
3. Supports teacher and audiologist by encouraging interaction and providing time in the school schedule for inservice and conferences.

CURRENT INVESTIGATIVE STUDIES

Although the curriculum and TAC have been used effectively in classrooms for the hearing impaired for several years, a number of questions were unresolved.

1. How valid is the sequence of performance objectives?
2. What is the relationship of the objectives in one strand of the curriculum to another?
3. What is the relationship of the TAC to curriculum objectives?
4. What effect does the ASIPS have on pupil's development of auditory skills?

The first three questions are primarily measurement problems and could conceivably be answered using classical analysis procedures. The constraint imposed by random sampling, coupled with the difficulty in controlling extraneous variables, makes it difficult to obtain data on large numbers of hearing-impaired pupils in various hearing loss and age groups. An alternate strategy for dealing with these measurement questions involves application of latent trait theory.

Latent trait theory specifies a relationship between the observable traits or abilities assumed to underlie performance on a test (Hambleton and Cook, 1977). Application of a latent trait procedure yields item statistics that are invariant when the item is given to a different set of examinees. It also yields person ability estimates that are invariant when a different set of items is administered to the same examinee. Removing sample dependency from test development eliminates the need for elaborate sampling designs and would appear to be a good solution to the ASIPS measurement problems.

Study I

To evaluate the feasibility of using a latent trait model with auditory skill items, the data from the 750 pupils from the original TAC standardization study were analyzed. Because the 139 items in the TAC were representative of the range and type of items needing further study, and because classical item analysis data were already available, it was hypothesized that if the latent trait procedures were valid for the intended application, the data yielded would be consistent with the classical analysis data. The latent trait procedure selected was the Rasch model described by Wright (1977). The BICAL program (Wright and Mead, 1977) was used for the analysis.

Findings   Median difficulty values are reported in Table 21.1 for each of the 10 subtests. Difficulty values were transformed to a 0 to 100 scale by multiplying by a factor of 6.25 and adding 50. The standard error estimates were similarly transformed. The Rasch scaling supports the sequence of the subtests. The greatest difference in difficulty for adjacent subtests occurred between subtests I and II. In subtest I, the

Table 21.1   Median Rasch difficulty estimates for items in TAC subtests

TAC subtest	Difficulty in logits	Transformed difficulty	Difference between subtests
I	-6.8	7.3	
			21.9
II	-3.3	29.2	
			10.9
III	-1.6	40.1	
			3.0
IV	-1.1	43.1	
			8.1
V	0.2	51.2	
			5.1
VI	1.0	56.3	
			2.9
VII	1.5	59.2	
			7.6
VIII	2.7	66.8	
			6.9
IX	3.8	73.7	
			5.1
X	4.6	78.8	

task involves a gross categorical discrimination task—speech versus nonspeech. In subtest II, a pupil must discriminate among various speech messages, human nonspeech, and environmental sounds.

The smallest differences occurred between subtests III and IV— discrimination of stereotypic speech messages versus single element core noun vocabulary; and between subtests VI and VII—recalling four critical elements versus sequencing three events.

Average P values obtained for each subtest by the 750 subjects in the original standardization study were compared with difficulty estimates from the Rasch scaling. The difficulty sequence was the same for both sets of data; however, difficulty tended to be underestimated for lower subtests and overestimated for higher subtests by average P values as opposed to Rasch scaling.

Table 21.2 reports statistics from the original item analysis as compared with statistics from the Rasch scaling. Because of the differences operating in the calculation of the standard errors, they cannot be directly equated; however, the standard error associated with the Rasch difficulty estimates appears to be significantly less than the estimates derived from the classical procedures, particularly for mid-range subtests.

Conclusions   The Rasch scaling procedure evaluated in the present study supports the sequential nature of the TAC subtests. More importantly, because the findings are congruent with available objective data, the procedure is a credible one for future development of related assessment tools in the content domain.

Table 21.2   Comparison of item analysis statistics for classical and Rasch procedures

	Classical item analysis				Rasch scaling	
	No. of items	SD	SE	KR_{20}	$\hat{SE}$	Median point biserial
I	10	1.2	0.54	0.86	2.17	0.26
II	15	3.5	1.16	0.89	1.22	0.49
III	15	4.8	1.73	0.87	0.96	0.60
IV	20	8.1	2.43	0.91	0.96	0.76
V	15	6.5	2.91	0.80	0.97	0.83
VI	15	5.8	2.25	0.85	0.97	0.77
VII	15	5.8	2.25	0.85	0.97	0.70
VIII	15	5.1	1.91	0.86	1.05	0.70
IX	9	2.2	1.03	0.78	1.30	0.56
X	10	2.1	1.21	0.67	1.99	0.50

A particularly noteworthy finding, depicted in Figure 21.1, is the difference between subtests VII and IX (simple stories) and VIII and X (complex stories). The tasks are identical for each story type except in IX and X the stories are accompanied by a competing message at 0 dB S/N. According to the obtained calibration there is a difference of 14 transformed units between VII and IX and 12 units between VIII and X. This would suggest that the noise condition has a similar magnitude of effect on both tasks, a question which has not been readily answered using a classical approach. The unique advantages available

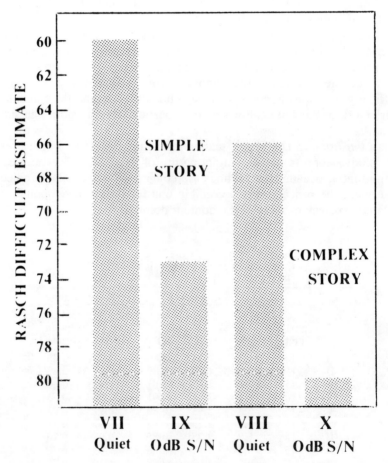

Figure 21.1.   Effect of competing message on item difficulty for simple and complex story tasks.

because of the ratio scaled data enable a more precise investigation of these kinds of differences.

Study II

Having established the credibility of a latent trait procedure for auditory skill items within a hearing-impaired population, the next step was to calibrate items from selected objectives in the Auditory Skills Curriculum. The purpose of the study was threefold: 1) to compare performance on TAC to curriculum objectives; 2) to evaluate the sequence of curriculum objectives; and 3) to evaluate the relative difficulty of items under varying competing message conditions.

In all, 13 objectives were chosen for study, eight from the discrimination strand and five from the memory-sequencing strand. In addition to an optimal S/N (no competing message), seven objectives were evaluated with a +6 dB S/N competing message and six of these seven also at a 0 dB S/N competing message. Five test items were constructed according to specifications in the curriculum for each of the objectives and for each competing message condition. All messages were presented on cassette tape to pupils under earphones at a pupil determined comfort level. Pupils were not permitted to change presentation level during the test administration.

Preliminary Findings   Although the intent is to collect data on a minimum of 200 pupils in order to insure reliability of the scaling procedure, a total of 65 pupils were tested and a preliminary scaling was carried out using the BICAL program.

The relative difficulty levels for TAC subtests and selected performance objectives are plotted in Figure 21.2. Items from the same objective which were tested in various competing message conditions are connected by solid lines. It can be seen that the +6-dB S/N level was indeed a good intermediate level between the optimum and 0 dB S/N conditions. The scaling generally supports the sequence of objectives within the discrimination and memory sequencing strands. Although the results are tentative because of the sample size, they give the first objective answers to the questions at hand.

Conclusion   The tentative conclusion is that Rasch scaling appears to have a great deal of potential in terms of answering the kinds of questions related to ASIPS. Because the procedure is not sample dependent, the findings should generalize to a full spectrum of hearing-impaired pupils regardless of age and degree of hearing loss. The procedure should be useful in verifying the sequence of objectives and provide a means for objectively charting the relative difficulty of a multitude of discrete auditory tasks. It is envisioned that the infor-

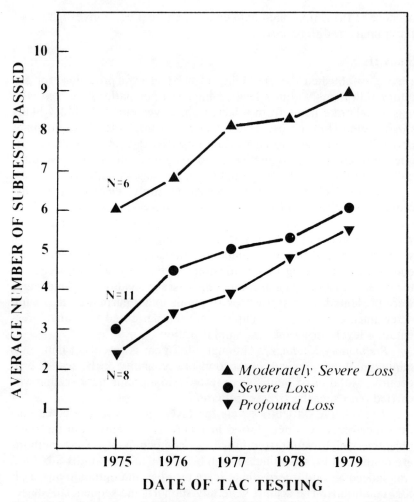

Figure 21.2.   Comparison of difficulty level for TAC and selected Auditory Skills Curriculum IPOs.

mation available from the scaling of TAC items will be useful as a means of anchoring future items to the continuum.

Study III

A third study was directed at measuring pupil's auditory skill growth over time. Since its preliminary development in 1975, the TAC has been administered yearly to pupils at the Southwest School for the Hearing Impaired. Concurrently, teachers have increased their use of the curriculum; from initially using the TAC in just a few classes during the 1975–1976 school year, to applying it in all classes in 1978. Longitudinal data were compiled for 25 pupils who had been on the curriculum since its inception and had been given the TAC annually over a 5-year period.

TAC scores for this group were analyzed by date of testing. The analysis showed an average total gain in raw scores from 1975 to 1979 of 38.4 points, with an average yearly increase of nearly 10 points. The largest gain in TAC scores (15 points) occurred between 1975 and 1976 when pupils were first exposed to the Auditory Skills Curriculum.

Averaged data can often obscure more significant relationships. The sample was divided into groups on the basis of degree of loss to examine whether changes in TAC scores were greater or less, depending on the degree of hearing impairment. Figure 21.3 shows the average TAC performance across years for the 25 pupils grouped according to degree of loss category—six pupils with moderately severe losses (55 to 70 dB), 11 pupils with severe losses (71 to 90 dB), and eight pupils with profound losses (91 dB and greater). When analyzed in this fashion, it is apparent that consistent gains in performance occurred, at each successive test date, for each of the degree of loss groups.

In order to determine what effect age might have had on performance, results were compared to data gathered in the standardization study. Based on the average age of the follow-up sample at the first date of TAC testing (6.2 years), comparisons were made between TAC performance at each year of testing (1975–1979) and average TAC scores for pupils in the standardization sample grouped by year of age (6 to 10).

Average raw scores and number of subtests passed for the longitudinal sample by date of TAC testing, and for the standardization sample by age, are presented in Table 21.3. Note that the follow-up sample size was 25 for test years 1975 through 1978, but that only 13

Table 21.3.   Comparison of TAC performance for longitudinal and standardization studies

	Longitudinal study				Standardization study		
Test date	N	Average age	Average raw score	No. subtests passed	N	Age	Average raw score	No. subtests passed
1975	25	6;2	59.9	3.6	77	6	65.7	4.0
1976	25	7;2	74.9	4.8	86	7	60.4	3.7
1977	25	8;2	84.4	5.4	68	8	66.5	4.1
1978	25	9;2	89.8	5.8	81	9	63.0	3.9
1979	13	9;2	98.3	6.4	76	10	62.4	3.9

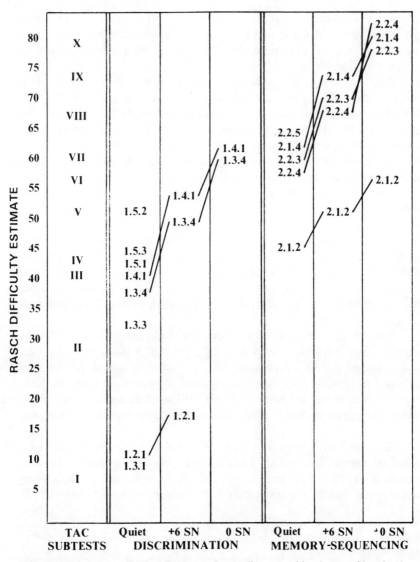

Figure 21.3.   Average TAC performance for pupils grouped by degree of hearing loss.

of those pupils were available for TAC administration in 1979. Of the
12 pupils not tested, most had moved out of the elementary program
at the Southwest School and into fully integrated educational settings.
This explains why the mean age was the same for the 1978 and 1979
groups. The pupils in the standardization sample were all tested during

the 1976–1977 school year, and are grouped by year of age at the test date. Comparison of TAC performance for the two groups shows systematic gains across years for the pupils in the longitudinal study.

SUMMARY

The TAC, Auditory Skills Curriculum, and Audio Worksheets are now in use in programs throughout the country. The inservice materials are in use in our own programs but have not been published. The authors are committed to further refinement of the system as well as continued evaluation with a broader audience. Although more definitive research into the effectiveness of the system is anticipated, existing data, primarily the result of evaluations by teachers and audiologists using the system, are highly supportive. The authors have collected a large amount of such information indicating that not only does ASIPS enable professionals to effect change in hearing-impaired pupils' auditory skills, it also results in changed expectation levels of the professional.

REFERENCES

Hambleton, R. K., and L. Cook. 1977. Latent trait models and their use in analysis of educational test data. J. Educ. Meas. 14:75–96.

Office of the Los Angeles County Superintendent of Schools. 1979a. Auditory Skills Curriculum. Foreworks, North Hollywood, Calif.

Office of the Los Angeles County Superintendent of Schools. 1979b. Test of Auditory Comprehension. Foreworks, North Hollywood, Calif.

Office of the Los Angeles County Superintendent of Schools. 1980. Audio Worksheets. Foreworks, North Hollywood, Calif.

Trammell, J. L., and S. L. Owens. 1981. The auditory skills instructional planning system at the secondary level. J. Acad. Rehab. Audiol. 14:198–207.

Wright, B. D. 1977. Solving measurement problems using the Rasch model. J. Educ. Meas. 14:97–116.

Wright, B. D., and R. J. Mead. 1977. BICAL: Calibrating rating scales with the Rasch model. Research Memorandum No. 23. Statistical Laboratory, Department of Education, University of Chicago, Chicago.

APPROACHES TO PERSONNEL PREPARATION: INSERVICE AND PRESERVICE EDUCATION

CHAPTER 22

THE USE OF QUESTIONNAIRE DATA AS A BASIS FOR INSERVICE PLANNING

Julia M. Davis and Neil T. Shepard

CONTENTS

In recent years increased pressure has been brought to bear on publicly funded educational systems to provide appropriate education and training for handicapped children. These state and federal laws have affected regular classroom teachers in several ways, significantly changing the teaching task they face. Teachers are now expected to teach classes in which one or more of the students may have one or more of a large variety of handicapping conditions. In the vast majority of cases, teachers have had no special training in the teaching of exceptional children, in coordinating classroom work with resource room efforts or other special support services, in curriculum modification for special students, or even in basic understanding of the characteristics and needs of handicapped children. As a result, there is considerable current interest in determining ways of providing effective and appropriate inservice training to the regular classroom teacher, as well as to other educational personnel who come in contact with handicapped students.

The most common approach to inservice training for personnel involved with impaired children in the public schools has been to provide a short-term workshop or continuing education program conducted by a selected "expert" in the field. Although this method can provide participants with a large body of information in a relatively short period of time, there are five major disadvantages.

1. In most cases inservice training is provided for a number of different professionals at the same time, such as regular classroom teachers, school psychologists, and school nurses. Although the various personnel have some common informational needs, this type of inservice training may lead to the provision of some unnecessary or irrelevant information to certain participants, resulting in confusion or boredom. For example, a discussion of methods for teaching specific classroom subjects to handicapped children would be appropriate only for instructional personnel.
2. The format of a 1- or 2-day inservice program involves the presentation of a large amount of information, often without sufficient time for synthesis of information or adequate follow-up discussions to occur.
3. More often than not, this format results in the presentation of information about the "average" child. There is rarely sufficient time for discussion of how the information presented relates to individual children with whom the participants are involved.
4. The experts providing the inservice program are usually hired from outside the school system and, therefore, may have little knowledge of the specific problems that exist, the resources available, or the feasibility of various training strategies in that particular setting. This can result in less appropriate specific suggestions for change or suggestions that are too general to implement without additional help from other expert consultants.
5. Finally, when the content of inservice training is determined solely by the expert involved, or at best, by the expert and one or two school personnel, it may not meet all of the needs of the trainees.

As a result of these disadvantages, alternative approaches to the development and implementation of inservice training for school personnel have been proposed. One of the most feasible involves the use of local school personnel as trainers in areas in which they have expertise. Training in hearing impairment could be provided by teachers of the hearing impaired, speech-language pathologists, or audiologists, depending on the specific needs of those to be trained. In the case of hard-of-hearing children, audiologists may offer the broadest perspective, but only if their preservice training has included coursework in the effects of hearing impairment on the development of children and strategies for remediating communication deficits. The emergence of educational audiology as a specialty reflects the need for such personnel in the school systems, and training programs are currently involved in efforts to provide broadly based training for audiologists who will be employed in the schools.

Recognizing the validity of this approach to meeting the inservice needs of school personnel, the Department of Speech Pathology and Audiology at the University of Iowa initiated a project designed to prepare audiologists to function as providers of inservice training to personnel in their local or district educational institutions. Audiologists were selected as the recipients of the training for several reasons. More than 60 audiologists are employed in Iowa's public schools at present. Many of them were trained at the University of Iowa, a trend that is likely to continue. The training program at this university is a broadly based one, including training in basic sciences, language development and disorders, diagnostic and habilitative audiology, and education.

In order to train audiologists to develop appropriate inservice materials, their preservice training must include three important sets of information directly related to the task at hand. First, they must have knowledge of the characteristics and needs of hearing-impaired children in general. Some of this information is available from textbooks and other course materials. Second, they must have knowledge of the demographic and educational status of the children to be served (in this case, the hearing-impaired children in Iowa's public schools). This information is available from school records; interviews with children, parents, and teachers; and observations or evaluations of the children being educated. Finally, they must have information regarding inservice needs as perceived by school personnel for whom training is to be provided. This information should be obtained directly from school personnel, but it does not appear to be standard practice to do so. The purpose of seeking input from the target population is to determine what they perceive to be the problems faced by hearing-impaired children and how they view their own roles in alleviating these problems.

These three sets of information can then be used to prepare inservice materials and procedures that will have a direct impact on the particular children being educated, insofar as this is possible when a heterogeneous group of children is involved.

The purpose of this chapter is to describe the methodological approach employed to obtain the last two sets of information described above. Both involved the use of a survey questionnaire with random samplings of a target population.

METHOD

Survey 1: Status of Hearing-Impaired Children

Information regarding the demographic and psychoeducational status of hearing-impaired children in Iowa's schools was obtained by use of an extensive survey questionnaire (Shepard et al., 1981). Audiologists employed in the public schools completed questionnaires on a random sample of 1,250 hearing-impaired children. This yielded data about age, sex, onset of hearing loss, hearing status, use of amplification, academic and language achievement, educational placement, and special support services as they related to various degrees and types of hearing loss. The results of the survey are reported elsewhere (Shepard et al., 1981; Davis et al., 1981) and will not be reported here. It is important, however, to indicate some of the problems encountered in collecting and using such data. Although the audiologists who collected that data were employed in the school systems in which the children were enrolled, they found it difficult to obtain the needed information. Children's files were often incomplete, containing only general information or test scores with inadequate descriptions of when and how they were obtained. Data for many children were kept in two or more separate files. In some school systems each child had a central file, a school file, and an individual file kept by a classroom teacher or clinician. Academic test scores, such as those yielded by the Iowa Test of Basic Skills, were sometimes filed separately by grade or class in administrative offices. Results of special testing, such as intellectual or language evaluations, were often kept by the individual psychologist or speech-language pathologist who was the examiner. As a result, obtaining comprehensive data about children was a difficult, time-consuming, and costly task. Most of the audiologists found it necessary to collect the data after hours and on weekends when school buildings were often locked, adding to the inconvenience of the experience. Because they were paid well for completing the questionnaires and because of a high level of professional commitment, the audiologists provided a 100% return of the questionnaires. They often followed up on missing data or were able to interpret information because of their specialized training in audiology. A key factor in the successful collection of these data was the use of these specialized personnel within the school system.

The advantages of the data collection method described above include the completeness of the data obtained, both in terms of the number of children reported and the amount of data reported for each, and its accuracy. It is doubtful that volunteers or nonprofessionals would have been able to collect as much data, even if they were motivated to do so. Unfortunately, this method is costly in terms of both money and time. The collection of the data on the 1,250 children involved in this study cost several thousand dollars and took a little more than a year to complete.

Table 22.1.   Professionals surveyed in opinion
questionnaire

Classroom teachers (3%)
  Regular classroom teachers
  Art teachers
  Music teachers
  Physical education teachers
  Shop instructors/teachers of industrial arts
Special teachers (3%)
  Special education teachers
  Reading specialists
  Learning disabilities teachers
Principals or assistant principals (3%)
Counselors (3%)
Work-study instructors (3%)
School nurses (10% of the state)
Speech-language pathologists (100% of the state)
Teachers of the hearing impaired (100% of the state)
Psychologists (100% of the state)

The percentages give the rate of sampling within any
given school district unless otherwise specified.

Survey 2: Inservice Needs of School Personnel

To determine the inservice needs of school personnel a questionnaire
was designed that provided information about previous training, understanding of hearing impairment, problems experienced with hearing-
impaired children, and desires regarding the content and format of
future inservice training. In addition to general demographic and experiential questions directed to all respondents, special questions were
designed for each of the following types of personnel: classroom teachers, special education teachers, principals, counselors, work-study instructors, school nurses, speech-language pathologists, teachers of the
hearing impaired, and psychologists.[1]

School personnel were sampled at different rates to insure a large
return and a small error rate. Table 22.1 lists the rate at which each
of the professional groups were sampled. The sampling was done via
school districts according to size. All school districts in Iowa were
divided into small (0 to 999 students), medium (1,000 to 2,999), and
large (3,000 and above) categories according to pupil enrollment. Because there are so many small school districts in Iowa, approximately
the same number of the various professionals were employed in each
of the three school sizes.

[1] The survey questionnaire is available on request from Julia M. Davis, Department
of Speech Pathology and Audiology, University of Iowa, Iowa City, Iowa 52242.

Twenty percent of the districts within each size were chosen randomly and questionnaires were sent to personnel in those districts. To insure a reasonable rate of return, cooperation was sought from the superintendents of each district to be sampled. Letters describing the need for the information being sought were sent to the administrators with the request that they endorse the project and encourage their employees to complete the questionnaires. Follow-up phone calls were made to answer questions and urge cooperation. As a result of these efforts, letters of endorsement were sent along with each of the questionnaires. Because the return rate was quite high for all the professional groups sampled (51% to 81%), the authors believe that this procedure enhanced the collection of these data significantly. Certain professional groups were sampled statewide rather than from selected districts because of the relatively small number of them within the state. The return rate for these groups (nurses, speech-language pathologists, teachers of the hearing impaired, and psychologists) ranged from 57% to 75%. A total of 999 individuals completed and returned the questionnaires.

Data from both surveys were coded for computer storage and analysis. The survey of professionals included some open-ended questions, the answers to which were also coded and grouped for analysis.

DISCUSSION

Although the two survey instruments were independently designed and provided different sets of information, they proved to be most informative when data from both were used jointly to clarify inservice needs. A few examples will illustrate the advantages of collecting empirical information about children as well as opinions from educators.

To illustrate the ways in which information from the two surveys can be combined to plan inservice, several pieces of data will be presented. Figure 22.1 shows the classroom placement status for the hearing-impaired children in this sample. Figure 22.2 shows the status of hearing aid use as it relates to classroom placement.

Table 22.2 shows the amount of training in hearing impairment received by classroom teachers. Table 22.3 gives the most common responses to the question regarding the need for further information about hearing impairment.

As can be seen from these figures and tables, most hearing-impaired children are being educated in regular classrooms. This is especially true for children whose losses do not exceed 50 dB hearing level (HL). Approximately 70% of those who wear hearing aids are

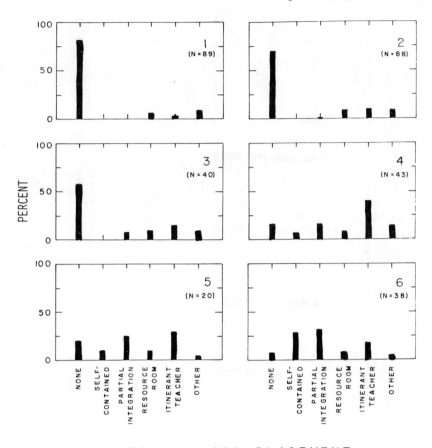

SPECIAL CLASS PLACEMENT

Figure 22.1.   Percentage of hearing-impaired children from one sample in various class-room placements in the Iowa public schools. Groups 1 through 6 represent an increasing degree of hearing impairment from mild (1) to profound (6). Groups 3 and 4 represent children with moderate losses of sensitivity. Data for children with conductive or high-frequency hearing losses are not included.

Table 22.2.   Percentage of classroom teachers who have received training designed to help serve hearing-impaired children

Training	%
Preservice courses or practicums	6
Inservice (associated with employment)	4
Regular personal contact with professionals trained to serve the hearing impaired	8
No training	82

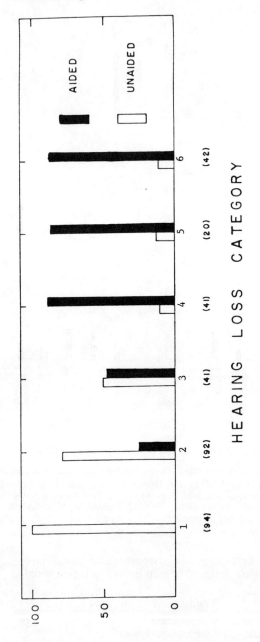

Figure 22.2. Percentage of children with bilateral hearing impairments wearing personal amplification as a function of degree of hearing loss. Groups 1 through 6 represent an increasing degree of hearing impairment from mild (1) to profound (6). The number of children in each group is indicated within the parentheses.

Table 22.3.   Inservice needs of professionals providing
services to hearing-impaired students

Area	%
Types and characteristics of hearing loss	61
Adaptation of curriculum for hearing impaired student	61
Overview of educational methods of teaching the hearing impaired	61
Effects of hearing loss on academic achievement	55
Effects of hearing loss on psychosocial development	52
Hearing aids and hearing aid use	28

doing so in regular classroom settings during some part of their day. However, only 20% of those children wearing hearing aids spend their entire day in a regular classroom with no special support. As a result, regular classroom teachers may see the monitoring of a particular child's hearing aid as being the responsibility of those providing the special support services. Therefore, they feel no need for inservice training regarding hearing aids and their use. Teachers are more likely to request information about curriculum modifications appropriate for hearing-impaired children. Until a greater proportion of hearing-impaired children routinely use amplification in the educational setting, the efficacy of providing extensive inservice training about hearing aids to classroom teachers or other general educational personnel is questionable. They will probably never need more than an introduction to what an aid can and cannot accomplish because they encounter them so infrequently.

Examination of the data yielded by teachers of the hearing impaired reveals a different picture. More than 80% of the children they serve wear hearing aids. Although 44% of these special teachers reported that they did not feel comfortable dealing with hearing aids, only 6% of them requested further training in this topic. The data on monitoring of amplication revealed that the most frequent monitoring (indeed, almost the only monitoring) was done by teachers of the hearing impaired. When all these pieces of information are added together, it seems important that a substantial portion of inservice for teachers of the hearing impaired should concentrate on the use of amplification. These data seem to indicate that these teachers view amplification as a minor factor in education of hearing-impaired children, an assumption that is not shared by the authors. One possible explanation for this may lie in the fact that training programs for teachers of the deaf concentrate on education of severely to profoundly hearing-impaired children, stressing the use of visual aids to communication. The population served in public schools tends to be made up of children with less severe hearing losses who therefore have a better prognosis for use of amplification. Inservice training in the use of amplification *by the target population* whom teachers serve in regular schools might enhance children's use of hearing aids in the educational setting.

The inservice topics requested by the classroom teachers surveyed (see Table 22.3) were quite similar to those named by teachers of the hearing impaired, counselors, speech-language pathologists, special education teachers, and psychologists. All expressed interest in the effects of hearing impairment on educational achievement and psychosocial development. The available literature on these topics involves so-called "deaf" children; information about less severely hearing-impaired children is scarce. The survey of children's files revealed no data regarding the psychosocial status of children and little data on educational achievement. Only 55% of the files of children with sensorineural or mixed losses (Groups 1 through 6) contained intelligence test scores; only 65% contained measures of academic achievement; and only 27% contained language assessment results. More complete psychoeducational information would seem essential if appropriate educational plans are to be developed for these children. It seems that the information most desired by public school personnel is not generally available to them, either from school records or existing research literature. This fact has several implications for the development of inservice training. First, there is an evident need to base inservice on the status of children, preferably those being served locally. This corroborates the assumption that the most effective inservice may be provided by local personnel who are familiar with the specific children, services, and personnel involved. Second, the relative scarcity of psychoeducational data in the children's files suggests that inservice for administrators may be necessary before funds are made available to insure the personnel and time necessary to evaluate hearing-impaired children adequately.

These examples illustrate the importance of obtaining the factual data about children and information about the interests of school personnel. Use of only one set of information is quite likely to lead to inservice efforts that are less than suitable.

SUMMARY

The need to improve inservice training for school personnel who come in contact with hearing-impaired children prompted a two-part study of the psychoeducational and demographic status of hearing-impaired children in the public schools and the perceived knowledge and needs of the educators who serve them. Two survey instruments were designed and information was obtained from 1,250 children's files and 999 school personnel representing various professional groups. Comparisons were made between the location, characteristics, and status of the children and the responses from school personnel regarding their inservice needs. As a result, the following recommendations for the development of inservice content and delivery are made:

1. Inservice should be provided by local personnel whenever possible.
2. Preservice training in the development of inservice models should be provided to those professionals who usually provide support services to hearing-impaired children. These include teachers of the hearing impaired, speech-language pathologists, and especially audiologists.
3. Inservice content should differ for various types of personnel, each of whom have different responsibilities and information gaps and needs. The needs of local personnel should be assessed before inservice content is planned.
4. Inservice content should be as specific to the children being served as possible. It may be necessary to collect psychoeducational data on individual children to obtain much of the information to be imparted.
5. There is a striking need for further research into the academic, language, and psychosocial status of children with varying degrees of hearing impairment.
6. The method used in this investigation is equally appropriate for collecting information about any facet of the effects of hearing impairment (on communication skills, for example) and the planning of inservice for personnel who seek to alleviate the deficits that exist.

REFERENCES

Davis, J. M., N. T. Shepard, P. Stelmachowicz, and M. Gorga. 1981. Characteristics of hearing impaired children in the public schools, Part II: Psychoeducational data. J. Speech Hear. Disord. 46:130–137.

Shepard, N. T., J. M. Davis, M. Gorga, and P. Stelmachowicz. 1981. Characteristics of hearing impaired children in the public schools, Part I: Demographic data. J. Speech Hear. Disord. 46:123–129.

CHAPTER 23

INSERVICE TRAINING FOR PUBLIC SCHOOL SPEECH-LANGUAGE PATHOLOGISTS IN THE MANAGEMENT OF MAINSTREAMED HEARING-IMPAIRED CHILDREN

Antonia B. Maxon and Diane Brackett

CONTENTS

The University of Connecticut (UConn) Mainstream Project is an inservice training program for speech-language pathologists in the public schools who have hearing-impaired children in their caseloads. Speech-language pathologists are eligible for participation in the project if they work with children in the public schools who have been identified as having a hearing loss and who are using amplification. The project has been in existence since September 1976, the first year functioning as a part-time pilot project and the last 3 years as a full-time program. The project co-directors are an audiologist and a speech language pathologist who carry out the various aspects of the program described below.

PROJECT DESCRIPTION

Each year, there are two full-day workshops, one in September and one in May, which allow for dissemination of information and sharing of techniques among the participants. During the initial workshop, the project is described, basic information about amplification trouble-shooting and speech-language assessment is provided, and initial school visits are scheduled. A packet of handouts, a battery tester, a hearing aid stethoscope, and an audio cassette of "Speech through a hearing aid and FM system" are distributed to the project partici-pants.[1] This audio cassette was developed to demonstrate the detri-mental effects of distance from the speaker and ambient noise when listening in the classroom. This is followed by a discussion of the de-mographic data collection process, which is described below. The final workshop is designed to collect demographic information and sum-marize the year's work. The project participants share their ideas and information concerning resources and materials, as well as suggest changes in the inservice program. Additionally, they pool suggestions for clinical audiologists who provide services to hearing-impaired chil-dren throughout the state.

The project co-directors also visit the speech-language patholo-gists at their schools approximately once a month. During these visits the following activities are performed: (1) troubleshooting amplification systems; (2) interpreting speech-language tests; (3) measuring noise levels in the classrooms and therapy rooms; (4) taping samples for speech production intelligibility testing; (5) making recommendations for auditory and speech-language management; and (6) meeting with other appropriate school personnel. The project co-directors also may observe in the mainstream classroom and make suggestions for edu-cational modifications.

A continuing education course was designed to convey the theo-retical material which is needed for the practical management of the mainstreamed hearing-impaired child in the public school. The course includes the following content areas: audiological assessment, ampli-fication assessment and management, speech acoustics, classroom acoustics, language development, speech-language assessment and management, psycho-educational assessment, social considerations in mainstreaming, and individual educational programming. All of the ma-terial is related to the hearing-impaired child in the public school and

[1] Information about handouts and other materials is available on request from the authors, Communication Sciences Department, U-85 University of Connecticut, Storrs, Connecticut 06268.

is presented in light of the demographic information collected through the project.

DEMOGRAPHIC DATA

The demographic data are collected to 1) describe the typical mainstreamed hearing-impaired child for the purpose of differentiating him or her from the child typically described in the literature; and 2) modify the existing inservice training program. Table 23.1 shows the means and ranges for the 165 hearing-impaired children in Connecticut who have been monitored through the project from 1977 to 1979.

These data demonstrate that even though the mean better ear pure tone average (500, 1000, 2000, 4000 Hz) is 60.1 dB hearing threshold level (HTL: ANSI, 1969), the hearing losses range from a pure tone average (PTA) of 5 dB HTL through greater than 110 dB HTL. This indicates that the hearing-impaired children who have to function in the regular classroom vary from those who have normal or nearly normal hearing in at least one ear to children who have bilateral profound hearing losses. Thus, the professionals who work with hearing-impaired children in public schools must be aware of the heterogeneity of this population, and the effects of the degree of hearing impairment upon the educational capabilities and behaviors of these children.

Although it is not apparent from the PTA, the aspect which typically distinguishes these children from the hearing-impaired children generally described in the literature (DiCarlo, 1968) is that they are highly dependent upon their hearing for reception of speech informa-

Table 23.1. Demographic data on 165 hearing-impaired children in 81 Connecticut public schools

	Mean	Range
Hearing levels (PTA better ear; dB HTL)[a]	60.1	5–110
Receptive speech discrimination (better ear; %)	78.0	0–100
Aided receptive discrimination (%)[b]		
Auditory only	58.4	0–100
Visual only	44.0	0–98
Auditory-visual	86.2	8–100
Receptive vocabulary (deviation from chronological age; years)	−3.3	−10.8–+4.8

[a] HTL, hearing threshold level.

[b] As measured by PBK word lists and presented in a face-to-face situation. The children were using either their personal hearing aids or wireless FM auditory trainers.

tion. This can be seen from the unaided receptive speech discrimination scores and the aided discrimination scores. The latter scores were obtained by presenting PBK lists in three conditions: auditory only, visual only, and auditory-visual. The mean better ear receptive discrimination score of 78% is good. A comparison of the aided receptive discrimination scores across modalities is fair for auditory only (58.4%) and poorer for visual only (44%); but when the children were allowed to function in a normal conversational manner (combined auditory-visual) their scores improved to 86.2%. There is a noticeable difference between the aided auditory discrimination score and that obtained in the clinic. This discrepancy is not unusual when one considers that these two sets of scores were obtained in different noise conditions, with different professionals performing the test, and with different amplification conditions. That is, some of the children were listening in considerable noise and with relatively poor amplification, which would adversely affect their performance in the aided condition.

In addition to the variability of degree of pure tone hearing loss among these children, their ability to use aided residual hearing to receive speech information varies considerably as well. The ranges for the receptive discrimination score (0% to 100%), the aided auditory receptive discrimination score (0% to 100%), and the aided auditory-visual receptive discrimination score (8% to 100%) are quite large and vary from poor to excellent. Although this may have had some effect on the differences between aided and unaided mean scores, it is believed that the greatest influences on scores were those listed above.

The difficulties in assessing the language abilities of the mainstreamed hearing-impaired child will not be discussed here. Due to the low age ceilings on most of the available spoken language tests, the psycholinguistic skills of older children are difficult to determine. Receptive vocabulary levels can be assessed with the Peabody Picture Vocabulary Test (PPVT) (Dunn, 1965). Hearing-impaired children generally have difficulty with vocabulary (Kretschmer and Kretschmer, 1978) and, as can be seen from Table 23.1, the hearing-impaired child in the public school is not particularly different. The mean deviation from chronological age (CA) for receptive vocabulary was 3.3 years, demonstrating a vocabulary deficit for these children. It is interesting to note, however, that the range of deviation scores (−10.8 to +4.8 years) demonstrates that although some of the children are functioning at quite a depressed level, there are some who are functioning at and above the levels of their hearing peers.

In general, the speech production intelligibility of the hearing-impaired child in the public school is relatively good, that is, the speech can be fairly well understood by an untrained listener. Several speech intelligibility measures have been used, including a rating scale procedure in which naive listeners rated the intelligibility with and without anchors (examples of the best and worst productions within which the listener heard may fall), a direct transcription procedure in which naive listeners wrote down each word in a list spoken by the hearing-impaired child, and a sentence procedure in which naive listeners wrote down the key word in a sentence spoken by the hearing-impaired child.

This last procedure, the Sentence Assessment of Speech Production Intelligibility (SASPI) was designed by Seewald (1981) to assess the more subtle production errors which affect the speech intelligibility of this population. He found that no more complete information was obtained with this technique than with the rating scale.

All of the data reported so far indicated that the average mainstreamed hearing-impaired child has and makes good use of his or her residual hearing, and has good language skills and speech production skills.

AMPLIFICATION

Because the mainstreamed hearing-impaired child is dependent on being able to use his or her hearing, it is important to assure that the amplification is functioning properly. During the project the speech-language pathologists are taught about troubleshooting amplification equipment, stressing the necessity for someone at the school to test the batteries and listen to the hearing aids and FM systems on a daily basis. If the speech-language pathologist is not present at the child's school every day, he or she is responsible for explaining how and why troubleshooting is necessary to someone else at the school, for example, the school nurse.

Because the speech-language pathologist is considered the most appropriate on-site professional to be case manager of the child, he or she should have a good understanding of how hearing aids and wireless FM auditory trainers work, how they differ from one another, and what can go wrong with them. An integral part of understanding the function and purpose of various types of amplification systems includes the knowledge of how comprehension of auditory information is affected by the interaction of classroom acoustics and the use of amplification. It is believed that in order for the speech-language pathologists to be able to make recommendations for such things as FM systems and physical or acoustic modifications of the classroom, they must know about the problems of distance, noise, and reverberation time in the average classroom. Audio and videotapes are used to demonstrate these difficulties and to enhance the theoretical information provided.

Because there is an emphasis on remediation through the auditory system for mainstreamed children, it becomes necessary to encourage the speech-language pathologists to understand how the child functions with amplification. This necessitates familiarizing the participants with the type of clinical audiological evaluation which must be carried out in order for them to know if the child's amplification is appropriate and the type of benefit received from it. The recommended audiological assessment includes:

1. *Routine pure tone, speech, and impedance measurements*
2. *Objective amplification evaluation: Electroacoustic and/or listening (troubleshooting) evaluation of the hearing aids and the wireless FM auditory trainer*   The electroacoustic analysis is the preferred method, but there are clinics that do not have the facility to do this.
3. *Subjective amplification evaluation: Speech discrimination and warble tone thresholds with hearing aids and with the wireless FM auditory trainer*   Although this aided information is critical for management, it is usually the most difficult for the speech-language pathologists to obtain and may not be carried out by the audiologists in the clinics.
4. *Reporting*   Type and degree of hearing loss are described, including how well the child is able to use his or her hearing for speech reception and discrimination; hearing aid and FM system, that is, settings, good volume, type of earmold; effects of classroom acoustics; and possible academic considerations.

It was discovered that the information listed above was not readily available to the public school speech-language pathologists and, initially, was often not even found in the child's folder. Once given the reasons for the practical need for this information, the participants often would obtain it by the end of the project.

SPEECH RECEPTION

In an additional effort to help understand how the child functions with amplification, an explanation of speech acoustics is presented to the project participants. Following the presentation of the theoretical material, the relationship between the acoustic cues for speech perception and a hearing-impaired child's aided and unaided hearing is explained.

This helps the speech-language pathologists understand which acoustic cues the children can acutally receive.

One of the critical examples of them is the difficulty that a child with a severe high frequency hearing loss will have hearing /s/. This is very important—not only for speech production, but also for conveying and receiving syntactic information (e.g., cat versus cats: pluralization when the final consonant of the word is voiceless). Some strategies, (e.g., having the child make use of the silence that he or she hears where the /s/ acutally occurs) are explained so that the speech-language pathologist can implement them when managing the child. Also conveyed is the observation that there are often acoustic cues available to the child within his or her range of useable residual hearing (e.g., some formant transitions). The acoustic information in the low frequencies, such as voicing, duration, and nasalization, is described and emphasized because most hearing-impaired people are able to perceive cues in this frequency region. The clinicians are encouraged to determine if at least these cues are perceptible to their children.

The speech-language pathologists should then be able to determine if the types of receptive errors that the children make are appropriate or inappropriate in light of their aided hearing and the available perceptual cues. The clinicians are urged to use this information as a basis for remediation. They are also urged to determine the extent of the speech information which the child can actually hear, which may be distorted and/or acoustically missing, and relate this to the child's speech production. As Fry (1978) pointed out, a child may be able to make use of distorted acoustic information in order to obtain a correct production, that is in order to match his or her production to that which is heard, the child must produce the correct sound. In addition to setting up more realistic goals for the children, this knowledge has made it easier for clinicians to know where and how to determine remediation for their children in relation to their use of hearing and speech.

SPEECH PRODUCTION

The data collected have shown that the mainstreamed hearing-impaired child can generally produce a phoneme in isolation, indicating knowledge of manner and place of articulation and voicing. Because a specific phoneme may not be audible to the child in certain contexts, he or she may not produce it in those contexts without training, but may do so in others, that is, those contexts in which the child actually hears that specific phoneme. Therefore, for the mainstreamed hearing-impaired child, problems in speech production are intricately related to the ability to perceive speech sounds in contexts which do not stress them as well as in stressed contexts.

One error so evident in the speech of the mainstreamed population is the omission of specific phonemes as morphological markers. Therefore, what may be taken as a syntactic problem (e.g., not using pluralization) may really be a speech production problem. The clinician must determine which it is, and then take appropriate remedial measures. The clinican must ascertain if the child actually understands pluralization, possession, and noun/verb agreement before a conclusion about speech production can be made. The mainstreamed child may often have little difficulty in producing /s/, /z/, /t/, or /d/ in isolation or in stressed syllables in words. The problem arises in unstressed contexts where the audibility of the cues is reduced. Examples of these phonemes as morphological markers can be seen in Table 23.2

With the theory that there are a variety of possible acoustic cues available to the hearing-impaired child, it is suggested that a remediation procedure for these speech production problems be developed which leads to self-monitoring and eventually automatic production. Many of these children have received traditional articulation therapy in which the emphasis is on the production of a phoneme; and in general, throughout therapy remain at a level at which they can produce the phoneme in isolation and in stimulus words, but never attain carryover to spontaneous speech. Often these children can skip these initial stages of therapy and go directly to working on carryover. Because speech perception, rather than production per se seems to be a problem, it would seem logical to work on improving the child's ability to use the acoustic cues available with amplification for monitoring his or her verbal output.

Most speech-language pathologists in the project have had training in designing and implementing articulation programs for children with

Table 23.2.   Phonemes used as morphologic markers that hearing-impaired children may have difficulty hearing

Phoneme	Morphologic use	Example
/s/	Pluralization	cats
/s/	Third person present possessive	its
/z/	Pluralization	cars
/z/	Third person present possessive	hers
/t/	Past tense	walked
/d/	Past tense	carried

functional articulation disorders. Some of the suggested adaptations of these programs emphasize self-monitoring through the use of multiple acoustic cues. Goal selection is based on analyses of the child's aided audiogram in combination with the knowledge of the frequency bands and intensity of consonant sounds. Therapy suggestions are made such as monitoring the clinician's production of gross and fine distinctions using live voice and audiotapes, and then monitoring these distinctions in linguistic contexts. A further move toward self-monitoring is made when the child begins to listen to his or her productions on audiotape, making the same fine distinctions. The final step is self-monitoring by the child as he or she produces the utterances.

The above information is conveyed to speech-language pathologists through monthly visits, two workshops, and the continuing education course. The materials and handouts used at various phases of the project demonstrate the auditory emphasis of the program and the attempt to apply the audiological and acoustic information to all aspects of communicative behavior.

SUMMARY AND CONCLUSIONS

The UConn Mainstream Project has provided inservice training concerning hearing-impaired children to public school speech-language pathologists over the last 5 years. The major focus of the project has been to make public school personnel more aware of the implications of hearing loss and its effects on speech production, speech perception, language, and academic and social skills. As is true of many educational situations, the project co-directors learned a great deal during the experience and changes have been and will continue to be made in the implementation of the project. Plans for the future include evaluating the present program by returning to the speech-language pathologists who have participated in the project in the past, and expanding the presently defined population of hearing-impaired children to include those who presently demonstrate or have a history of conductive hearing loss. The possibility of adding personnel to the project to deal with the complex issues of the bilingual hearing-impaired child in the public school is also being considered.

ACKNOWLEDGMENT

The UConn Mainstream Project has been made possible through the continued support of the Office of Special Education, U. S. Department of Education.

REFERENCES

American National Standards Institute. 1969. American National Standard Specifications for Audiometers, ANSI-S3.6-1969. American National Standards Institute, Inc., New York.

DiCarlo, L. M. 1968. Speech, language and cognitive abilities of the hard-of-hearing. Proceedings of the Institute of Aural Rehabilitation (SRA Grant No. 212-T-68). University of Denver, Denver.

Dunn, L. M. 1965. Peabody Picture Vocabulary Test (PPVT). American Guidance Service, Circle Pines, Minn.

Fry, D. B. 1978. The role and primacy of the auditory channel in speech and language development. In M. Ross, and T. G. Giolas (eds.), Auditory Management of Hearing-Impaired Children. University Park Press, Baltimore.

Kretschmer, R. R., and L. W. Kretschmer. 1978. Language Development and Intervention with the Hearing Impaired. University Park Press, Baltimore.

Seewald, R. C. 1981. The interrelationships among hearing level, utilization of auditory and visual cues in speech reception and speech intelligibility in children. Doctoral dissertation, University of Connecticult, Storrs, Conn.

CHAPTER 24

A MODEL INSERVICE-PRESERVICE TRAINING PROGRAM TO IMPROVE THE SPEECH OF HEARING-IMPAIRED CHILDREN

Irving Hochberg and Joanna L. Schmidt

CONTENTS

The failure of many hearing-impaired children to acquire intelligible speech has been related to the relative quantity and quality of speech training that is being delivered to these children. It has been argued by a number of leading educators (among others, Boothroyd, this volume; Hogan, 1980; Ling, 1976;) that teachers are inadequately prepared to engage in the difficult task of providing effective speech services to severely and profoundly hearing-impaired children, and consequently do not meet their oral communicative needs. The emergence of large numbers of inadequately trained professional personnel who lack the requisite commitment, do not possess the fundamental knowledge, and have not acquired the necessary skills to teach speech effectively has been observed as well (Ling, 1976; Northcott, 1971). The unhappy consequence of these circumstances is that speech is not being taught, being taught minimally, or being taught poorly. The growing awareness of this prevailing situation has led to a recognition of the need to develop inservice training programs to supplement preservice personnel preparation (Bishop, 1980; Boothroyd, this volume). An educational project conceptualized to meet this challenge was conducted at the City University of New York Graduate School.

DESIGN OF THE INSERVICE-PRESERVICE TRAINING PROJECT

To make a significant and long-term impact on the more effective delivery of speech services to hearing-impaired children, the design of the educational program needed to incorporate both inservice and preservice training components. It was important that both the symptoms and the presumed cause of the widespread failure of hearing-impaired children to acquire useful speech be addressed.

The first year of the project was devoted to an assessment of the inservice training needs of professional personnel providing speech services to hearing-impaired children. Information was gathered in relation to the needs of preservice training programs in both education of the hearing impaired and speech-language pathology and audiology with respect to speech for the hearing impaired. Task force meetings were held with (1) teachers of the hearing impaired; (2) speech pathologists working with hearing-impaired children; (3) preservice training program directors; (4) state education consultants; (5) administrators of service programs for hearing-impaired children; and (6) supervisors of speech services in programs for the hearing impaired. In addition, site visits were made to selected school programs, and a national survey was carried out relative to the inservice needs of professional personnel.

Based on the accumulated data, a locally based inservice training program was designed, which included voluntary participation of schools in the New York City area. The purpose was to prepare local school personnel to subsequently train colleagues in their respective school programs.

The third year of the project focused on two major activities: (1) the implementation of inservice training programs within each of the participating schools; and (2) the initiation of a 5-day summer workshop on the speech of hearing-impaired children for faculty in preservice training programs. The latter involved a number of college and university training programs in both hearing impairment education and speech-language pathology and audiology.

The recommendations that emerged from the various task forces and the data obtained from the national survey further emphasized the need to develop a systematic program of inservice training for both classroom teachers of the hearing impaired and speech-language pathologists working with such children (Hochberg, Levitt, and Osberger, 1980). The information obtained from these and other sources formed the basis for the activities that are described below.

REGIONAL INSERVICE TRAINING PROGRAM

Although it was recognized that a dual approach was necessary in meeting both inservice and preservice needs, practical considerations dictated that initial efforts should concentrate on the development of a locally-based inservice training program. This would facilitate ongoing evaluation and monitoring.

The program was based on the following considerations:

1. Local school personnel were to provide subsequent inservice training to their colleagues at their respective employment settings. Each participating school was represented by both a teacher of the deaf and a speech-language pathologist.
2. The inservice training curriculum was based on the expressed needs of professional personnel, and reflected the theoretical base of information that underlies the effective application of instructional skills. The integration of theory and practice was stressed.
3. The curriculum facilitated the implementation of various inservice training models appropriate to the particular needs and capabilities of various school programs.
4. Participating school programs included both total and oral-aural modes.
5. Because the ultimate objective was to establish a resident inservice training program in each school, the major responsibility for its continued development following its establishment was assumed by school personnel.

Each school was represented by one classroom teacher and one speech-language pathologist, although several programs included a resource room teacher as well. The participating institutions and programs included the Lexington School for the Deaf, St. Francis de Sales School for the Deaf, St. Joseph's School for the Deaf, Mill Neck Manor Lutheran School for the Deaf, the programs for the hearing impaired of the Bureau of Cooperative Services in Nassau and Westchester Counties, and the programs of both the Bureau for Hearing Handicapped Children and the Bureau for Speech Improvement of the Board of Education of the City of New York.

The participants included six classroom teachers, six speech-language pathologists, and three resource room teachers, all of whom attended weekly, 4-hour, lecture-discussion-demonstration sessions over a 15-week period for a total of 60 hours of inservice training. Didactic material was supplemented with relevant readings, demonstrations, and audio-visual instructional materials. The latter, for example, included audiotapes illustrating various errors of speech of the hearing impaired, the display of the acoustics of speech employing the Speech Spectrographic Display (Spectraphonics Corp.), a videotaped demonstration of the effects of background noise and the effect of the speaker-listener relationship on speech intelligibility,[1] and videotaped instruction of various speech assessment and speech training procedures.[2]

Assessment of Inservice Training

The degree to which inservice training increased the level of information on the part of the recipients was assessed by a five-point rating scale (i.e., on a continuum of minimal to extensive knowledge), which was used to compare baseline knowledge before training with acquired knowledge after training. The difference between pre- and post-training ratings was considered to be the extent to which knowledge was acquired. For the purpose of comparison, the 55 questions on the rating questionnaire were classified into seven major content areas (Figure 24.1).

According to the mean pre- and post-training ratings for (1) classroom teachers and resource room teachers; (2) speech-language pathologists; and (3) the two groups combined, the teachers had less baseline information as a group than did the speech-language pathologists before training across the seven content areas. After inservice training, however, they appeared to have acquired a greater amount of information than did the speech-language pathologists. It would appear that the amount of knowledge was increased as a result of this 15-week training program as assessed by this rating-scale.

The pre- and post-training ratings for each of the seven content areas are presented in Figure 24.2. With one exception, that of hearing aids, speech-language pathologists had relatively more baseline information on all remaining content areas than did classroom and resource room teachers. It is not unreasonable to expect that coursework and

---

[1] Courtesy of Drs. Antonia Maxon, Diane Brackett, and Mark Ross, of the University of Connecticut Mainstream Project.

[2] These videotapes were developed in cooperation with Janet Head and Margot Cusack of the Lexington School for the Deaf.

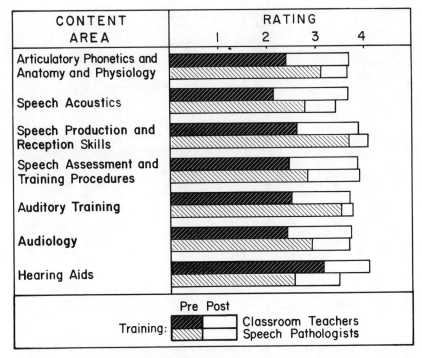

Figure 24.1. Ratings of pre- and post-inservice knowledge on major content areas by classroom teachers and speech-language pathologists.

practicum experiences with hearing aids and other amplification systems are more likely to be included as part of preservice training in education of the hearing impaired as opposed to speech-language pathology. Secondly, there was a general tendency for content areas that received extreme ratings of most or least knowledge before training to receive similar ratings after inservice training. Speech acoustics received the lowest or nearly the lowest ratings before and after training, whereas hearing aids received the highest pre- and post-training ratings by teachers, and speech production and reception skills received the highest ratings by speech-language pathologists before and after training. Thirdly, an inverse relationship was observed in terms of relative gain among content areas rated high and low. For example, for teachers, speech acoustics, which received the lowest ratings, obtained the greatest gain in acquired information; whereas hearing aids, which received the highest rating, made the least gains. Finally, it seems that inservice training proved to be most effective in those areas in which the participants had the least amount of baseline information as re-

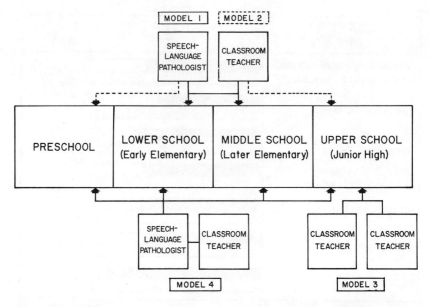

Figure 24.2.   Alternative inservice training models in participating day school programs.

flected by the maximum gains made in those content areas, as determined from the mean group ratings (i.e., speech acoustics, speech assessment, audiology). At the very least, systematic inservice training over a protracted period of time can increase knowledge in areas of particular weakness.

    An assessment of the degree of self-confidence on the part of the participants after inservice training was conducted. Each teacher completed a 3-point rating scale which sought to identify the relative degree of confidence (very, somewhat, or not confident) for various activities. The participants as a group felt more confident in those activities that were related to the provision of services and less confident in presenting didactic material and demonstrating the application of such material to their professional colleagues. Because pretraining baseline rankings were not available, comparisons cannot be made with respect to the relative increase of self-confidence as a result of inservice training.

ALTERNATIVE INSERVICE TRAINING MODELS

The participating school programs represented two types of educational settings: day schools for the deaf and public school resource room or itinerant service programs. Within each setting a variety of inservice training models emerged, each of which was designed according to the needs of the respective professional staff, the resource capabilities of the program, and the inherent limitations imposed by each setting. The original inservice training curriculum was modified to contain a core of 10 instructional modules that could be implemented in each of the participating schools (see Hochberg, 1980, for the core curriculum and the characteristics of the various programs).

Model School Programs

Day Schools for the Deaf A day school is defined as a self-contained school providing educational services to children whose primary handicap is hearing impairment. Hearing-impaired children with other handicapping conditions (e.g., mental, emotional, visual, or orthopedic impairments) also may be enrolled in day schools. In New York State, children between 3 and 21 years of age attend day schools, with some schools maintaining infant programs for children between 0 and 3 years of age. Not all day schools, however, provide services for children between 15 and 21 years of age.

Figure 24.2 depicts a composite of the four day schools that participated in the inservice training project. For the purpose of illustration, these day schools are collapsed into one continuous school program characterized by the four divisions shown. Four distinct inservice training models were developed in each of the day schools. One speech-language pathologist and one classroom teacher from each school (or two classroom teachers in Model 3) were trained to be inservice providers. The major distinguishing features of the inservice training models that were developed are described.

Model 1 In Model 1, participation by staff members was voluntary. Together the speech-language pathologist and the classroom teacher presented two 6-week inservice courses for continuing education credit, first to 15 members of the lower school and then to a group of 15 teachers from the middle school. One inservice provider presented the lectures and prepared the accompanying materials, while the other supervised the recipient teachers as they practiced speech maintenance activities with their students. A primary objective during these practice sessions was to provide repeated opportunities for these essentially naive listeners (the staff members receiving inservice training) to evaluate their students' speech production of various target phonemes in words. During the following year a special topics inservice course attended by 30 staff members was conducted by project staff in response to expressed needs. The staff also participated in a research study with project staff.

Model 2   In Model 2, participation by staff members was voluntary. The speech-language pathologist, whose caseload was drawn from the preschool and lower school divisions, presented inservice training to three classroom teachers from these divisions. The classroom teacher provided inservice training to two teachers from the upper school, and to one speech-language pathologist who worked with children from these two classrooms. The inservice providers presented essentially the same information to their respective groups, although they modified the presentations relative to the ages of the children. They provided additional inservice speech training in a similar format during the following school year.

Model 3   In Model 3, the two classroom teachers who provided inservice training were selected from a special upper school program which was designed to meet the individualized communication needs of individual children and embraced oral and manual modes of communication. The target audience receiving training included 9 teachers of the hearing impaired and instructional aides. Because the latter participants had no formal preparation in the education of the hearing impaired, the inservice curriculum was suitably modified to accomodate their lack of background and permit them to proceed at their own pace.

Model 4   In Model 4, participation in the inservice training program was mandatory for all classroom teachers. In addition, one assistant, nine speech-language pathologists, and two supervisors also attended the inservice sessions. Although both a speech-language pathologist and a classroom teacher became inservice providers, the latter left the school after the first semester. Inservice training subsequently was provided by the remaining speech-language pathologist on a weekly basis. The inclusion of all divisions in the training program established an improved continuity among divisions. During the following year, the inservice was continued for 25 staff members on a voluntary, biweekly basis with greater emphasis on practical applications.

Concurrent with the provision of inservice training was the implementation of a daily speech period in the classrooms of the upper three divisions of the school. During this period, speech department staff members circulated among designated classrooms to assist teachers as they provided individualized reinforcement of specific speech targets that were developed during weekly individual or small group speech sessions (Schmidt et al., 1981).

The major advantage of providing inservice training in day school settings appears to be two-fold: (1) the continuity of educational services in one physical location; and (2) the facilitation of opportunities for ongoing communication among professional personnel and between departments. On the other hand, an apparent limitation that exists within such educational settings relates to the absence of exposure to the normal speech models that ordinarily are available from hearing students in a public school setting.

If it can be supposed that an "ideal" model for inservice speech training exists among those described it might well be the one developed in Model 1. The responsibility for the preparation of training was shared by the inservice providers, participation by staff members was voluntary, and the target groups were sufficiently small to facilitate discussion of the needs of individual children. The latter is considered to be rather critical for the assimilation of the theoretical foundations of speech and for the application of information in the classroom activities. Large-group, mandatory participation exemplified in Model 4 (and in Model 1 below) proved to be an insurmountable limitation to accomplish the objective of assimilation and application.

Public School Programs Programs for hearing-impaired children within the public schools typically provide resource room and/or itinerant services, and are usually located in different buildings throughout a school district. Such decentralized placement of services appears to facilitate the mainstreaming of hearing-impaired children with normally hearing children. However, the limitation imposed by this type of organization concerns the facilitation of the linkage mechanism wherein all school personnel providing educational services to hearing-impaired children within a school district may interact and communicate. In Figure 24.3 resource rooms for hearing-impaired children are depicted and represent a composite of the participating public school settings.

Model 1 In Model 1, inservice training was incorporated into the regular monthly meetings of all (40 to 45) resource room teachers from the five boroughs of New York City. Of this group, 26 teachers completed the entire sequence of inservice training. Practical limitations dictated the organization of this type of inservice model, and resulted in several notable disadvantages. These included (1) limited communication and interaction among participants because of widely dispersed school programs; (2) minimal reinforcement of learning because of monthly intervals of time; and (3) limited interaction between recipients and instructor due to the large target group.

Model 2 Originally in Model 2, a classroom teacher, an itinerant teacher, and a speech-language pathologist were trained from this suburban county-wide program. The classroom teacher who left the day school in Model 4 was hired as a resource room teacher by this program, and became involved as an additional inservice provider. Consequently, four trained individuals were capable of providing inservice training to an original group of nine teachers from preschool through grade 12 classes. Of these, five teachers completed the entire inservice training program. The obvious practical advantages of having such a large number of inservice providers were the distribution of responsibility for the overall training program and the small-group interaction between instructors and recipients. The resource room teacher has gone on to provide inservice training to parents, mainstream teachers, and hospital staff.

Several factors have practical consequences upon the success or failure of inservice programs based in the school setting. The nature and availability of incentives for the voluntary or mandatory participation of teachers becomes critical, and must be determined at the outset. In several schools various incentives were available; in other schools the professional agreements (union contracts) defined the organization of training. The support services that are necessary for the preparation and duplication of instructional materials, audio-visual assistance, and so on were more readily available in day schools than in the decentralized public school programs. The amount of regularly scheduled time slots provided for instruction, the number of sessions

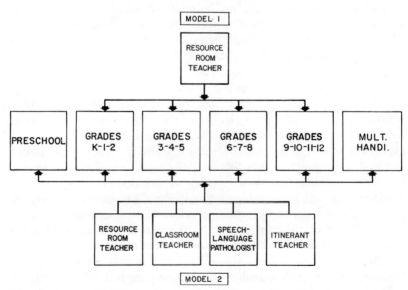

Figure 24.3.   Alternative inservice training models in participating public school programs for the hearing impaired.

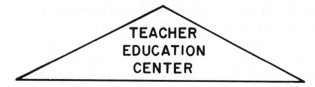

LABORATORY RESOURCE FACILITY

Information Storage Retrieval
Instructional Materials Production
Instructional Materials Center
Demonstrations of Teaching
Instructional Systems Development

TEACHER
EDUCATION
CENTER

PRESERVICE PROGRAMS

SERVICE PROGRAMS

Hearing Impairment Ed.
Speech-Language Path.
and Audiology

School Programs
for the
Hearing Impaired

competency-based modules
professional field experiences
microteaching
independent study
evaluation and testing

independent study
seminars
courses
workshops
institutes
consultant services

Figure 24.4.   A consortium model of preservice and inservice education converging on the development of a teacher education center (after Mallan, 1974).

available, the duration of the overall inservice program, and the availability of released time for the inservice providers to prepare materials are all critical variables to consider. Demonstrations of theoretical information in classroom situations with individual children requires extensive time commitment as well, and a determination should be made as to whether there is sufficient time allotted for including these essential activities. The data obtained from the evaluations of those receiving inservice training revealed a general desire for such experiences. The realization of the interests and needs on the part of the teaching staff in connection with these and other inservice activities has prompted one day school to consider a staff position in inservice training so that individualized classroom application can be expanded. The feedback received from all school programs is that individualized classroom instruction demonstrating theoretical principles of speech training in practical situations should be emphasized.

REGIONAL PRESERVICE TRAINING WORKSHOP

To address the preservice component of the project, eight training programs in education of the hearing-impaired and/or speech-language pathology and audiology participated in a 5-day workshop at the Graduate School during July, 1979. The participating institutions included Bloomsburg State College, Hunter College of CUNY, New York University, State University College at Geneseo, University of Northern Illinois, University of Pittsburgh, Western Maryland College, and William Paterson State College.

The workshop was designed to: (1) update participants on recent developments in research and research-related educational strategies relevant to the speech of hearing-impaired children; (2) identify present and future needs believed to be most critical in personnel preparation; (3) facilitate interaction among the participants of the disciplines of education of the hearing-impaired and speech-language pathology and audiology; and (4) consider alternative strategies for incorporating recent information and research findings about speech and speech training into preservice curricula.

An evaluation of daily activities and at the termination of the workshop revealed the following observations. Personal and professional needs which were either unmet during the workshop, emerged as a consequence of workshop activities, or required additional information were cited. These included (1) live demonstrations of teachers teaching hearing-impaired children; (2) a consideration of the competencies needed by teachers of hearing-impaired children to teach speech; (3) the use of speech and sign; (4) opportunities for hands-on experiences with sensory aids, and their application to speech training; and (5) further information on the relationship between the total communication philosophy and the development and improvement of speech skills.

In general, virtually all of the needs among teacher trainers correspond to the needs of professional personnel providing services to hearing-impaired children. That the workshop proved to be successful in meeting many of the professional needs of the participants, and that there emerged an expression of a continuing need to acquire information about current research related to the speech of hearing-impaired children, to observe demonstrations of specific teaching techniques, to obtain hands-on experiences with modern sensory aids, and to further understand the role of speech training in the total communication philosophy further emphasizes the need for systematic and relevant continuing professional education as well as inservice training.

To ascertain what, if any, impact the workshop may have had upon subsequent curriculum modification among the training programs, a follow-up questionnaire was distributed approximately 7 months later. Seven participants responded, indicating that the material presented was useful and that in every instance some or all of the material has been variously incorporated during classroom teaching, student teaching, graduate clinical practicum, and staff development. Table 24.1 shows the order in which the content areas were ranked from most to least useful by questionnaire respondents.

The experiences obtained during the workshop already have had some impact upon several of the training programs, and there are indications that further impact will be made in the near future. What is equally clear, however, is that although certain gains have been made among the participants in the inservice training program, and among the college training programs involved in the workshop, our experiences suggest that a more coordinated effort on the part of preservice and inservice programs within local geographic areas would contribute substantially towards greater long-term impact than the initiation of activities exclusively in either type of program. The following section describes a plan that involves the resources of preservice, inservice,

Table 24.1.   Rank order of content areas reported most to least useful by workshop participants

Rank	Content Area
1	Speech acoustics
2	Classroom acoustics and amplification systems
3	Systematic speech training procedures
4	Assessment procedures
5	Speech production and reception abilities of hearing-impaired children
6	Student teaching and practicum in speech
7	Maintenance and carry-over of speech skills
8	Sensory aids and auditory training
9	Speech physiology
10	Mainstreaming hearing-impaired children

and research laboratory capabilities as a potentially effective approach in meeting the challenge of improving the delivery of speech services to hearing-impaired children.

A CONSORTIUM MODEL OF INSERVICE-PRESERVICE TRAINING

The authors have substantiated the original hypothesis regarding the prevailing need to improve the delivery of speech services to hearing-impaired children. Yet the magnitude of the problem is even more widespread and critical than was initially supposed. It is evident that speech-language pathologists working with hearing-impaired children are equally as frustrated as are classroom teachers in meeting the speech training needs of these children, and attest to the need for systematic inservice training in this area. Moreover, it became clear that there is an equally pressing need for continuing professional education for teacher trainers if substantive changes are to be made within existing preprofessional training programs in education of the hearing-impaired and speech-language pathology and audiology. An approach that incorporates both preservice and inservice education is inescapable.

The approach conceptualized herein is based upon the collaborative efforts among the members of three component programs: the preservice training program, the programs delivering services to hearing-impaired children, and the laboratory resource facility. The establishment of cooperation and interaction among the three components is essential to the success of this approach. At its optimum level of operation such a "consortium" model of education can result in a variety of mutually beneficial advantages.[3]

1. The laboratory facility and the college training programs can assist school service programs with needs assessment (program priorities) and role analyses (teacher effectiveness and teacher-clinician interaction) to determine both preservice and inservice training needs.
2. The school service programs can identify appropriate and realistic ways of providing input into preservice college training programs.
3. The constituent programs could render mutual assistance in relating initial training to continuing training. Such assistance can be supplemented by activities from the laboratory resource facility.

---

[3] A number of these advantages have been paraphrased from those presented by Howey (1977).

4. The college training programs might contribute to the transitional and continuing phases of teacher and clinician renewal in the school programs.
5. The college training and school service programs can assist the laboratory resource facility in identifying and evaluating the development of teaching strategies and materials.
6. The programs can assist in reviewing systematically the combined training resources of college, laboratory, and school service programs to identify possible complementary, shared, and pooled personnel resources.
7. Assigned personnel from the respective constituent programs can periodically evaluate one another's programs.
8. Short-term, critical problem-solving task forces can be developed, composed of personnel from each of the three component programs.

Figure 24.4 depicts the way in which the consortium model is conceptualized and converges upon the notion of a Teacher Education Center (Mallan, 1974). Each component has the individual responsibility of developing and implementing a variety of activities that characterize its capabilities and inherent objectives. The contributions of each component are enhanced as a consequence of its participation in the consortium, with the ultimate goal of these mutually assisted activities merging within the Teacher Education Center. With reference to the present project, the establishment of such a center may involve teachers of the hearing impaired, resource room teachers, speech-language pathologists, teacher trainers, supervisors of clinical practicum, supervisors of speech services in school programs, staff members of the laboratory resource facility, and others whose functions and responsibilities relate to the activities of the consortium.

Such a center serves as the linking mechanism among the constituent programs, wherein the resources of these programs are facilitated. The concept of the Teacher Education Center reflects an expanding approach to inservice education, and is applicable to the consortium model being considered. The notion of such a center is related to the need on the part of professional staff to interact with colleagues in an informal environment, outside of the school setting, for the purpose of relating to others whom they perceive understand their own work (Howey, 1977). Optimally, the operation of the Teacher Education Center can result in a series of activities that serve the needs of professional personnel in a variety of ways, and in so doing, may realize the presumed benefits cited earlier.

It is important to emphasize the ongoing collaboration between the preservice programs in education of the hearing impaired and speech-language pathology and audiology. Their participation is critical because their respective graduates will be responsible for the education and management of the hearing-impaired child. The development of communication and cooperation among these disciplines is a critical first step toward the implementation of this model.

IMPLEMENTATION OF THE CONSORTIUM MODEL

An experimental consortium model was implemented during the 1980–1981 academic year and involved the CUNY Center for Research in Speech & Hearing Sciences (research facility), the training programs in hearing impairment education and speech-language pathology and audiology at SUNY-Geneseo (preservice programs), the City School District of Rochester (service programs for the hearing impaired), and more recently, the Rochester Oral School for the Deaf. This satellite consortium was developed as a demonstration project incorporating the fundamental principles of collaboration and interaction outlined above. The approach afforded an opportunity to make major impact upon both preservice and inservice education, and to demonstrate its replication in the other local regions.

Both preservice and inservice activities evolved as a result of this collaborative framework (see Hochberg et al., 1981). Undergraduate courses within each of the respective preservice programs were modified to integrate current research into useful clinical practices and to include the study of the communicative needs of hearing-impaired children. At the graduate level, an interdepartmental course was developed to include recent research in the speech sciences and the clinical implications of such information on the speech of hearing-impaired children; more extensive information on sensory aids was included in coursework; and the development of summer workshops applicable to students in both programs was initiated.

These modifications were easily effected because of the ongoing interdepartmental cooperation that existed, and the concern on the part of the respective faculties for the need to monitor, evaluate, and respond to changing needs of personnel preparation. Furthermore, the programs previously had been involved in the planning and delivery of inservice training programs in the local geographic area, and thus were familiar with the needs of graduates entering service delivery programs for the hearing impaired.

The inservice activities involved a group of 27 school personnel, including teachers of the hearing impaired, speech clinicians, regular classroom teachers, and resource personnel. An 8-week program of 90-minute lecture/demonstrations was conducted in one of the Rochester schools, and was based on a preliminary assessment of the needs of the professional personnel.

A 3-week program was developed to follow up and expand upon the activities of the initial 8-week inservice program, and was held at SUNY-Geneseo during the 1981 summer session. It was designed to maximize demonstration and practice with specific materials and techniques so that theoretical information could be meaningfully integrated with application.

In addition to these activities the consortium has provided a unique framework for (1) the evaluation and subsequent modification of an audio-tape program of listening training with segmental and suprasegmental errors common in the speech of hearing-impaired children; (2) field testing of an assessment procedure to profile the speech communication that takes place within a classroom; and (3) the development, evaluation, and refinement of innovative teaching methods that could be employed during clinical practicum and delivery of services. Future consortium activities will include long-term assessment of the way in which both modified preservice education and inservice training have affected intervention strategies in the delivery of speech services to hearing-impaired children.

CONCLUDING COMMENT

The provision of effective speech services to hearing-impaired children demands the highest level of commitment and expertise on the part of professional personnel involved in such acitivity. It requires the knowledge, skills, and competencies to be acquired over an extended period of time, beginning with undergraduate studies, followed by more intensive graduate education, and supplemented by systematic professional continuing education. Employing this premise as a working principle, the inservice-preservice training program described in this paper was designed to meet such a challenge. It was conceptualized from the very start that if long-term impact were to be realized, both the cause and symptoms of inadequate preparation needed to be addressed; and in so doing, a series of integrated instructional activities for both teachers of the hearing impaired and speech-language pathologists would have to be developed that would upgrade knowledge, develop effective skills, and improve specific competencies in the more effective delivery of speech services to hearing-impaired children.

The model of inservice training incorporated those educational principles that appeared to us to be both sound and practicable within the constraints imposed by our resources, capabilities, and personnel. Although adjustments and modifications were necessary during various phases of the project, they did not appear to be detrimental to the realization of the objectives that had to be accomplished.

The consortium model that emerged from the activities that were developed, and the one that we advocate, is by no means the only approach that is possible. It was adopted because its inherent character provides the kind of collaborative framework that facilitates the accomplishment of the goals of the present project. We believe that it contains a number of attributes that cannot be duplicated by other models, and that these far outweigh whatever disadvantages may exist. As a model to be replicated elsewhere, the basic design of the triad can be approximated by whatever local resources may be available in a given geographic area. Exact duplication of the model may not be possible, and under certain circumstances, not altogether desirable. However, it is our belief that it does afford both personnel preparation and service delivery programs a unique opportunity for long-term interaction and collaboration for the mutual benefit of both.

ACKNOWLEDGMENTS

The authors wish to acknowledge with appreciation the contributions of the following individuals during various phases of this project: Harry Levitt, Mary Joe Osberger, Jean Schultz, and Linda Hoffnung. Appreciation is also extended to the participating classroom teachers and speech-language pathologists who have implemented the inservice training programs at their schools, and to their respective supervisors and administrators for their continued support of the project. To the members of the original task forces, the respondents to the national survey, the participants in the preservice workshop, and the various individuals who have been called upon for their particular expertise, the authors are grateful indeed. Finally, acknowledgment is given to the Office of Special Education of the U.S. Department of Education for their continued support of this project.

REFERENCES

Bishop, M. E. 1980. Summary and recommendations of the chairman. In J. D. Subtelny (ed.). Speech Assessment and Speech Improvement for the Hearing Impaired. A. G. Bell Association for the Deaf, Washington, D.C.
Hochberg, I. 1980. A model inservice training program to improve the speech of hearing impaired children. Volta Rev. 82:419–429.

Hochberg, I., H. Levitt, and M. J. Osberger. 1980. Improving speech services to hearing impaired children. Asha 22:480–484.

Hochberg, I., J. L. Schmidt, L. M. Solomon, B. Godsave, N. Schiavetti, and E. Burgess. Improving speech services for hearing-impaired children in the schools: A consortium model for meeting continuing education and preservice training needs. Lang. Speech Hear. Serv. Schools. In press.

Hogan, Sr., J. L. 1980. Pre-conference recommendations. In J. D. Subtelny (ed.), Speech Assessment and Speech Improvement for the Hearing Impaired. A. G. Bell Association for the Deaf, Washington, D.C.

Howey, K. R. 1977. A framework for planning alternative approaches to inservice teacher education. Paper prepared for the American Association of Colleges for Teacher Education, May.

Ling, D. 1976. Speech and the Hearing Impaired Child: Theory and Practice. A. G. Bell Association for the Deaf, Washington, D.C.

Mallan, J. T. 1974. Teaching centers: Utopia, eutopia or kakotopia? Paper presented at the annual meeting of the American Association of Colleges for Teacher Education, Chicago.

Northcott, W. 1971. Competencies needed by teachers of hearing-impaired infants (birth to three years of age) and their parents. Doctoral dissertation, University of Minnesota, Minneapolis.

Schmidt, J. L., L. M. Solomon, A. Martello, and I. Hochberg. 1981. Modifications of classroom speech training prompted by systematic inservice education. J. Acad. Rehabil. Audio. 14:17–32.

CHAPTER 25

SKILLS + KNOWLEDGE + X-FACTORS = EFFECTIVE SPEECH TEACHING

Janet M. Head

CONTENTS

SPEECH TEACHING: AN INTERACTION

Teaching is an elusive act. Dictionaries use multiple phrases to define its meaning. The World Book Dictionary (Barnhart, 1968) states: "Teaching: to give lessons in; to give instructions about; to help to learn; to give knowledge of; to make known to" (p. 1112). These five definitions present two different views: the first two focus on sending information and the last three on receiving information. There is clearly within this multiple definition an effort to identify an interaction between the teacher/sender and the learner/receiver. Effective teaching involves this interaction and implies an increment of knowledge or skill on the part of the learner.

This interactive nature of teaching warrants careful examination by those who would teach. Each student enters the learning arena with a unique set of attributes that strongly influence the potential for change as a result of a particular teaching/learning interaction. Teachers, too, arrive with idiosyncratic attitudes, skills, and knowledges. The multitude of variables that accrue make it impossible to accurately predict the learning outcome of any teacher-student interchange. It is possible for appropriate and creative teacher behavior to result in zero learning by a particular student; it is just as possible for a student to learn in spite of incompetent teaching techniques. Teaching-learning is clearly not a mathematical event. This principle can be applied to the teaching of speech to hearing-impaired children with one exception: the variables involved are multiplied many times over.

STUDENT ATTRIBUTES AS VARIABLES

There are essentially three tiers of behaviors that constitute communicative speech:

Tier I   Production of the motor acts that result in the acoustic speech signal

Tier II   Employment of these motor acts within a linguistic system

Tier III   Use of these motor acts within a linguistic system in verbal communicative interchange

Although speaking involves the use of organs, muscles, and nerves associated with involuntary life supporting functions, speech behavior on all three tiers is voluntary. This applies to a student's willingness to engage in syllable repetition practice at the Tier I level, to the use of such a skill as producing an intonation contour with a terminal fall to signal the end of a statement at the Tier II level, and to the personal decision to initiate or respond to verbal communication at the Tier III level. Specific sets of variables regarding student/learner speech behavior apply at each tier and virtually dictate an individual's present functioning and potential for future functioning.

Tier I

Variables for Tier I motor acts involve all the following components of motor speech behavior:

1. *Structural fidelity*   Are the student's physical structures within a range of normality that allows for production of the acoustic and visual properties of the speech signal without extreme compensation?
2. *Musculature*   Is there adequate muscular range and control?
3. *Motor coordination*   Do the structures and muscles operate cooperatively and with sufficient speed?
4. *Motor memory*   Can both specific motor acts and sequences of motor acts be remembered and reliably repeated?
5. *Imitative skills and propensity to imitate*   Can the student/learner translate behavior observed in others through audition, vision, or

taction into similar motor acts? Does the student/learner enjoy, tolerate, or reject this activity?

6. *Perceptual skills* Are the senses developed to a point at which the student/learner can employ them efficiently in first observing, then imitating, and finally, automatizing speech behavior? A student's ability to use residual hearing in receiving and producing speech will be influenced by such familiar factors as degree and configuration of hearing loss; age at which appropriate amplification is provided; auditory attention ability; perceptual function involving figure-ground interpretation, auditory closure, and directionality; and level of auditory comprehension. How efficiently the student/learner uses vision in the reception and production of speech is dependent on adequacy in the areas of ocular functioning, visual attention skill, perception of figure-ground and spatial relationships, visual closure, and visual comprehension. Student use of tactual skills in the speech production and reception task will involve tactual attention ability, sensitivity to tactile input, and skill in interpreting and relating vibrotactile information to the appropriate aspects of the speech signal.

Tier II

Tier II involves the application of physical production skills to the generation of phonemic strings with syntactic and semantic integrity. The variables that affect this behavior include: mental factors such as integrative processing; comprehension of auditory, visual, and tactual signals; code acquiring skills including memory for sequences and processing for meaning; and reliability of motor act production to the degree that these acts can be reproduced at will and within a system.

Tier III

Tier III behavior involves the use of motor acts within a linguistic system in verbal communicative interchange. Variables include all the forces that contribute to human communicative behavior. Some are internal and stem from the depths of the individual. Among these are: communicative need and desire to reach out to others; the manner in which this need is translated into behavior; personality organization; emotional health, stability, and stamina; impulse control; ability to concentrate and focus attention; flexibility of thought processes; and the ability to automatize mental and motor behavior. Other variables are external and accrue from the environment. They affect the opportunities a particular individual has to communicate and the reinforcements received for communicating. The style and amount of interaction among family members, the number of languages used, and the level of syntactic and semantic sophistication employed all impact on an individual child.

TEACHER SKILLS AND KNOWLEDGE AS VARIABLES

The dynamics of the speech teaching act involve an array of teacher behaviors that flow from one to the other at a rapid rate. They include locking into communicative engagement with the student, eliciting speech from the student, correcting the student's speech, and reinforcing student "tries" at improving speech. This sequence of behaviors is repeated many times in even a brief speech tutoring session. Competence in making the lightning-fast decisions that are required in each of these behaviors stems from the bank of skills and knowledge the teacher possesses. Essential areas are discussed below.

The teacher requires knowledge about those child behaviors that are prerequisites for traditional speech tutoring. Among these is the child's ability to relate in a one-to-one setting with an adult, including the maintenance of eye contact and the attention to and participation in something other than a self-initiated activity. Knowledge is needed about the normal developmental pattern of verbal communicative competence, about assessing a student's current level of functioning in this area, and about the use of these two bodies of information to identify appropriate learning goals for that student. Additionally, a teacher must be knowledgeable about the nature of conversation and skilled in engaging students in such verbal and/or vocal interchange. Appropriate teacher behaviors include vocal or verbal turn-taking, establishing a context, employing syntactic variations, and incorporating a variety of visual and situational clues that enhance meaning.

Knowledge of the multisensory characteristics of the raw materials of the speech signal is needed, including the body of information subsumed under the broad areas of physiological phonetics and acoustic phonetics. The teacher must be skilled in applying this information to teaching techniques involved in the interweaving of perceptual training with speech teaching and the highlighting of selected auditory, tactile, or visual parameters in demonstrating corrections for students. Additional skill is required in the use of a standard transcription system such as the International Phonetic Alphabet (IPA) for purposes of record keeping and in reading the literature.

The integral relationship between the production of intelligible speech and the student's grasp of the language must be understood. An example of this is the dramatic increase in the intelligibility that occurs when, in spite of deviant articulation, the correct number of syllables for the intended message is produced. Related to this is the skill of eliciting corrections from students including: identifying the error made; deciding what is a reasonable correction; communicating the expected correction to the student; and reinforcing the student's attempt. Behavior management techniques can be employed that allow the teacher to avoid power battles by seeing clearly whether particular behaviors interfere with the tasks at hand. For instance, whether a child stands up or sits at a table while he or she practices a syllable string makes little difference to the speech task. Some teachers, however, seem to focus on the unimportant standing behavior rather than the very important speech behavior. Identifying a reward system for each student that will keep him or her working at a productive level can enhance the learning potential in any situation.

Finally, skill is needed to guide the student through the leap from motor skill acquisition to the use of these skills in his or her spoken language system. This involves understanding that before motor skills can be productively applied to phonology, they must be accurate, fast, facile, and flexible; that phonetic contexts vary in production difficulty, some being easy enough for practice in early stages of skill acquisition and others being more appropriate in later stages; that speech production skills even though adequately developed will most likely not transfer automatically into meaningful use without the teacher systematically providing opportunities for use and expecting gradual improvement in use.

THE X-FACTORS AS VARIABLES

The teacher skills and knowledge identifed above as being requisites for effective speech teaching are currently being addressed to varying degrees in teacher training programs; to a large degree, they can be taught. Many of the variables described as student attributes can also be taught. In addition, there are other powerful factors that come into play in the speech teaching interaction about which much less is known. Although these "X-factors" are eternally operating, it is not clear at the present time whether they can be taught. Some of these factors relate specifically to the individual student/learner: the strength of the student's communicative need, for instance, and the drive to reach out to others will affect motivation for becoming facile in this area. Student aptitude for language and tolerance for the repetition that is a necessary ingredient for skill acquisition will also vary among individuals.

Other X-factors are associated with the particular teacher involved. Intellectual and behavioral flexibility will shape the teacher's ability to empathize with the student and to act on supervisory suggestions. Synthetic thinking ability will determine teacher talent for relating theory to practice, translating learning principles into teaching activities, applying behavioral development facts to management techniques, and channeling personality dynamics into effective interactive teaching style. The need to nurture will influence the degree to which a teacher interacts with the student in ways that lead to student independence. Setting standards for behavior is a function that is transferred from teacher to student as the student matures and of necessity involves some student discomfort. Teachers with strong needs to nurture may find it hard to witness student frustration, even though it may be appropriate to the situation and an impetus toward learning. Such teachers are prone to allow students to lean on them past the time when it is productive. An example of this behavior is the teacher who continues to provide correction models past the time when it would be reasonable to expect the student to have internalized the model and be ready to self-correct. Tolerance for systematic behavior involving repetitive acts will predict whether the teacher tests hearing aids regularly and efficiently; updates expectations regarding student speech accuracy on the basis of current skill acquisition; and is firm, fair, and consistent in holding students to standards of communicative behavior.

The power of these X-factors to enhance or negate speech teaching efforts justifies their consideration in some way by all who are involved in this task. The X-factors might be examined as part of standard preservice course work or through on-the-job inservice programs. Those items that relate to teachers' personal qualities might best be addressed during some type of individual or group counseling. Self-awareness in these areas can be as important a competence for teaching speech as theoretical knowledge and technical skills.

SUMMARY

Effective speech teaching involves an interplay of forces, events, and abilities associated with what learners and teachers bring *to* the situation; what happens during the teaching-learning interchange; and what attitudes, skills, and knowledge learners subsequently incorporate into their personal functions. Knowledgeable management of those areas that can be ameliorated will increase the occurrence of effective speech teaching.

REFERENCE

Barnhart, C. (ed.). 1968. The World Book Dictionary. Field Enterprises, Chicago.

Author Index

Subject Index

Fundamental frequency variation,
25, 41–43, 47–48, 76, 78, 81, 93,
121
intelligibility and, 38–39
perception of, 123
spectrograms, 26–31, 46, 187
vocal fold tension and, 36

Genioglossus (GG) muscles, 77, 84–
92
Glide consonants, 62–63, 65, 67,
123, 126–127, 219, 222–224, 342
Glottalization, 44, 47, 49, 67
Glottal opening, improper posture
of, 36–37, 98, 113–115
Glottal stops, 57, 64, 190, 244, 260–
262, 279

Head Start programs, 6
Hearing aids, 131, 261, 263–265, 285
acoustic cues from, 133, 135, 138–
139
classroom type related to use of,
372–374
degree of hearing loss, 147
demographic data using, 381
design of, 8
evaluation using, 156, 178, 225,
382, 384
preservice training using, 392–393
see also Amplification
Helen test, 173, 177
Hudgins Word Intelligibility Tests,
181

Imitation, 141–142, 344
of auditory signals, 24, 32–34, 123
of vibrotactile signals, 32–34, 154
of visual signals, 32–34
Implosives, 28, 66, 212
Inservice training, 192, 353, 363,
367–377, 379–387, 389–406, 414
Instructional objectives, 14, 350–
355, 359–360, 380
Intensity of speech, 154, 336–337
International Phonetic Alphabet
(IPA), 412

Intonation patterns of phonology,
11, 354
Iowa Test of Basic Skills, 370
IPA, see International Phonetic
Alphabet

Labial consonants, 271
Labial fricatives, 260
Laryngeal function and posture, 45–
47, 76, 114, 120, 185, 190
fundamental frequency, 36–37,
123–124
voiced implosive production, 28–
29
Laryngoscopy, 191, 236
Latent trait theories, 355–359
Lateral consonants, 62, 65, 67
Linguistic organization, 33
Lipreading, 132–133, 135–138, 143,
155–156, 163, 171–173, 199, 298
see also Imitation
Lung volume, 97–98, 102–103, 107–
108, 111–115

Magner Intelligibility Test, 183–184
Magnetometers, 97, 99
Mainstreaming, 13–14, 367–369,
381–387
Measurement
acoustic, 77–84, 92–93, 185
air flow, 191
esophageal air pressure, 191
physiological, 92
Modified Rhyme Test, 217, 225–226
Motor theory of speech perception,
120

Nasal consonant production
correct, 259, 261, 342
substitution errors in, 63, 67, 271,
273
testing of, 205, 207, 220–224, 268–
269
Nasality, 135, 138–139, 171, 190,
316
Nasalization deviation, 36, 43, 54,
65, 219–221, 385